The Theory of Optical Activity

INTERSCIENCE MONOGRAPHS ON PHYSICAL CHEMISTRY

EDITOR: I. Prigogine
FACULTÉ DES SCIENCES
UNIVERSITÉ LIBRE DE BRUXELLES
BRUSSELS, BELGIUM

Insoluable Monolayers at Liquid-Gas Interfaces
BY G. L. GAINES (EDITOR)

Chemistry of Dissociated Water Vapor and Related Systems
BY M. VENUGOPALAN AND R. A. JONES

The Theory of Optical Activity
BY DENNIS J. CALDWELL AND HENRY EYRING

The Theory of Optical Activity

by **DENNIS J. CALDWELL**
and **HENRY EYRING**

DEPARTMENT OF CHEMISTRY
UNIVERSITY OF UTAH
SALT LAKE CITY

WILEY-INTERSCIENCE
a Division of John Wiley & Sons, Inc.
New York • London • Sydney • Toronto

Library of Congress Catalog Card Number: 74-144331
ISBN 0-471-12980-1

Printed in the United States of America

10 9 8 7 6 5 4 3 2 1

Preface

This book develops the theory of the interaction of electromagnetic waves with matter, which provides information particularly valuable to the study of molecular structure. Ultraviolet and infrared spectroscopy are now supplemented by circular dichroism, the result of the difference between the absorption coefficients for left and right circularly polarized light. Traditionally the optical rotation of molecules has been measured at specific wavelengths. It later became evident that the continuous dispersion over the range of the instrument was even more useful, particularly in absorption regions. Just as the circular dichroism of a molecule measures the difference in absorption coefficients, optical rotatory dispersion measures the difference in indices of refraction for right and left circularly polarized light. These properties measure dissymmetry, which arises when a molecule or crystal is nonsuperimposable on its mirror image.

The amino acids found in the proteins of all living things are exclusively of the L-type, and the sugars in the chromosomes are all D. This impressive evidence for the ability of enzymes to select one molecule and reject its mirror image indicates that optical acitvity is a tool useful in unraveling many biological questions. A magnetic field along a light beam causes magnetic circular dichroism and optical rotation. This property is called the Faraday effect, and it is exhibited by all substances. Although it is less sensitive to molecular structure than natural optical activity, it is a valuable diagnostic tool in classifying electronic transitions. A rudimentary knowledge of electromagnetism and quantum mechanics will greatly facilitate an understanding of the theory. References at the end of the book suggest useful supplementary reading.

Emil Fischer, using classical organic chemical methods, was able to establish the relative configuration of many compounds by synthesizing one from the other. Bijvoet and others then established the absolute configuration of various molecules by preparing crystals of their salts containing heavy metal atoms such as rubidium. Ordinarily X-rays serve to establish the distances between planes of similarly situated atoms through the application of the familiar Bragg equation. If X-rays having frequencies near the absorption edge of the rubidium atom are used, they suffer a phase change as they pass by the rubidium. One is thereby enabled to tell whether a plane containing rubidium is in front of or behind one that does not. This establishes the absolute configuration of the molecules in the crystal. The circular dichroism of such molecules of known configuration is of great importance in the comparison of calculation with experiment.

Starting from basic electromagnetic and quantum theory, we present a complete development of all the fundamentals of optical activity theory, both modern and classical. There are many excellent texts covering the experimental and empirical aspects of the problem; accordingly considerably less space will be devoted to these questions than would otherwise be merited.

Since departure from symmetry is being measured, group theory, the study of the consequences of symmetry, is basic to our considerations. Electronic transitions in a chromophore are affected by its environment. As a result much can be learned about the shape of the intramolecular force field and its dependence on distance. We strongly believe that this powerful means of studying the configuration and conformation of molecules is worth the effort required to master it. Perhaps this book will transmit to the reader some of the excitement that comes from exploring in an untamed land. Much remains to be done both theoretically and experimentally.

Our indebtedness to others will be apparent from our published papers which, however, are not in general reviewed here. These papers also express our appreciation to the National Institute of Health, the National Science Foundation, and the U.S. Army for their support of work related to the book. We wish to express our appreciation to Carol Farnsworth for typing the manuscript, to Alexis Kelner for the illustrations, and to Karin Dahlgren and K. K. Cheong for reading parts of the manuscript.

Dennis J. Caldwell
Henry Eyring

Salt Lake City, Utah
March 1971

Contents

The Theory of
Optical Activity

CHAPTER 1

The Classical Theory

1.1. The General Phenomenon

When a beam of polarized light is rotated upon passage through matter, the substance is said to be *optically active.* The term *optical rotation* describes this phenomenon in general, and *optical rotatory power* refers to the ability of a substance to rotate the plane of polarized light.

Since it has primarily been the task of chemists to amass the great wealth of data on optically active substances, the convention for determining the sign of rotation has been chosen from the point of view of the observer. If the plane of polarization* as seen by an observer looking toward the light source is rotated clockwise, the medium is said to be dextrorotatory (+); if the plane is rotated counterclockwise, the medium is levorotatory (−).

The opposite convention more suited to theoretical parlance has sometimes been employed by physicists: If the tip of the electric vector, which is perpendicular to the direction of propagation and parallel to the plane of polarization, traces out a right-handed helix, the medium is said to be dextrorotatory (+). Since the majority of papers, both experimental and theoretical, have employed the chemist's convention, it will be used throughout this book.

Unlike absorption, which has an exponential dependence on path length, the amount of rotation is directly proportional to the path length. In the case of absorption the amount of photons absorbed in a given infinitesimal path length dl is $k\,dl$ and the total number is constantly diminished with the resulting exponential dependence of intensity on path length. When the rotation of the plane of polarization is being measured, the polarization of each photon is on the average changed by a constant amount by each reflection in the medium, the number of reflections being proportional to the path length. Thus the proportionality of rotation to path length applies equally well to absorbing and nonabsorbing media.

Pasteur was the first to associate the phenomenon of optical activity with structural dissymmetry. In his celebrated work on the subject he noticed that

* In this context the term "plane of polarization" will refer to that plane determined by the electric vector $\mathbf{E}$ and the direction of propagation $\mathbf{k}$.

there were two types of crystals of an optically active substance, which could be separated mechanically under a microscope. A careful inspection of the two crystals found them to be mirror images of one another; solutions thereof gave equal and opposite rotations.

A necessary condition for optical activity is that the smallest characteristic unit of a substance not be superimposable on its mirror image. Although this criterion covers the vast majority of cases, it is not a sufficient condition, as will be shown subsequently. The general requirement is that the symmetry group of the unit structure contain no improper rotations, which include reflection planes, rotation-reflection axes, and a center of inversion. In the case of true liquids and gases the characteristic units will be molecules or ions. In solids the unit cell as a whole must be considered; if the various ions, atoms, or molecules in the unit cell are arranged in a dissymmetric pattern, the crystal will be optically active. It will be seen that it is not necessary for a crystal to contain molecules or ions optically active in solution in order to rotate the plane of polarized light as, for example, an examination of crystalline sodium chlorate will show.

To a certain degree it may be expected that the optical rotation of a substance will be proportional to the number of dissymmetric characteristic units per unit volume. In dilute solutions the rotation should be proportional to the concentration of optically active substance with departures from linearity occurring with increasing concentrations owing to intermolecular interactions. In principle one may envision an inactive crystal lattice with dissymmetric unit cells imbedded in it at regular intervals. For sufficiently large intervals the rotation will be proportional to the concentration of dissymmetric unit cells; however, in practice an optically active crystal will be composed of identical adjacent unit cells with no room for varying "concentration."

The rotation of optically active substances is generally expressed in degrees per decimeter. For crystals, which exhibit larger rotations than liquids, the results are often given in degrees per centimeter.

It is desirable to gain a comparison of the rotatory power of the individual characteristic units of different compounds. The amount of rotation due to a given thickness of active medium is inversely proportional to the average volume occupied by the characteristic unit; therefore, the observed rotation in degrees per decimeter (denoted by the symbol ϕ*) multiplied by the molecular weight divided by the density will be a measure of the rotatory power of the individual units. For convenience this figure is divided by 100 to give the molecular rotatory power $[M]$:

$$[M] = \frac{\phi M}{100d}. \tag{1.1.1}$$

* We have followed the practice of E. U. Condon [*Rev. Mod. Phys.*, **9**, 432 (1937)] in expressing the rotation by the symbol ϕ, reserving the customary α for the polarizability.

Another quantity quite often used is the specific rotation $[\phi]$, which is defined as the rotation ϕ divided by the density. In fact a great many workers in the field report their results in terms of the specific rotation.

1.2. The Electromagnetic Field

Before investigating the quantum mechanical theory there is much that can be learned from the phenomenological electromagnetic approach. From this one is able to gain a fundamental insight into the nature of optical activity.

Classically an oscillating charged particle will produce an electromagnetic radiation field which may be described by two vectors, the electric vector **E** and the magnetic induction **B**. The force field is propagated in the form of a wave which travels in free space with a velocity c. A precise physical interpretation of the vectors **E** and **B** is not easily given in general, although they may be defined in terms of definite physical quantities.

In the electromagnetic wave **E** and **B**, which are functions of space and time, form a right-handed coordinate system with **k**, the unit vector along the direction of propagation, such that $\mathbf{E} \times \mathbf{B}$ is along the positive **k**-direction.

In free space **E** and **B** have a simple interpretation: $\mathbf{E} = \mathbf{E}(\mathbf{r}, t)$ is the force on a unit charge at time t located at position **r**; $\mathbf{B} = \mathbf{B}(\mathbf{r}, t)$ is the force on a fictitious unit magnetic pole at time t located at position **r**. In the wave both the spatial and temporal parts of **E** and **B** have a sinusoidal dependence which may be written

$$\mathbf{E} = \mathrm{Re}(\mathbf{E}_0 e^{-i\psi}) \tag{1.2.1a}$$

$$\mathbf{B} = \mathrm{Re}(\mathbf{B}_0 e^{-i\psi}), \tag{1.2.1b}$$

where $\psi = \omega(t - \mathbf{k} \cdot \mathbf{r}/c)$ and $\omega = 2\pi\nu$ is the circular frequency of the wave.

The nature of the vectors $\mathbf{E}_0$ and $\mathbf{B}_0$ depends on the source and history of the radiation. In the most general case the light is elliptically polarized, and the vectors **E** and **B** will trace out a helical path with an elliptical cross section. In any plane perpendicular to **k**, the direction of propagation, the instantaneous values of **E** and **B** will be uniform.

There are two special cases of interest: If one may write $\mathbf{E}_0 = E_0\mathbf{i}$ and $\mathbf{B}_0 = B_0\mathbf{j}$, where $\mathbf{i} \times \mathbf{j} = \mathbf{k}$ and E_0 and B_0 are real, the light will be *plane polarized*, and the vectors vibrate in constant directions at right angles to one another. On the other hand, if $\mathbf{E}_0 = E_0(\mathbf{i} \pm i\mathbf{j})$ and $\mathbf{B}_0 = B_0(\mathbf{i} \pm i\mathbf{j})$, the light is circularly polarized: $\mathrm{Re}[(\mathbf{i} \pm i\mathbf{j})e^{-i\psi}] = \mathbf{i}\cos\psi \pm \mathbf{j}\sin\psi$. When $\psi = 0$ the vector **E** is along the **i**-direction, and as ψ increases a component is produced along the positive **j**-direction for the upper sign and the negative **j**-direction for the lower. Since $\mathbf{i} \times \mathbf{j} = \mathbf{k}$, this means that the upper sign will by our convention describe left circularly polarized light and the lower sign right circularly polarized light.

In plane polarized light the vectors are constant in direction but change in magnitude. For circularly polarized light the vectors are constant in magnitude but change in direction, whereas for elliptically polarized light the vectors change both in magnitude and direction. Only with plane polarized light can the electromagnetic field have an instantaneous value of zero.

All the effects observed when electromagnetic radiation passes through matter are due to the impressed oscillation of charges contained therein. Each charge acted upon by the field oscillates and accordingly gives rise to an electromagnetic radiation field of its own. Inside the region occupied by matter the amplitudes of these oscillations with their individual phases are added to that of the impinging wave to produce a modified wave traveling through the medium.

The net result outside of absorption regions is a change in phase, which means that for plane polarized light **E** and **B** reach their maximum values at intervals of $c/n\nu$, where n, the index of refraction, is a function of the medium. The expression for the phase ψ becomes $\psi = 2\pi\nu(t - n\mathbf{k} \cdot \mathbf{r}/c)$.

1.3. The Velocities of Light

Although the optical phenomena to be described in this book are governed by the phase velocity through a medium, it is of interest to discuss the various definitions for the velocity of light in material media. When an electromagnetic wave impinges upon a layer of matter the charges therein do not instantaneously reach their dynamic equilibrium condition of forced oscillation. The preceding layers have tended to resist the passage of the wave by oscillating out of phase with it.

According to Brillouin, inside the medium the main pulse of radiation is preceded by a precursor wave starting with zero amplitude which grows slowly and finally decays into a second precursor having the natural period of the electrons. Finally the amplitude rises very rapidly to that of the principle train of forced oscillations, which carries the main body of energy.

Now it is true that the first manifestation of the disturbance at a distance z from the surface will be made at a time z/c after the wave reaches the surface, and thus in all material media the wave front velocity of light is equal to c, the free space velocity. From the above discussion it is apparent that the signal velocity, which is the rate of flow of the main body of energy, will be less than the wave front velocity.

In optical rotation we are concerned with phase velocity. In a nondispersive medium the phase ψ may alternatively be written for propagation along the z-direction as

$$\psi = kz - \omega t,$$

where k is the wave number $2\pi\nu/c$.

The surfaces with a given constant phase ψ' are determined by requiring that

$$\psi' = kz - \omega t.$$

The velocity of propagation of phase is then

$$c_p = \frac{dz}{dt} = \frac{\omega}{k}. \tag{1.3.1}$$

In a dispersive medium there will be a superposition of waves with differing frequencies and wave numbers. The combined amplitudes of these waves comprise an aggregate wave train. For a given frequency of incident light the wave numbers will be a known function of ω, and the group velocity is defined by

$$c_g = \frac{d\omega}{dk}. \tag{1.3.2}$$

The signal velocity may never exceed c, the vacuum velocity of light, but both the phase and group velocities may be either greater or less than c. At very high frequencies the electrons are unable to follow the undulations of the incident wave, and all the above defined velocities approach c. At lower frequencies outside regions of absorption these velocities approach the phase velocity c/n, and one may properly say that for all practical purposes the "velocity" of light in matter is equal to c, the vacuum velocity, divided by n, the index of refraction.

Ideally the rotatory power of a substance would be investigated with a completely monochromatic beam of light having frequency ω and wave number k with a phase velocity ω/k. In practice one has a collimated beam with a narrow range of frequencies. Strictly speaking a phase velocity cannot be assigned to this beam, and the group velocity must be employed; however, if the range of frequencies is narrow enough the group velocity will be very close to the phase velocity of a wave with its frequency at the center of the spread.

1.4. Maxwell's Equations

The cause of optical activity is dissymmetric electronic motion. The forced oscillations of even randomly oriented molecules will cause a dissymmetric coherent scattering. The salient features of the problem may be displayed in two ways. The simplest models consist of one or two electrons whose motion is governed by dissymmetric constraints. In the first a single electron moves along a helical path under a harmonic restoring force. The nature of the constraint makes this model more difficult to deal with than appears at first sight. At any particular instant the charge behaves like a simple linear oscillator with no dissymmetric scattering. Only when a time average of the scattered radiation is computed does the dissymmetry make itself evident. Since the calculation would follow a drastically different path from the more profitable routes toward understanding the problem, this model will be somewhat modified. For this reason the second alternative, the system of coupled linear oscillators, will best serve as an introduction to the subject.

A simple model will be discussed in a qualitative manner to help clarify the subsequent mathematical development. The steps in understanding the phenomenon are as follows:

1. The fields acting on the molecules must be characterized.

2. The motion of the electrons caused by these fields must be determined. For classical models this entails the solution of the Lagrangian or Hamiltonian equations of motion, which give the positions and momenta as functions of time. In the actual wave mechanical case the probability of a given state for the molecule is determined as a function of time.

3. Once the classical or quantum mechanical solutions are known it is a simple matter to obtain the electric and magnetic dipole moments of the system as a function of time.

4. One may proceed in one of two ways to obtain the scattered radiation. Conceptually attractive but mathematically more difficult is the process of averaging over all molecular orientations and adding the amplitudes of the scattered electric and magnetic dipole radiation at a given field point. The variation in direction of the resultant electric vector from point to point along the beam path may then be determined.

Alternatively, the powerful methods of continuum electrodynamics will provide the most convenient approach to the problem. Once the significance of the four vectors **B**, **H**, **D**, and **E** has been grasped along with the relations connecting them, $\nabla \times \mathbf{E} = -(1/c)\dot{\mathbf{B}}$ and $\nabla \times \mathbf{H} = (1/c)\dot{\mathbf{D}}$, it is much simpler to solve the electromagnetic equations for material media. It happens that in optically active media only elliptically polarized waves are transmitted. If the driving frequency is far from an absorption band the waves will be circularly polarized. A plane wave impinging upon the medium can be resolved into left- and right-handed circularly polarized components. Inside the medium these are transmitted with different phase velocities. The emergent wave will have its plane of polarization rotated with respect to the original direction.

In free space the electromagnetic field is traditionally defined by two vectors **E** and **B** which determine the forces on static and moving charges according to the equation $\mathbf{F} = e[\mathbf{E} + (\mathbf{v} \times \mathbf{B})/c]$. In the absence of sources (charge density equals zero) the divergence of the vector fields must be zero:

$$\nabla \cdot \mathbf{B} = 0,$$
$$\nabla \cdot \mathbf{E} = 0.$$

A familiar theorem in the calculus of vector fields states that

$$\int_V \nabla \cdot \mathbf{U}\, d\tau = \int_S \mathbf{U} \cdot d\boldsymbol{\sigma},$$

where the integral on the left is taken over any volume V and the one on the right taken over its bounding surface S, whose vector element of area is $d\boldsymbol{\sigma}$.

The equation $\nabla \cdot \mathbf{E} = 0$ thus requires the flux of $\mathbf{E}$ through any closed surface to be zero. This is a direct consequence of the distance dependence of the field from a collection of point charges. In Figure 1.1 the two situations of a charge e outside and inside a sphere are shown. The field is given by $\mathbf{E} = e\mathbf{r}/r^3$.

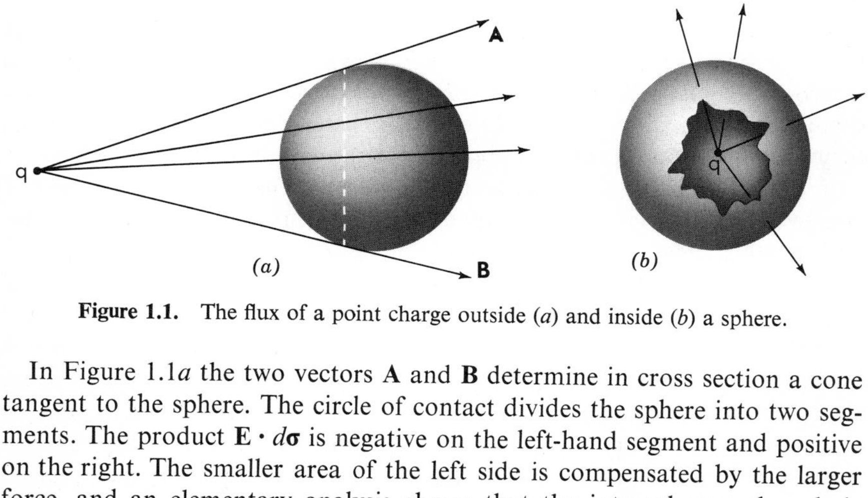

Figure 1.1. The flux of a point charge outside (*a*) and inside (*b*) a sphere.

In Figure 1.1*a* the two vectors **A** and **B** determine in cross section a cone tangent to the sphere. The circle of contact divides the sphere into two segments. The product $\mathbf{E} \cdot d\boldsymbol{\sigma}$ is negative on the left-hand segment and positive on the right. The smaller area of the left side is compensated by the larger force, and an elementary analysis shows that the integral over the whole sphere is indeed zero; that is, in differential form $\nabla \cdot \mathbf{E} = 0$.

In Figure 1.1*b* **E** and $d\boldsymbol{\sigma}$ are parallel at all points, and

$$\mathbf{E} \cdot d\boldsymbol{\sigma} = (e\mathbf{r}/r^3) \cdot \mathbf{r}r\, d\Omega = e\, d\Omega,$$

where $d\Omega$ is the element of solid angle. This immediately gives $\int \nabla \cdot \mathbf{E}\, d\tau = 4\pi e$. If instead of a single isolated charge there is a continuum with density ρ, $e = \int_V \rho\, d\tau$, whence $\nabla \cdot \mathbf{E} = 4\pi\rho$.

In a material medium the uncertainty in electronic positions and their large number makes it impossible to apply the laws of vacuum electrodynamics to individual charges. The fields **E** and **B** are now redefined on a macroscopic level to be the average quantities over a region large enough to contain a great many molecules.

In the case of time dependent fields a statistical averaging must be performed, which implies a time averaging over times large compared with the intervals of microscopic change but small with regard to macroscopic observation. It is to be emphasized at the outset that **E** and **B** are not necessarily the fields acting on specific regions of a particular molecule. This may be seen by considering a cubic lattice and comparing the average field over the space of a unit cell with that at a lattice point. The first quantity is the average field **E** and the second is the effective field $\mathbf{E}_{\text{eff}}$.

In any microscopic region that is known not to contain charges the equation $\nabla \cdot \mathbf{E}_{\text{mic}} = 0$ is satisfied, where $\mathbf{E}_{\text{mic}}$ is a local microscopic field. If we concentrate on a volume element large enough to contain an appreciable number of molecules but small enough to be a differential element of volume on a macroscopic scale, a medium of neutral molecules may be regarded as having zero average charge density in any such region.

The application of an external field will cause a polarization of charge from one part of the molecule to another. The net effect may be treated on a macroscopic scale by regarding each molecule as an *impenetrable* point dipole. The formation of these dipoles will change the average field **E**, since they tend to produce fields in opposition to the impressed field.

If the polarization is uniform throughout the medium, the amount of charge in any internal volume element is still zero. If the polarization is nonuniform there may be a net accumulation. For example, a charge e placed at the center of a dielectric sphere will produce a dipole at a distance r of magnitude $\alpha e/r^2$, where α is the polarizability of the molecule. In any spherical shell the amount of charge leaving the outer surface is exactly compensated by the amount entering the inner surface, since the area of the surface varies as r^2 and the induced dipole moments as $1/r^2$. At the very center there is an uncompensated accumulation of opposite charge which reduces the value of the field everywhere in the medium. Here $\nabla \cdot \mathbf{E}$ has a singularity; the equation $\nabla \cdot \mathbf{E} = 0$ is still satisfied everywhere else in the medium.

The role of a volume distribution of dipole moment can be assessed by the standard mathematical analysis which postulates a dipole moment volume density **P**. The potential energy at a field point $\mathbf{r} = \mathbf{r}(x, y, z)$ arising from the dipoles in a volume element $d\tau'$ at $\mathbf{r}' = \mathbf{r}'(x', y', z')$ is $\mathbf{P} \cdot \nabla'(1/R)d\tau'$, where $R = \sqrt{(x' - x)^2 + (y' - y)^2 + (z' - z)^2}$ and differentiation is with respect to the coordinates of the source point.

The total potential energy at an arbitrary field point due to a volume distribution of dipole moment is $\phi = \int \mathbf{P} \cdot \nabla'(1/R) d\tau'$. Integration by parts is equivalent to using the vector formula

$$\nabla' \cdot \left(\frac{\mathbf{P}}{R}\right) = \left(\frac{1}{R}\right)\nabla' \cdot \mathbf{P} + \mathbf{P} \cdot \nabla'\left(\frac{1}{R}\right);$$

this gives

$$\phi = -\int_V \frac{\nabla' \cdot \mathbf{P}}{R} d\tau' + \int_V \nabla' \cdot \left(\frac{\mathbf{P}}{R}\right) d\tau.'$$

The transformation of the last term by means of the divergence theorem gives

$$\phi = -\int_V \frac{\nabla' \cdot \mathbf{P}}{R} d\tau' + \int_\sigma \frac{\mathbf{P} \cdot d\boldsymbol{\sigma}}{R}.$$

This leads to the interpretation that $-\nabla' \cdot \mathbf{P}\, d\tau'$ is the polarization charge which has accumulated in the volume element $d\tau'$ owing to the inhomogeneous dipole moment distribution and $\mathbf{P} \cdot d\boldsymbol{\sigma}$ is the charge on the surface element $d\boldsymbol{\sigma}$.

Therein lies the formal justification for the analysis of the dielectric between two condenser plates. Inside the medium the positive and negative ends of the dipoles cancel except on the surface where a net charge per unit area of $+P$ accumulates at one end and $-P$ at the other. Inside the medium there results an opposing field equal to $-4\pi\mathbf{P}$.

It is worth emphasizing the conditions under which this result is valid. If the actual microscopic distribution of the dipoles is truly random, the cancellations occur as proposed; however, when each dipole occupies a well-defined lattice site as in a crystal, the field in the center due to the surface dipoles is negligible while the better part of it comes from those dipoles in the neighborhood of the plane perpendicular to the impressed field and containing the observation point.

It is clear that the method of measuring charge density in free space must be modified in the presence of matter to take into account local accumulations of charge from inhomogeneous polarization. The equation $\nabla \cdot \mathbf{E} = 4\pi\rho$ becomes $\nabla \cdot \mathbf{E} = 4\pi(\rho_t + \rho_p) = 4\pi(\rho_t - \nabla \cdot \mathbf{P})$, where ρ_t is the true charge density and ρ_p is the polarization excess or deficiency from inhomogeneous polarization. A new vector quantity is defined as $\mathbf{D} = \mathbf{E} + 4\pi\mathbf{P}$ such that $\nabla \cdot \mathbf{D} = 4\pi\rho_t$.

The magnetic field can be analyzed along the same lines in terms of magnetic dipoles; however, it is more generally appropriate to consider the magnetic field from the standpoint of its ultimate cause, moving charge, or current. The simple fact that a conducting wire with current density $\mathbf{J}$ is surrounded by concentric lines of magnetic force is expressed mathematically through the relation $\nabla \times \mathbf{B} = (4\pi/c)\mathbf{J}$. In material media it is necessary to divide the current into microscopic and macroscopic contributions. For our purposes microscopic currents will be those arising from the forced oscillations of individual molecules. The oscillating dipoles constitute a polarization current which may be regarded as a continuum of current density within the limits of the macroscopic observation of the medium. The circular or magnetic dipole currents do not give an additive effect in the same way as do the polarization currents, as may be seen from Figure 1.2. The small loops represent adjacent molecules with clockwise current distributions. When these are all equal in magnitude the interior currents cancel, leaving only the outer loop. This is the formal justification for regarding a uniformly magnetized medium as arising from an equivalent exterior current carrying coil.

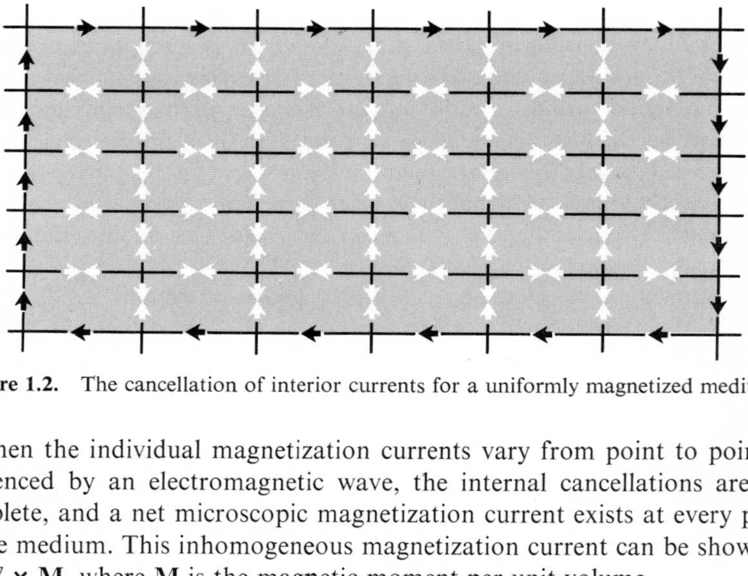

Figure 1.2. The cancellation of interior currents for a uniformly magnetized medium.

When the individual magnetization currents vary from point to point as influenced by an electromagnetic wave, the internal cancellations are not complete, and a net microscopic magnetization current exists at every point of the medium. This inhomogeneous magnetization current can be shown to be $c\nabla \times \mathbf{M}$, where $\mathbf{M}$ is the magnetic moment per unit volume.

In brief, the types of waves transmitted by a medium will depend upon the nature of the oscillating electric dipole moments and the degree of inhomogeneity of the magnetic currents.

In charge and current free space the electric and magnetic flux vectors $\mathbf{E}$ and $\mathbf{B}$ satisfy the relations

$$\nabla \times \mathbf{B} = \frac{1}{c}\frac{\partial \mathbf{E}}{\partial t}, \tag{1.4.1a}$$

$$\nabla \times \mathbf{E} = -\frac{1}{c}\frac{\partial \mathbf{B}}{\partial t}. \tag{1.4.1b}$$

Equation 1.4.1*b* is Faraday's law of magnetic induction, which was originally discovered by observing the currents produced in wires moving through a magnetic field. It is also satisfied in material media provided **E** is the statistically averaged electric field and **B** is the magnetic field arising from all types of currents.

The form of (1.4.1*a*) appears to differ from the original relation, $\nabla \times \mathbf{B} = (4\pi/c)\mathbf{J}$. This implies that in free space $\mathbf{J} = (1/4\pi)(\partial \mathbf{E}/\partial t)$, which is the convection current postulated by Maxwell to satisfy the requirement of charge conservation needed for the theory of radiation.

Our discussion may be summarized by the two equations for material media

$$\nabla \times \mathbf{E} = -\frac{1}{c}\frac{\partial \mathbf{B}}{\partial t}, \tag{1.4.2a}$$

$$\nabla \times \mathbf{B} = \frac{4\pi}{c}\mathbf{J}_{\text{total}} = \frac{4\pi}{c}\left(\mathbf{J}_{\text{mac}} + c\nabla \times \mathbf{M} + \frac{\partial \mathbf{P}}{\partial t} + \frac{1}{4\pi}\frac{\partial \mathbf{E}}{\partial t}\right)$$

$$= \frac{4\pi}{c}\,\text{(macroscopic current + inhomogeneous magnetization current + polarization current + free space convection current).} \tag{1.4.2b}$$

Equation 1.4.2*b* is generally rewritten in terms of the usual definition as

$$\nabla \times \mathbf{H} = \frac{1}{c}\frac{\partial \mathbf{D}}{\partial t} + \frac{4\pi}{c}\mathbf{J},$$

where $\mathbf{H} = \mathbf{B} - 4\pi\mathbf{M}$, $\mathbf{D} = \mathbf{E} + 4\pi\mathbf{P}$, and **J** is now the macroscopic or "true" current density.

In the subsequent derivations of the relations governing optical rotatory power nothing is particularly gained by using the vectors **H** and **D**, and equations 1.4.2 will be written in their original extended form.

To determine the desired electromagnetic properties of a substance it will be necessary to relate **M** and **P** to **E** and **B**. This is done in two stages. First a molecule may be considered to occupy an isolated region in which the equations

$$\nabla \times \mathbf{E}' = -\frac{1}{c}\frac{\partial \mathbf{B}'}{\partial t}$$

and

$$\nabla \times \mathbf{B}' = \frac{1}{c}\frac{\partial \mathbf{E}'}{\partial t}$$

are satisfied, where **E**′ and **B**′ are the effective electric and magnetic fields, which as we have seen are not the same as the statistically averaged quantities, **E** and **B**.

Again, following convention, it is found that the force equation on a charged particle,

$$\mathbf{F} = e\left(\mathbf{E}' + \frac{\mathbf{v} \times \mathbf{B}'}{c}\right),$$

is put into a form necessary for the Lagrangian and Hamiltonian formulations of mechanics if a scalar potential ϕ' and a magnetic potential $\mathbf{A}'$ are defined such that

$$\mathbf{E}' = -\nabla\phi' - \frac{1}{c}\frac{\partial \mathbf{A}'}{\partial t}$$

and

$$\mathbf{B}' = \nabla \times \mathbf{A}'.$$

The above equations are then satisfied provided that

$$\nabla\left(\nabla \cdot \mathbf{A}' + \frac{1}{c}\frac{\partial \phi'}{\partial t}\right) = 0.$$

In radiation scattering problems $\partial\phi'/\partial t$ is generally set equal to zero. Since ϕ' depends on the charge density, this entails the assumption that the radiation leaves the charge density unaltered. Then $\nabla \cdot \mathbf{A}'$ is a constant, which may be set equal to zero.

This phase of the calculation will give atomic electric and magnetic polarization vectors **p** and **m** in terms of the effective field quantities and their time derivatives. Finally, either $\mathbf{E}'$ or $\mathbf{B}'$ may be related to **E** or **B** by a detailed analysis of the structure of the medium, by no means a simple task. It has often been the practice to relate $\mathbf{E}'$ to **E** and $\mathbf{B}'$ to **B** separately. The electrostatic relation, $\mathbf{E}' = \mathbf{E} + (4\pi/3)\mathbf{P}$, has been quite popular. The whole question needs closer examination, particularly in light of the fact that the electromagnetic field is described by four, not six, independent functions.

1.5. Qualitative Discussion

Before developing the phenomenological equations of optical activity it is worth while to discuss some classical models in detail, since a great insight into the problem may be obtained which is not available quantum mechanically.

The prototype of many molecular systems consists of two one-dimensional oscillators whose motion is coupled. The steps in the subsequent development will appear more clearly if the various forces at work are first analyzed from a qualitative standpoint by considering a conveniently constituted model in several orientations. The degrees of freedom of the oscillators will be at right angles to each other and to the line connecting them. It should be mentioned that if they are considered as dipoles formed by small oscillations the dipole-dipole interaction term given by

$$V_{12} = \frac{e^2 q_1 q_2}{R^3} [\mathbf{b}_1 \cdot \mathbf{b}_2 - 3(\mathbf{b}_1 \cdot \mathbf{b}_{12})(\mathbf{b}_2 \cdot \mathbf{b}_{12})] \tag{1.5.1}$$

will be zero, where

q_1, q_2 = displacements from equilibrium,
$\mathbf{b}_1, \mathbf{b}_2$ = respective directions of motion,
$\mathbf{b}_{12}$ = unit vector from 1 to 2,
R = distance of separation.

It happens that this is the most favorable orientation for dissymmetric scattering but the least favorable for dipole coupling. Since we are at the moment concerned with the mechanism of the scattering, the other difficulty may be remedied for the moment by considering the two oscillators as being joined by a suitable system of springs such as to render the overall motion dissymmetric. Strictly speaking, the uncoupled system has two planes of symmetry. In this case it is the manner of coupling which destroys the symmetry.

Consider the six representative orientations in the electromagnetic field determined by the vectors **k**, **E**, and **B** in Figure 1.3. The vectors determine the directions of positive coordinate measurement, and it is assumed that there is a potential energy of coupling given by $Q_{12}q_1q_2$. In the orientation A_1 the motion of the second oscillator is determined by the electric field, whereas that of the first occurs solely by virtue of its coupling to the second. The form of the coupling $Q_{12}q_1q_2$ indicates that an increase in q_2 tends to make q_1 decrease.

If there were no difference in phase between $\mathbf{b}_1$ and $\mathbf{b}_2$ the motion of q_2 would cause q_1 to reach its maximum negative value when q_2 was at its maximum positive value. The motion of q_2 is in phase with **E** and that of q_1 is in phase with $-\mathbf{B}$. A similar analysis indicates that for the orientation A_2, q_1 is in phase with **E** and q_2 is in phase with **B**. The net result is complete destructive interference of the oscillations perpendicular to **E**.

The phase difference must now be invoked. If at some instant in both orientations **E** reaches its maximum at the origin, q_1 will also be a maximum in the A_2 orientation; but in the A_1 case q_1 will be a maximum at some other instant since its motion is in phase with q_2. The net result is that at any time the interference of the perpendicularly polarized radiation is incomplete. The

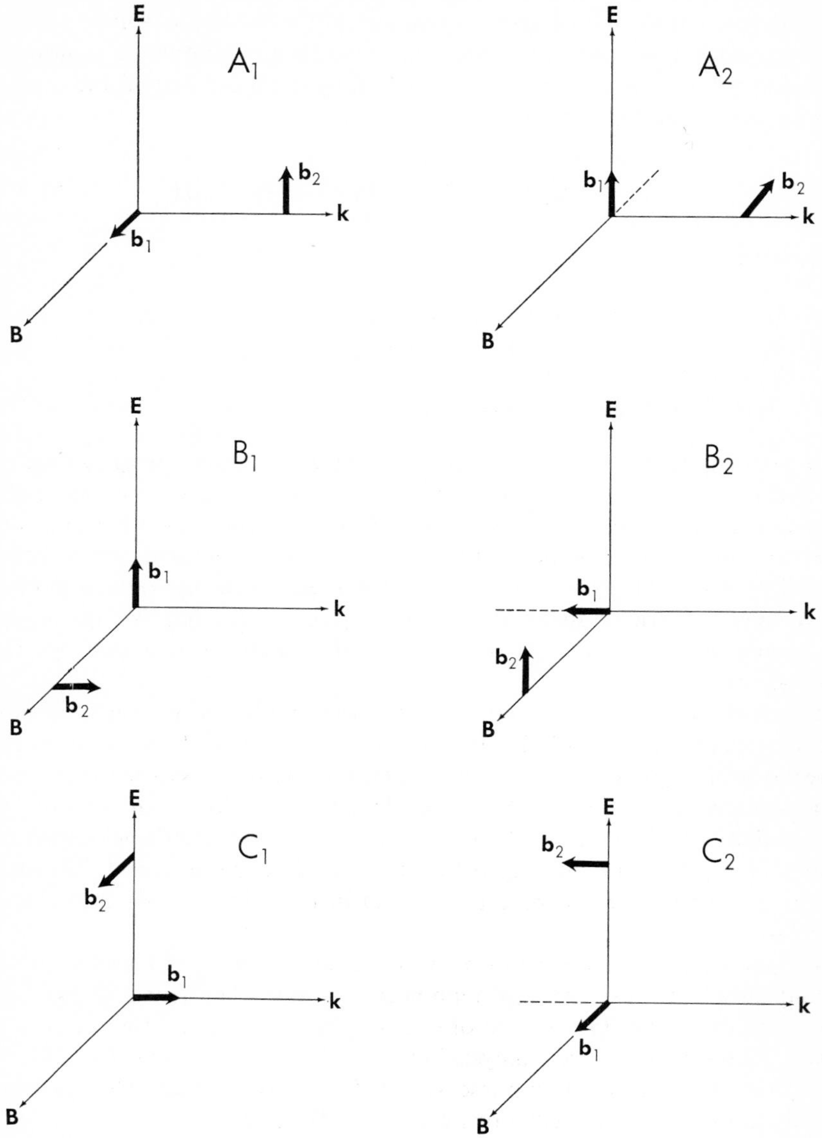

Figure 1.3. The coupled oscillator model.

detailed analysis which follows shows that the oscillations perpendicular to **E** are in phase with and in fact proportional to $\partial \mathbf{B}/\partial t$.

In the second pair of orientations B_1 and B_2 the coupled oscillations are in phase with **E**, and by the preceding analysis the components of scattered radiation polarized along the direction of propagation undergo complete destructive interference. Finally the orientations C_1 and C_2 exhibit no motion at all, since the vectors $\mathbf{b}_1$ and $\mathbf{b}_2$ are perpendicular to the electric field.

The magnetic dipole radiation arising from the system will be calculated from the detailed model. This illustration is merely meant to set the stage for the theory of dissymmetric scattering.

1.6. Coupled Linear Oscillators

The general classical treatment of two coupled oscillators may now be presented. The three vectors $\mathbf{b}_1$, $\mathbf{b}_2$, and $\mathbf{b}_{12}$ will have an arbitrary configuration, as shown in Figure 1.4. The molecule can be considered to lie in a cavity

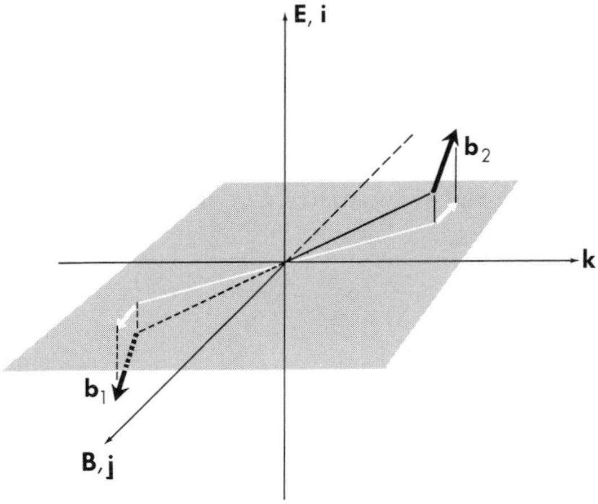

Figure 1.4. The orientation of two coupled oscillators in the laboratory coordinate system.

where the effective field quantities satisfy the free space form of the Maxwell equations

$$\nabla \times \mathbf{E} = -\frac{1}{c}\frac{\partial \mathbf{B}}{\partial t} \tag{1.6.1a}$$

$$\nabla \times \mathbf{B} = \frac{1}{c}\frac{\partial \mathbf{E}}{\partial t}, \tag{1.6.1b}$$

where the primes have been dropped.

The Newtonian equation of motion for one of the oscillators may be written

Force = mass × acceleration = (harmonic restoring force) + (coupling force) + (damping force) + (impressed field). (1.6.2)

For the first oscillator the restoring force is $V_1 = -k_1 q_1$. The potential energy of coupling is $V_{12} = Q_{12} q_1 q_2$, where Q_{12} is determined from a relationship such as (1.5.1). The coupling force is given by $-(\partial V_{12}/\partial q_1) = -Q_{12} q_2$. The damping force arises from several origins. The accelerated charge radiates energy at a rate given by

$$-\frac{dW}{dt} = \frac{2}{3}\frac{e^2(\ddot{q}_1)^2}{c^3}. \tag{1.6.3}$$

This may be equated to the rate of work done by the system against a force F_{rad}, which is $F_{\text{rad}}\dot{q}_1$. Generally the velocity and acceleration of a particle are uncorrelated and the radiation force must be determined on a time average basis; but in the special case of forced oscillations q_1 obeys the simple relation $q_1 = q_1^{(0)} e^{-i\omega t}$. The complex formulation will be used in this and all succeeding development. It has the advantage that both in phase and out of phase motions are described by the same complex function without the need for encumbering the differential equations with separate sine and cosine terms. All quantities will be assumed complex and any desired physical quantity can be obtained from the real part of the appropriate expression. The radiation force satisfies the relation

$$\begin{aligned} F_{\text{rad}}\dot{q}_1 &= \frac{2}{3}\frac{e^2}{c^3}(\ddot{q}_1)^2 \\ &= -i\omega F_{\text{rad}} q_1 = \frac{2}{3}\frac{e^2}{c^3}\omega^4 q_1^2, \end{aligned}$$

from which it follows that

$$F_{\text{rad}} = \frac{2}{3}\frac{e^2}{c^3} i\omega^3 q_1 = -\frac{2}{3}\frac{e^2}{c^3}\omega^2 \dot{q}_1. \tag{1.6.4}$$

If $\frac{2}{3}(e^2/c^3)\omega^2 = \gamma_\omega$, the radiation force may be written like a viscous damping force, $F_{\text{rad}} = -\gamma_\omega \dot{q}_1$.

The motion of the electron is also modified by molecular collisions, which may invalidate the assumptions under which the above simple result is obtained. For example, a slightly more general discussion involving time averages shows $F_{\text{rad}} = \frac{2}{3}(e^2/c^3)\dddot{q}_1$, which reduces to (1.6.4) for forced harmonic oscillations. This result is valid provided the motion is periodic, which is not exactly the case for an electron in a molecule undergoing random collisions.

For the sake of flexibility the damping constants of the two electrons will be taken as unequal, $\gamma_1 \neq \gamma_2$; furthermore, since these constants are small, the damping will only be effective in the respective absorption regions where accelerations are at a maximum. The mathematical development is occasionally simplified by making use of this fact and setting $\gamma_1 = (e^2/c^3)\omega_1^2$, $\gamma_2 = (e^2/c^3)\omega_2^2$. The more general damping constants will be left unspecified but assumed for the above reason to be independent of the driving frequency.

Although the damping force bears a formal resemblance to a viscous drag the two behave quite differently. A viscous force opposes any motion, uniform or not, whereas the radiation damping force opposes only nonuniform or accelerated motion. Since periodic motion is always accompanied by acceleration, the two forces play much the same role in this case.

The insertion of the proper mathematical expressions into (1.6.2) for both coordinates gives

$$m\ddot{q}_1 + k_1 q + Q'_{12} q_2 + \gamma_1 \dot{q}_1 = e\mathbf{b}_1 \cdot \mathbf{E}_0(1) e^{-i\omega t} \tag{1.6.5a}$$

$$m\ddot{q}_2 + k_2 q + Q'_{12} q_1 + \gamma_2 \dot{q}_2 = e\mathbf{b}_2 \cdot \mathbf{E}_0(2) e^{-i\omega t}, \tag{1.6.5b}$$

where the electric field at any point has been written as $\mathbf{E} = \mathbf{E}_0(\mathbf{r}) e^{-i\omega t}$.

Since optical activity arises from a difference in phase over the extent of the system, it will be necessary to reflect this in the two quantities $\mathbf{b}_1 \cdot \mathbf{E}_0(1)$ and $\mathbf{b}_2 \cdot \mathbf{E}_0(2)$. The electric field is constant over the **i**, **j**-plane; if an expansion is made about the origin, one obtains

$$\mathbf{b}_1 \cdot \mathbf{E}_0(1) = \mathbf{b}_1 \cdot \mathbf{E}_0(0) - (\mathbf{b}_1 \cdot \mathbf{i})(\mathbf{b}_{12} \cdot \mathbf{k}) \frac{R}{2} \frac{\partial E_0(0)}{\partial z}$$

$$\mathbf{b}_2 \cdot \mathbf{E}_0(2) = \mathbf{b}_2 \cdot \mathbf{E}_0(0) + (\mathbf{b}_2 \cdot \mathbf{i})(\mathbf{b}_{12} \cdot \mathbf{k}) \frac{R}{2} \frac{\partial E_0(0)}{\partial z}.$$

Insertion of this into (1.6.5) and division by m gives

$$\ddot{q}_1 + \omega_1^2 q_1 + Q_{12} q_2 + \Gamma_1 \dot{q}_1 = Q_1 e^{-i\omega t} \tag{1.6.6a}$$

$$\ddot{q}_2^2 + \omega_2^2 q_2 + Q_{12} q_1 + \Gamma_2 \dot{q}_2 = Q_2 e^{-i\omega t}, \tag{1.6.6b}$$

where

$$Q_{12} = Q'_{12}/m, \qquad \Gamma_1 = \gamma_1/m, \qquad \Gamma_2 = \gamma_2/m,$$

$$Q_1 = \frac{e}{m} \left[\mathbf{b}_1 \cdot \mathbf{E}_0(0) - (\mathbf{b}_1 \cdot \mathbf{i})(\mathbf{b}_{12} \cdot \mathbf{k}) \frac{R}{2} \frac{\partial E_0(0)}{\partial z} \right],$$

$$Q_2 = \frac{e}{m} \left[\mathbf{b}_2 \cdot \mathbf{E}_0(0) + (\mathbf{b}_2 \cdot \mathbf{i})(\mathbf{b}_{12} \cdot \mathbf{k}) \frac{R}{2} \frac{\partial E_0(0)}{\partial z} \right].$$

The steady state solution to these simultaneous equations may be obtained by setting

$$q_1 = q_1^{(0)} e^{-i\omega t} \tag{1.6.7a}$$

$$q_2 = q_2^{(0)} e^{-i\omega t}, \tag{1.6.7b}$$

where $q_1^{(0)}$ and $q_2^{(0)}$ are complex and time independent. The differential equations now become a pair of linear algebraic equations

$$(-\omega^2 + \omega_1^2 - i\omega\Gamma_1)q_1^{(0)} + Q_{12}q_2^{(0)} = Q_1$$

$$Q_{12}q_1^{(0)} + (-\omega^2 + \omega_2^2 - i\omega\Gamma_2)q_2^{(0)} = Q_2,$$

with solutions

$$q_1^{(0)} = \frac{(-\omega^2 + \omega_2^2 - i\omega\Gamma_2)Q_1 - Q_2 Q_{12}}{(-\omega^2 + \omega_1^2 - i\omega\Gamma_1)(-\omega^2 + \omega_2^2 - i\omega\Gamma_2) - Q_{12}^2} \tag{1.6.8a}$$

$$q_2^{(0)} = \frac{(-\omega^2 + \omega_1^2 - i\omega\Gamma_1)Q_2 - Q_1 Q_{12}}{(-\omega^2 + \omega_1^2 - i\omega\Gamma_1)(-\omega^2 + \omega_2^2 - i\omega\Gamma_2) - Q_{12}^2}. \tag{1.6.8b}$$

As will be recalled from (1.4.2) and the preceding discussion, the electromagnetic properties of a medium are determined by the time dependent magnetic and electric dipole moments. These are given by

$$\mathbf{M} = N\langle \mathbf{m} \rangle_{\text{av}} = \frac{e}{2c} N\left\langle \sum_i \mathbf{r}_i \times \mathbf{b}_i \dot{q}_i \right\rangle_{\text{av}} \tag{1.6.9a}$$

$$\mathbf{P} = N\langle \mathbf{p} \rangle_{\text{av}} = eN\left\langle \sum_i \mathbf{b}_i q_i \right\rangle_{\text{av}}, \tag{1.6.9b}$$

where N is the number of systems per unit volume, $\mathbf{r}_i$ is the vector distance from the origin to the ith electron, and the average is taken over all orientations with respect to the fixed vectors **k**, **E**, and **B**.

Use of the relations,

$$\mathbf{r}_1 = -\frac{R}{2}\mathbf{b}_{12} \qquad \text{and} \qquad \mathbf{r}_2 = \frac{R}{2}\mathbf{b}_{12},$$

in (1.6.9a) along with (1.6.7) and (1.6.8) gives

$$\mathbf{M} = -i\omega\frac{eNR}{4c}\left[\left\langle \frac{(-\mathbf{b}_{12} \times \mathbf{b}_1)(\Delta_2 Q_1 - Q_2 Q_{12})}{\Delta_1\Delta_2 - Q_{12}^2} + \frac{(\mathbf{b}_{12} \times \mathbf{b}_2)(\Delta_1 Q_2 - Q_1 Q_{12})}{\Delta_1\Delta_2 - Q_{12}^2} \right\rangle_{\text{av}} e^{-i\omega t}\right] \tag{1.6.10a}$$

$$\mathbf{P} = eN\left[\left\langle \frac{\mathbf{b}_1(\Delta_2 Q_1 - Q_2 Q_{12}) + \mathbf{b}_2(\Delta_1 Q_2 - Q_1 Q_{12})}{\Delta_1\Delta_2 - Q_{12}^2} \right\rangle_{\text{av}} e^{-i\omega t}\right], \tag{1.6.10b}$$

where

$$\Delta_1 = -\omega^2 + \omega_1^2 - i\omega\Gamma_1,$$
$$\Delta_2 = -\omega^2 + \omega_2^2 - i\omega\Gamma_2.$$

This will require the averaging of quantities with the form

$$(\mathbf{i}\cdot\mathbf{A})\mathbf{B} \quad \text{and} \quad (\mathbf{i}\cdot\mathbf{A})(\mathbf{k}\cdot\mathbf{B})\mathbf{C},$$

where **i**, **j**, **k** are the orthogonal unit vectors of a fixed coordinate system and **A**, **B**, **C** are to be averaged over all orientations subject to a fixed relative configuration. The calculation may further be implemented by writing

$$(\mathbf{i}\cdot\mathbf{A})\mathbf{B} = (\mathbf{i}\cdot\mathbf{A})(\mathbf{i}\cdot\mathbf{B})\mathbf{i} + (\mathbf{i}\cdot\mathbf{A})(\mathbf{j}\cdot\mathbf{B})\mathbf{j} + (\mathbf{i}\cdot\mathbf{A})(\mathbf{k}\cdot\mathbf{B})\mathbf{k}$$

and

$$(\mathbf{i}\cdot\mathbf{A})(\mathbf{k}\cdot\mathbf{B})\mathbf{C} = (\mathbf{i}\cdot\mathbf{A})(\mathbf{k}\cdot\mathbf{B})(\mathbf{i}\cdot\mathbf{C})\mathbf{i} + (\mathbf{i}\cdot\mathbf{A})(\mathbf{k}\cdot\mathbf{B})(\mathbf{j}\cdot\mathbf{C})\mathbf{j} + (\mathbf{i}\cdot\mathbf{A})(\mathbf{k}\cdot\mathbf{B})(\mathbf{k}\cdot\mathbf{C})\mathbf{k}.$$

Consider the identity element I of a three-dimensional space along with the general orthogonal transformation T:

$$I = \begin{bmatrix} 1 & 0 & 0 \\ 0 & 1 & 0 \\ 0 & 0 & 1 \end{bmatrix}, \qquad T = \begin{bmatrix} a_{11} & a_{12} & a_{13} \\ a_{21} & a_{22} & a_{23} \\ a_{31} & a_{32} & a_{33} \end{bmatrix}.$$

The rows and columns of T are the components of orthogonal unit vectors with $a_{11}^2 + a_{12}^2 + a_{13}^2 = 1$, $a_{11}a_{21} + a_{12}a_{22} + a_{13}a_{23} = 0$, etc., and $\det(T) = 1$. Starting from I the matrix T assumes all possible values in the averaging process consistent with the orthogonality requirements. The isotropy of space requires that the average of all permuted quantities be equal except for sign. The relation

$$\begin{aligned}\langle\det(T)\rangle_{\text{av}} &= \langle a_{11}a_{22}a_{33}\rangle_{\text{av}} + \langle a_{21}a_{32}a_{13}\rangle_{\text{av}} \\ &\quad + \langle a_{12}a_{23}a_{31}\rangle_{\text{av}} - \langle a_{31}a_{22}a_{13}\rangle_{\text{av}} - \langle a_{11}a_{32}a_{23}\rangle_{\text{av}} \\ &\quad - \langle a_{33}a_{12}a_{21}\rangle_{\text{av}} = 1\end{aligned}$$

indicates that

$$\begin{aligned}\langle a_{11}a_{22}a_{33}\rangle_{\text{av}} &= \langle a_{21}a_{32}a_{13}\rangle_{\text{av}} = \langle a_{12}a_{23}a_{31}\rangle_{\text{av}} \\ &= -\langle a_{33}a_{12}a_{21}\rangle_{\text{av}} = \langle a_{31}a_{22}a_{13}\rangle_{\text{av}} \\ &= -\langle a_{11}a_{32}a_{23}\rangle_{\text{av}} = \tfrac{1}{6}.\end{aligned}$$

The combination of the orthogonality conditions and the isotropy requirement gives

$$\langle a_{11}a_{12}\rangle_{\text{av}} = \langle a_{21}a_{22}\rangle_{\text{av}} = \langle a_{31}a_{32}\rangle_{\text{av}} = 0, \text{ etc.}$$

The relations

$$a_{11}^2 + a_{12}^2 + a_{13}^2 = 1$$

give

$$\langle a_{11}^2 \rangle_{\text{av}} = \langle a_{12}^2 \rangle_{\text{av}} = \langle a_{13}^2 \rangle_{\text{av}} = \tfrac{1}{3};$$

and finally the isotropy and orthogonality conditions give

$$\langle a_{11} a_{12} a \rangle_{\text{av}} = \langle a_{21} a_{22} a \rangle_{\text{av}} = \langle a_{31} a_{32} a \rangle_{\text{av}} = 0,$$

where a is any matrix element, since

$$\langle (a_{11} a_{12} + a_{21} a_{22} + a_{31} a_{32}) a \rangle_{\text{av}} = 0.$$

The product $(\mathbf{i} \cdot \mathbf{A})(\mathbf{j} \cdot \mathbf{B})(\mathbf{k} \cdot \mathbf{C})$ may be written $A_1 B_2 C_3$. The application of the orthogonal transformation T to these vectors transforms this quantity into

$$(a_{11} A_1 + a_{12} A_2 + a_{13} A_3)(a_{21} B_1 + a_{22} B_2 + a_{23} B_3)(a_{31} C_1 + a_{32} C_2 + a_{33} C_3).$$

Only six of the 27 terms survive the averaging process, giving

$$\begin{aligned}
&\langle A_1 B_2 C_3 \rangle_{\text{av}} \\
&\quad = \tfrac{1}{6}(A_1 B_2 C_3 + A_2 B_3 C_1 + A_3 B_1 C_2 - A_3 B_2 C_1 - A_1 B_3 C_2 - A_2 B_1 C_3) \\
&\quad = \tfrac{1}{6} \begin{vmatrix} A_1 & A_2 & A_3 \\ B_1 & B_2 & B_3 \\ C_1 & C_2 & C_3 \end{vmatrix} = \tfrac{1}{6} \mathbf{A} \cdot \mathbf{B} \times \mathbf{C}.
\end{aligned}$$

A similar analysis yields the relations

$$\begin{aligned}
\langle A_1 B_1 C_2 \rangle_{\text{av}} &= \langle A_1 B_2 C_2 \rangle_{\text{av}} = 0, \text{ etc.} \\
\langle A_1 B_1 \rangle_{\text{av}} &= \tfrac{1}{3} \mathbf{A} \cdot \mathbf{B}, \\
\langle A_1 B_2 \rangle_{\text{av}} &= \langle A_2 B_1 \rangle_{\text{av}} = 0, \text{ etc.}
\end{aligned}$$

The appropriate averages in (1.6.10) are found to be

$$\begin{aligned}
&\langle (\mathbf{b}_{12} \times \mathbf{b}_1)(\mathbf{b}_2 \cdot \mathbf{E}_0(0)) \rangle_{\text{av}} \\
&\quad = \tfrac{1}{3}(\mathbf{b}_{12} \times \mathbf{b}_1) \cdot \mathbf{b}_2 \mathbf{E}_0(0), \qquad \langle (\mathbf{b}_{12} \times \mathbf{b}_1)(\mathbf{b}_1 \cdot \mathbf{i})(\mathbf{b}_{12} \cdot \mathbf{k}) \rangle_{\text{av}} \\
&\quad = \langle (\mathbf{b}_1 \cdot \mathbf{i})[\mathbf{b}_{12} \times \mathbf{b}_1 \cdot (\mathbf{ii} + \mathbf{jj} + \mathbf{kk})](\mathbf{b}_{12} \cdot \mathbf{k}) \rangle_{\text{av}} \\
&\quad = \tfrac{1}{6} \mathbf{j}[\mathbf{b}_1 \cdot (\mathbf{b}_{12} \times \mathbf{b}_1) \times \mathbf{b}_{12}] \\
&\quad = \tfrac{1}{6}(\mathbf{b}_{12} \times \mathbf{b}_1)^2, \qquad \langle (\mathbf{b}_{12} \times \mathbf{b}_1)(\mathbf{b}_2 \cdot \mathbf{i})(\mathbf{b}_{12} \cdot \mathbf{k}) \rangle_{\text{av}} \\
&\quad = \tfrac{1}{6} \mathbf{j}(\mathbf{b}_{12} \times \mathbf{b}_2) \cdot (\mathbf{b}_{12} \times \mathbf{b}_1), \qquad \langle (\mathbf{b}_{12} \times \mathbf{b}_2)(\mathbf{b}_1 \cdot \mathbf{E}_0(0)) \rangle_{\text{av}} \\
&\quad = \tfrac{1}{3}(\mathbf{b}_{12} \times \mathbf{b}_2) \cdot \mathbf{b}_1 \mathbf{E}_0(0), \qquad \langle (\mathbf{b}_{12} \times \mathbf{b}_2)(\mathbf{b}_1 \cdot \mathbf{i})(\mathbf{b}_{12} \cdot \mathbf{k}) \rangle_{\text{av}} \\
&\quad = \tfrac{1}{6}(\mathbf{b}_{12} \times \mathbf{b}_1) \cdot (\mathbf{b}_{12} \times \mathbf{b}_2), \qquad \langle (\mathbf{b}_{12} \times \mathbf{b}_2)(\mathbf{b}_2 \cdot \mathbf{i})(\mathbf{b}_{12} \cdot \mathbf{k}) \rangle_{\text{av}} \\
&\quad = \tfrac{1}{6}(\mathbf{b}_{12} \times \mathbf{b}_2)^2.
\end{aligned}$$

This gives the result

$$\mathbf{M} = -i\omega \frac{e^2NR}{4mc} \frac{1}{\Delta_1\Delta_2 - Q_{12}^2}$$

$$\times \left\{\tfrac{2}{3}(\mathbf{b}_{12} \cdot \mathbf{b}_1 \times \mathbf{b}_2)Q_{12}\,\mathbf{E}_0^{(0)} + \tfrac{1}{12}R[(\mathbf{b}_1 \times \mathbf{b}_{12})^2(\Delta_1 + \Delta_2)\right.$$

$$\left. + 2Q_{12}(\mathbf{b}_1 \times \mathbf{b}_{12}) \cdot (\mathbf{b}_2 \times \mathbf{b}_{12})]\mathbf{j}\frac{\partial E_0^{(0)}}{\partial z}\right\} e^{-i\omega t}. \quad (1.6.11a)$$

$$\mathbf{P} = \frac{e^2N}{m} \frac{1}{\Delta_1\Delta_2 - Q_{12}^2} \left\{\tfrac{1}{3}[(\Delta_1 + \Delta_2) - 2Q_{12}(\mathbf{b}_1 \cdot \mathbf{b}_2)]\mathbf{E}_0^{(0)}\right.$$

$$\left. + \tfrac{1}{6}Q_{12}\,R(\mathbf{b}_{12} \cdot \mathbf{b}_1 \times \mathbf{b}_2)\mathbf{j}\frac{\partial E_0^{(0)}}{\partial z}\right\}. \quad (1.6.11b)$$

The electrodynamical equations are best solved in complex form. As will be recalled from (1.4.2), $\mathbf{M}$ and $\mathbf{P}$ are written in terms of the effective field quantities and their derivatives. These in turn are assumed to be linear functions of the quantities $\mathbf{E}$ and $\mathbf{B}$ themselves. The vector $\mathbf{B}$ will have the form $\mathbf{B}_0 e^{-i\omega(t - n\mathbf{k}\cdot\mathbf{r}/c)}$, where $\mathbf{B}_0$ is a complex amplitude constant and n is in general a complex quantity whose value is determined from the algebraic equations resulting from (1.4.2). The real part of n is the ordinary index of refraction equal to the ratio of the phase velocity of light *in vacuo* to that in the medium. The complex part of n is proportional to the absorption coefficient for the type of light transmitted.

The complex method is nothing more than a shorthand way of handling quantities with a sinusoidal time dependence. If G is such a time dependent quantity, it may be written $G = G_0 e^{-i\omega t}$, where the real part is understood. Differentiation gives $\partial G/\partial t = -i\omega G$. Consider an expression like $\alpha\mathbf{E}$, where $\mathbf{E} = \mathbf{E}_0 e^{-i\omega t}$ and $\alpha = \alpha_r + i\alpha_i$, with $\mathbf{E}_0$ real. Then $\mathrm{Re}(\alpha\mathbf{E}) = (\alpha_r \cos \omega t + \alpha_i \sin \omega t)\,\mathbf{E}_0 = \alpha_r\,\mathrm{Re}(\mathbf{E}) - (\alpha_i/\omega)\,\mathrm{Re}(\partial\mathbf{E}/\partial t)$; thus, the multiplication of $\mathbf{E}$ by a single complex quantity is equivalent to the summation of two independent quantities proportional to $\mathbf{E}$ and $\partial\mathbf{E}/\partial t$.

The relation $\nabla \times \mathbf{E} = -(1/c)(\partial\mathbf{B}/\partial t)$ applied to the vector $\mathbf{E} = \mathbf{i}E$ gives

$$\nabla \times \mathbf{E} = \mathbf{j}\frac{\partial E}{\partial z} = -\frac{1}{c}\frac{\partial \mathbf{B}}{\partial t} = \frac{i\omega}{c}\mathbf{B}.$$

Equations 1.6.11 may now be written as

$$\mathbf{M} = N\kappa\mathbf{B}' - N\beta^{\ddagger}\mathbf{E}' \quad (1.6.12a)$$

$$N\mathbf{P} = \alpha\mathbf{E}' + N\beta^{\ddagger}\mathbf{B}', \quad (1.6.12b)$$

where the effective fields are now indicated. The appropriate optical constants are given by

$$\kappa = \frac{e^2R^2\omega^2}{48mc^2}\left[\frac{1}{\Delta_1\Delta_2 - Q_{12}^2}(\mathbf{b}_1 \times \mathbf{b}_{12})^2(\Delta_1 + \Delta_2) + 2Q_{12}(\mathbf{b}_1 \times \mathbf{b}_{12})\cdot(\mathbf{b}_2 \times \mathbf{b}_{12})\right] \quad (1.6.13a)$$

$$\alpha = \frac{e^2}{3m}\frac{1}{\Delta_1\Delta_2 - Q_{12}^2}[(\Delta_1 + \Delta_2) - 2Q_{12}(\mathbf{b}_1 \cdot \mathbf{b}_2)] \quad (1.6.13b)$$

$$\beta^{\ddagger} = \frac{i\omega e^2 R Q_{12}(\mathbf{b}_{12} \cdot \mathbf{b}_1 \times \mathbf{b}_2)}{6mc(\Delta_1\Delta_2 - Q_{12}^2)}. \quad (1.6.13c)$$

The quantity κ may be called the complex magnetic susceptibility and α the complex polarizability. In the absence of damping, these quantities are real and provide an in phase contribution to **M** and **P**. Damping always gives an out of phase contribution, which is maximum at resonance. Likewise $\beta^{\ddagger}$ is imaginary in the absence of damping and the quantities $\beta^{\ddagger}\mathbf{E}$ and $\beta^{\ddagger}\mathbf{B}$ may be written as $-\beta'\dot{\mathbf{E}}$ and $-\beta'\dot{\mathbf{B}}$, where $\beta' = -(i/\omega)\beta^{\ddagger}$. The damping will provide components proportional to **E** and **B** which are a maximum at resonance. Equations 1.6.12 may then be written in their usual form:

$$\mathbf{M} = N\left(\kappa\mathbf{B}' + \frac{\beta\dot{\mathbf{E}}'}{c}\right) \quad (1.6.12a)'$$

$$\mathbf{P} = N\left(\alpha\mathbf{E}' - \frac{\beta\dot{\mathbf{B}}'}{c}\right), \quad (1.6.12b)'$$

where the constants are in general complex and $\beta/c = \beta'$.

1.7. Relation of Microscopic To Macroscopic Parameters

The relations between the macroscopic average and effective field quantities must be studied next. A precise formulation is particularly difficult, since local fields vary drastically within a molecule. If there is group degeneracy, the time dependent fields will vary in a similar manner, being large in the vicinity of the identical chromophores. A reasonable assumption for isotropic media is that there exists a linear relationship between the average and effective field quantities. In view of the Maxwell equations it is best to represent this relation in terms of the vector potential

$$\mathbf{A}' = S\mathbf{A}. \quad (1.7.1)$$

This in turn leads to the relations

$$\mathbf{E}' = -\frac{1}{c}\frac{\partial \mathbf{A}'}{\partial t} = S\mathbf{E} \tag{1.7.2a}$$

$$\mathbf{B}' = \nabla \times \mathbf{A}' = S\mathbf{B}. \tag{1.7.2b}$$

For a truly isotropic electrostatic field the Lorentz result has been useful in certain cases:

$$S_L = \left(1 - \frac{4\pi N\alpha}{3}\right)^{-1}. \tag{1.7.3}$$

Equations 1.4.2, 1.6.12′, and 1.7.1 may now be combined to give

$$\nabla^2\mathbf{A}(1 - 4\pi NS\kappa) - \frac{1}{c^2}\frac{\partial^2\mathbf{A}}{\partial t^2}(1 + 4\pi NS\alpha) = \frac{8\pi NS\beta}{c^2}\nabla \times \frac{\partial^2\mathbf{A}}{\partial t^2}. \tag{1.7.4}$$

The macroscopic current density $\mathbf{J}$ has been set equal to zero; and the relation $\nabla \times \nabla \times \mathbf{A} = -\nabla^2\mathbf{A}$, which is valid when $\nabla \cdot \mathbf{A} = 0$, has been used.

When $N = 0$ this reduces to the free space equation

$$\nabla^2\mathbf{A} = \frac{1}{c^2}\frac{\partial^2\mathbf{A}}{\partial t^2}. \tag{1.7.5}$$

The solution is

$$\mathbf{A} = \mathbf{A}_0\, e^{-i\omega(t - \mathbf{k}\cdot\mathbf{r}/c)}, \tag{1.7.6}$$

where $\mathbf{k}$ is a unit vector along the direction of propagation. In an inactive medium ($\beta = 0$, $N \neq 0$) one obtains a similar solution:

$$\mathbf{A} = \mathbf{A}_0\, e^{-i\omega(t - \bar{n}\mathbf{k}\cdot\mathbf{r}/c)}, \tag{1.7.7}$$

where the index of refraction is given by

$$\bar{n} = \left(\frac{1 + 4\pi NS\alpha}{1 - 4\pi NS\kappa}\right)^{1/2}. \tag{1.7.8}$$

The polarizability α is related to the intensity of electric dipole radiation, and the magnetic susceptibility κ is governed by magnetic dipole radiation, which is always several orders of magnitude lower in intensity. The denominator of this expression may therefore be set equal to unity. When $\beta \neq 0$ a solution may be assumed of the form

$$\mathbf{A} = \mathbf{A}_0\, e^{-i\omega(t - n\mathbf{k}\cdot\mathbf{r}/c)}.$$

This leads to the algebraic relation

$$\left(\frac{\omega^2 n^2}{c^2} - \frac{\omega^2\bar{n}^2}{c^2}\right)\mathbf{A} = \frac{i8\pi NS\beta\omega^3 n}{c^3}\mathbf{k} \times \mathbf{A}. \tag{1.7.9}$$

The vanishing of $\nabla \cdot \mathbf{A}$ requires that $\mathbf{k} \cdot \mathbf{A} = 0$; that is, $\mathbf{A}$ is perpendicular to the direction of propagation. One may write

$$\mathbf{A}_0 = \mathbf{i}A_1 + \mathbf{j}A_2,$$

and (1.7.9) becomes

$$(n^2 - \bar{n}^2)A_1 + ihnA_2 = 0 \tag{1.7.10a}$$

$$-ihnA_1 + (n^2 - \bar{n}^2)A_2 = 0, \tag{1.7.10b}$$

where $h = 8\pi NS\beta\omega/c$.

The determinant of this pair of homogeneous equations must vanish, with the result that

$$(n^2 - \bar{n}^2)^2 - h^2n^2 = 0. \tag{1.7.11}$$

To first order in the small quantity h the two positive solutions are

$$n_\pm = \bar{n} \mp \tfrac{1}{2}h. \tag{1.7.12}$$

The corresponding solutions to the linear equations are $A_1/A_2 = \mp i$. There will be two distinct forms of wave propagated in the optically active medium with the vector potentials

$$\mathbf{A}_+ = A_0(\mathbf{i} - i\mathbf{j})e^{-i\omega(t - n_+\mathbf{k}\cdot\mathbf{r}/c)} \tag{1.7.13a}$$

$$\mathbf{A}_- = A_0(\mathbf{i} + i\mathbf{j})e^{-i\omega(t - n_-\mathbf{k}\cdot\mathbf{r}/c)}. \tag{1.7.13b}$$

From (1.2.1) and the ensuing discussion it follows that $\mathbf{A}_-$ and $\mathbf{A}_+$ respectively describe left and right circular polarization.

Conventional plane polarized waves are excluded from an optically active medium by Maxwell's equations, the simplest solutions to which are opposite-handed circularly polarized waves with unequal phase velocities. The steady state solution to an optical activity problem will consist of plane polarized light in the regions outside the medium and a continuum of progressively rotated vectors inside, starting from the incident direction at one end and terminating at the emergent direction at the other. This continuum may be considered the result of the resolution of the incident plane polarized ray into opposite-handed circularly polarized rays with unequal phase velocities.

It will be recalled that β is real outside of absorption regions but acquires a sizable imaginary component inside. The phase is determined by the real part of $n_\pm$ and the absorption by the imaginary part. If one writes $n_\pm = n'_\pm + in''_\pm$, equations 1.7.13 become for propagation along the z-axis

$$\mathbf{A}_\pm = A_0(\mathbf{i} \mp i\mathbf{j})e^{-\omega n_\pm'' z/c}e^{-i\omega(t - n_\pm' z/c)}. \tag{1.7.14}$$

After traversing a distance z in the medium the phase difference is $(\omega z/c)(n_- - n_+)$. If $n_- > n_+$, the phase velocity of the right circularly polarized component is greater, which leads to dextrorotation. If two equal vectors have azimuthal angles ϕ_1 and ϕ_2, their sum will have the angle $\frac{1}{2}(\phi_1 - \phi_2)$. The angle of rotation in radians per unit path length will be

$$\phi = \frac{1}{2}\frac{\omega}{c}(n'_- - n'_+) = 4\pi NS\frac{\omega^2}{c^2}\beta', \qquad (1.7.15)$$

where β' is the real part of β.

The intensity of the radiation is found in the conventional manner by considering Maxwell's equations in the form

$$\nabla \times \mathbf{E} = -\frac{1}{c}\frac{\partial \mathbf{B}}{\partial t} \qquad (1.7.16a)$$

$$\nabla \times \mathbf{H} = \frac{1}{c}\frac{\partial \mathbf{D}}{\partial t} + \frac{4\pi}{c}\mathbf{J}. \qquad (1.7.16b)$$

An energy equation will be forthcoming by recognizing that the rate of energy expenditure on moving charge per unit volume is given by $\mathbf{J} \cdot \mathbf{E}$. Multiplication of the first of these equations by $\mathbf{H}$ and the second by $\mathbf{E}$ followed by the subtraction of the first from the second gives

$$\frac{c}{4\pi}\nabla \cdot (\mathbf{H} \times \mathbf{E}) = \frac{1}{4\pi}\mathbf{E} \cdot \frac{\partial \mathbf{D}}{\partial t} + \frac{1}{4\pi}\mathbf{H} \cdot \frac{\partial \mathbf{B}}{\partial t} + \mathbf{J} \cdot \mathbf{E}. \qquad (1.7.17)$$

Integration over a volume V bounded by a surface S gives upon use of the divergence theorem

$$\frac{c}{4\pi}\int_S \mathbf{H} \times \mathbf{E} \cdot d\mathbf{S} = \frac{1}{4\pi}\int_V \mathbf{E} \cdot \frac{\partial \mathbf{D}}{\partial t}\,dV + \frac{1}{4\pi}\int_V \mathbf{H} \cdot \frac{\partial \mathbf{B}}{\partial t}\,dV + \int_V \mathbf{J} \cdot \mathbf{E}\,dV. \qquad (1.7.18)$$

The terms on the right apparently represent the dissipation of energy within the volume, and the term on the left is the flow of energy through the surface. Since energy is conserved, this verifies the expected fact that any net loss within the volume is compensated by an equivalent amount passing through the surface.

For an isotropic medium the electromagnetic vectors are connected by the linear relations

$$\mathbf{D} = \varepsilon\mathbf{E} \qquad (1.7.19a)$$

$$\mathbf{B} = \mu\mathbf{H}. \qquad (1.7.19b)$$

Equation 1.7.18 may be written

$$-\frac{c}{4\pi}\int_S \mathbf{E} \times \mathbf{H} \cdot d\mathbf{S} = \frac{\varepsilon}{8\pi}\int_V \frac{\partial \mathbf{E}^2}{\partial t}\,dV + \frac{\mu}{8\pi}\int_V \frac{\partial \mathbf{H}^2}{\partial t}\,dV + \int_V \mathbf{J} \cdot \mathbf{E}\,dV. \qquad (1.7.20)$$

The minus sign has been introduced, since a negative rate of energy change on the right corresponds to a flow of energy out of the surface. If one considers a volume element in free space, the last term will be zero and the terms $\varepsilon \mathbf{E}^2/8\pi$ and $\mu \mathbf{H}^2/8\pi$ will be interpreted as energy densities; the vector $(c/4\pi)\mathbf{E} \times \mathbf{H}$, known as the Poynting vector, represents the flow of energy per unit time across the unit area.

Since **E**, **D**, **H**, and **B** are proportional to the time and space derivatives of **A**, the intensity of the radiation, which is a measure of its energy, will be proportional to **A**. From (1.7.14) one may write

$$I = I_0 e^{-\varepsilon_\pm z} = I_0 e^{-2\omega n_\pm'' z/c}, \tag{1.7.21}$$

from which it follows that $\varepsilon_\pm = (2\omega/c)n_\pm''$. The difference in extinction coefficients is called the circular dichroism and is given by

$$\theta = \varepsilon_- - \varepsilon_+ = 16\pi NS \frac{\omega^2}{c^2} \beta''. \tag{1.7.22}$$

This quantity can be measured directly with current instrumentation by shining alternate pulses of left and right circularly polarized light through the medium and electronically measuring the difference in absorption. In the following chapter the Kronig-Kramers transformations, which relate the real and imaginary parts of β, will be derived.

When circularly polarized components with different phase velocities are absorbed differentially, the resultant beam is elliptically polarized with a rotating principal axis. The progressive polarization upon the passage of initially plane polarized light through an optically active medium is shown in Figure 1.5. For a sufficiently long path length the ratio of the more strongly

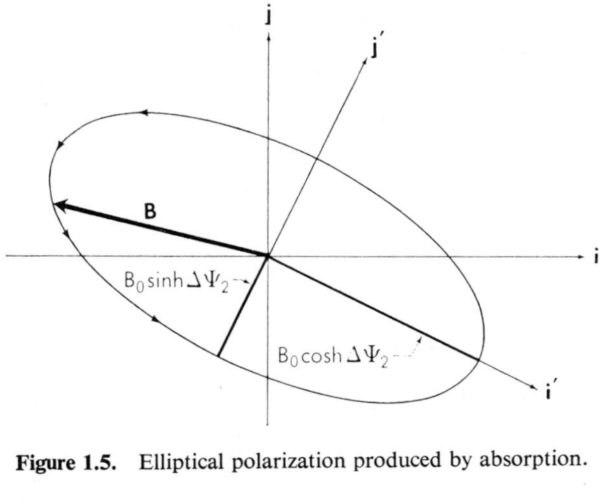

Figure 1.5. Elliptical polarization produced by absorption.

absorbed circular component to the lesser can be made arbitrarily small, and circular polarization finally results. In practice this is generally not realized, and most substances can be measured with small ellipticities by controlling the concentration and the path length.

1.8. Lorentzian Dispersion and Absorption

A considerable amount of qualitative information can be obtained from classical models like the coupled oscillator. In (1.7.15) and (1.7.22) the rotation and dichroism are proportional to the real and imaginary parts of $\beta = -(i/\omega)\beta^{\ddagger}$. From (1.6.13$c$) it follows that

$$\phi = AN\omega^2 RQ_{12}(\mathbf{b}_{12} \cdot \mathbf{b}_1 \times \mathbf{b}_2) \operatorname{Re}\left[\frac{1}{(\omega_1^2 - \omega^2 - i\Gamma_1\omega)(\omega_2^2 - \omega^2 - i\Gamma_2\omega) - Q_{12}^2}\right] \tag{1.8.1a}$$

$$\theta = 4AN\omega^2 RQ_{12}(\mathbf{b}_{12} \cdot \mathbf{b}_1 \times \mathbf{b}_2) \operatorname{Im}\left[\frac{1}{(\omega_1^2 - \omega^2 - i\Gamma_1\omega)(\omega_2^2 - \omega^2 - i\Gamma_2\omega) - Q_{12}^2}\right], \tag{1.8.1b}$$

where A depends only on fundamental constants and the effective field corrections.

The dispersion term may be written

$$\frac{1}{(\omega_1^2 - \omega^2 - i\Gamma_1\omega)(\omega_2^2 - \omega^2 - i\Gamma_2\omega) - Q_{12}^2} = \frac{\{[(\omega_1^2 - \omega^2)(\omega_2^2 - \omega^2) - Q_{12}^2] - \Gamma_1\Gamma_2\omega^2 + i\omega[\Gamma_1(\omega_2^2 - \omega^2) + \Gamma_2(\omega_1^2 - \omega^2)]\}}{\{[(\omega_1^2 - \omega^2)(\omega_2^2 - \omega^2) - Q_{12}^2]^2 + \omega^2\Gamma_1^2(\omega_2^2 - \omega^2)^2 + \omega^2\Gamma_2^2(\omega_1^2 - \omega^2)^2 + \Gamma_1^2\Gamma_2^2\omega^4 + 2Q_{12}^2\Gamma_1\Gamma_2\omega^2\}}. \tag{1.8.2}$$

This expression may be greatly simplified by observing that the damping constants Γ_1 and Γ_2 will be quite small and only of importance near resonance. In the absence of damping the denominator will be zero when $(\omega_1^2 - \omega^2)(\omega_2^2 - \omega^2) - Q_{12}^2 = 0$, which gives

$$(\omega_1'^2, \omega_2'^2) = \frac{\omega_1^2 + \omega_2^2}{2} \pm \tfrac{1}{2}\sqrt{(\omega_1^2 - \omega_2^2) + 4Q_{12}^2}. \tag{1.8.3}$$

These are to be interpreted as the new resonance frequencies arising from the coupling. When $\omega_1 = \omega_2$, as would be the case for two identical groups in a molecule, the "exiton" splitting is given by

$$\omega_1'^2 = \omega_1^2 - Q_{12} \tag{1.8.4a}$$

$$\omega_2'^2 = \omega_1^2 + Q_{12}. \tag{1.8.4b}$$

Since Γ_1 and Γ_2 are only important at resonance, the dependence on those terms containing powers of these quantities need not be stressed, and there is little error in rewriting the denominator as

$$[(\omega_1'^2 - \omega^2)^2 + \Gamma_1'^2\omega^2][(\omega_2'^2 - \omega^2)^2 + \Gamma_2'^2\omega^2].$$

This is identical in form to the result of setting $Q_{12} = 0$ in (1.8.2). When the coupling is weak there will be no need to distinguish between the primed and unprimed quantities. Equations 1.8.1 may now be written as

$$\phi = AN\omega^2 RQ_{12}(\mathbf{b}_{12} \cdot \mathbf{b}_1 \times \mathbf{b}_2) \times \frac{(\omega_1'^2 - \omega^2)(\omega_2'^2 - \omega^2)}{[(\omega_1'^2 - \omega^2)^2 + \Gamma_1'^2\omega^2][(\omega_2'^2 - \omega^2)^2 + \Gamma_2'^2\omega^2]} \tag{1.8.5a}$$

$$\theta = \frac{4AN\omega^2 RQ_{12}(\mathbf{b}_{12} \cdot \mathbf{b}_1 \times \mathbf{b}_2)\omega[\Gamma_1(\omega_2^2 - \omega^2) + \Gamma_2(\omega_1^2 - \omega^2)]}{[(\omega_1'^2 - \omega^2)^2 + \Gamma_1'^2\omega^2][(\omega_2'^2 - \omega^2)^2 + \Gamma_2'^2\omega^2]}, \tag{1.8.5b}$$

where the small factor $-\Gamma_1\Gamma_2\omega^2$ in the numerator of ϕ has been incorporated into ω_1' and ω_2'. Since $\omega_1'^2 + \omega_2'^2 = \omega_1^2 + \omega_2^2$, there is little error in replacing ω_1^2 and ω_2^2 in (1.8.5*b*) with $\omega_1'^2$ and $\omega_2'^2$. The primes may then be dropped; and the frequencies ω_1 and ω_2 will refer to the actual frequencies of the coupled system, which can be equal only in the limit of weak interactions.

If ω_1 and ω_2 are sufficiently different the behavior of these two curves is shown in Figure 1.6. The ORD curve has zeros at ω_1 and ω_2, which correspond very nearly to the extremum positions of the CD curve. This behavior may be considered as representative of all molecular systems. Traditionally the monotonic regions outside the absorption band are described as ordinary rotatory dispersion, and the behavior within the band is termed anomalous rotatory dispersion. By convention an ORD curve which reaches a maximum on the low frequency side of the absorption band is said to exhibit a positive Cotton effect.

The problem of identical oscillators is of central importance in high polymers such as helical proteins. It is therefore of interest to see what the simple classical theory has to say on this subject. There are two cases to consider; weak and strong coupling. In the former case the two frequencies are virtually equal. The curves are shown in Figure 1.7*a*. The intermediate case of moderately strong coupling is shown in Figure 1.7*b*. Here the splitting is large enough to give negative rotations in a small region. In practice it would be hard to distinguish between the two situations depicted in Figure 1.7, since there is always a background rotation which obscures the sign changes

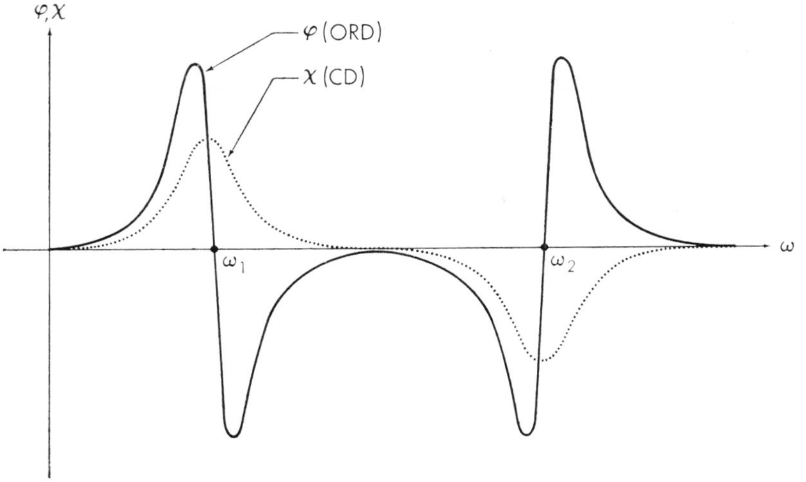

Figure 1.6. Optical rotatory dispersion (ORD) and circular dichroism (CD) curves for a pair of coupled oscillators.

within a given band; in addition the behavior of ORD and CD curves in an absorption band is strongly governed by other factors such as molecular vibration. In short, the classical theory predicts the behavior actually observed in these systems but gives no reliable method for correlating the data with the splitting of a degenerate frequency.

It should also be mentioned that the behavior exhibited here is of the so-called Lorentzian type associated with natural line widths. This would be expected from isolated atoms at rest in a rarified gas. Generally the molecules are undergoing frequent collisions which allow the system to attain the steady state for only a fraction of the time. The scattered radiation is the sum of damped wave trains from a statistical distribution of molecules in various states of transient motion. Under any fixed set of external conditions there is indeed a macroscopic steady state but one arising from a statistical distribution of microscopic transient states. The mathematical form of absorption or dichroism curves is often altered from Lorentzian to Gaussian behavior. There are reasons for believing that the qualitative behavior of the ORD and CD curves is substantially unaltered by the collision process. For the present the simple classical theory of natural line widths will suffice as an introduction to the subject.

From (1.7.8) the average complex index of refraction, which determines the ordinary absorption and dispersion properties of the medium, is given by

$$\bar{n} = \bar{n}' + i\bar{n}'' = \tfrac{1}{2}(n_+ + n_-) = \sqrt{1 + 4\pi NS\alpha} \cong 1 + 2\pi NS\alpha, \qquad (1.8.6)$$

where κ has been set equal to zero and the medium presumed to be sufficiently dilute for $\bar{n}$ to be nearly unity. The index of refraction is given by the real

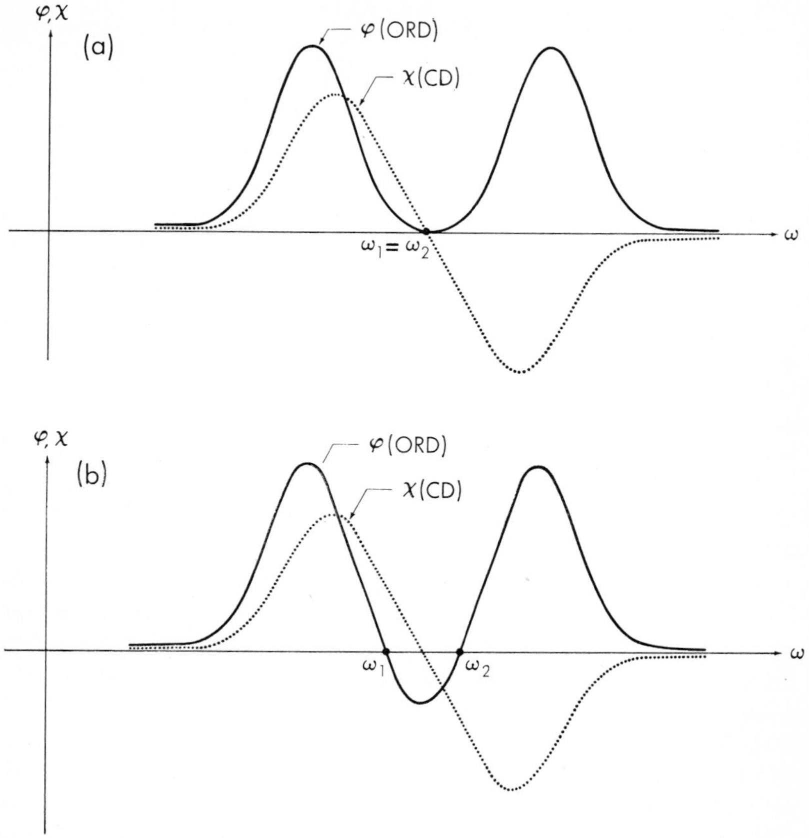

Figure 1.7. The degenerate case, with curves for weak (*a*) and moderately strong (*b*) coupling.

part of $\bar{n}$; the extinction coefficient ε is related to the complex part of $\bar{n}$ by the relation $e^{-\varepsilon z} = |e^{-i\omega(t - \bar{n}z/c)}|^2 = e^{-2\omega\bar{n}''z/c}$.

When it is borne in mind that the damping constants Γ_1 and Γ_2 are quite small and only of importance in absorption regions, (1.6.13*b*) may be rearranged to give

$$\bar{n}' - 1 = 2\pi NS \operatorname{Re}(\alpha)$$

$$= \frac{2\pi Ne^2 S}{3m}\left[\frac{\omega_1^2 - \omega^2}{(\omega_1^2 - \omega^2)^2 + \Gamma_1^2\omega^2}\left(1 - \frac{2Q_{12}\,\mathbf{b}_1 \cdot \mathbf{b}_2}{\omega_2^2 - \omega_1^2}\right) + \frac{\omega_2^2 - \omega^2}{(\omega_2^2 - \omega^2)^2 + \Gamma_2^2\omega^2}\left(1 + \frac{2Q_{12}\,\mathbf{b}_1 \cdot \mathbf{b}_2}{\omega_2^2 - \omega_1^2}\right)\right] \qquad (1.8.7a)$$

$$\varepsilon = \frac{2\omega \bar{n}''}{c} = \frac{4\pi\omega}{c} NS \operatorname{Im}(\alpha) = \frac{4\pi N e^2 \omega^2 S}{3mc}$$

$$\times \left[\Gamma_1\left(1 - \frac{2Q_{12}\,\mathbf{b}_1 \cdot \mathbf{b}_2}{\omega_2^2 - \omega_1^2}\right) \frac{1}{(\omega_1^2 - \omega^2)^2 + \Gamma_1^2\omega^2}\right.$$

$$\left. + \Gamma_2\left(1 + \frac{2Q_{12}\,\mathbf{b}_1 \cdot \mathbf{b}_2}{\omega_2^2 - \omega_1^2}\right) \frac{1}{(\omega_2^2 - \omega^2)^2 + \Gamma_2^2\omega^2}\right]. \tag{1.8.7b}$$

In the limit of weak coupling these equations reduce to the familiar ones for dispersion and Lorentzian absorption. When the original frequencies are equal, the two frequencies of the coupled system are related by $\omega_2^2 - \omega_1^2 = 2Q_{12}$; thus when the oscillations are parallel only one absorption band should be observed in this ideal case no matter what the splitting. When the oscillations are perpendicular, two bands of equal intensity are possible if the splitting is large enough. Intermediate orientations lead to bands of unequal intensity. Such behavior could only be observed in the event of strong coupling. It must also be remembered that when $\mathbf{b}_1$ and $\mathbf{b}_2$ are parallel the optical activity vanishes. There is no tendency toward unequal bands in the ORD or CD.

From a comparison of (1.8.5) and (1.8.7) it can be seen that the shapes of the curves for the average index of refraction and those for the difference $n_- - n_+$ are closely related. Just as the average index of refraction is related to the absorption coefficient by the Kronig-Kramers transform, the real and imaginary parts of the difference are connected by a similar relation; however, there is in general no simple relation connecting the average index of refraction to the difference. The above example merely appears to give a simple relation between the two arising from the simplicity of the model.

When the usual approximations are made (1.8.5*a*) may be written in the more familiar form

$$\phi = AN\omega^2 RQ_{12} \frac{\mathbf{b}_{12} \cdot \mathbf{b}_1 \times \mathbf{b}_2}{\omega_2'^2 - \omega_1'^2}$$

$$\times \left[\frac{\omega_1'^2 - \omega^2}{(\omega_1'^2 - \omega^2)^2 + \Gamma_1'^2\omega^2} - \frac{\omega_2'^2 - \omega^2}{(\omega_2'^2 - \omega^2)^2 + \Gamma_2'^2\omega^2}\right]. \tag{1.8.8}$$

The frequency dependence of the individual bands for $\bar{n}'$ and ϕ is governed by the factor $(\omega_1^2 - \omega^2)/[(\omega_1^2 - \omega^2)^2 + \Gamma_1^2\omega^2]$; the ORD contains the additional factor ω^2. In principle it should be possible to relate the width at half maximum of these two curves in a simple manner. The detailed discussion of these possibilities will be postponed until after the presentations of the quantum mechanical theory.

In coupled oscillator theories the dipole-dipole interaction is often used to obtain the constant Q_{12}. The angular dependence then has the form

$[\mathbf{b}_1 \cdot \mathbf{b}_2 - 3(\mathbf{b}_1 \cdot \mathbf{b}_{12})(\mathbf{b}_2 \cdot \mathbf{b}_{12})]\mathbf{b}_{12} \cdot \mathbf{b}_1 \times \mathbf{b}_2$. The configuration of the system may be specified by three angles: θ_1, the angle between $\mathbf{b}_1$ and $\mathbf{b}_{12}$; θ_2, the angle between $\mathbf{b}_2$ and $\mathbf{b}_{12}$; and γ, the dihedral angle between the planes determined by $(\mathbf{b}_1, \mathbf{b}_{12})$ and $(\mathbf{b}_2, \mathbf{b}_{12})$. It is not difficult to show that the maximum value of the above expression is attained when

$$\theta_1 = \theta_2, \qquad \cos^3 \gamma - 4 \cos^2 \gamma + 2 = 0, \qquad \cos \gamma = 2 \cot \theta_1.$$

The solutions are approximately $\theta_1 = 68°30'$, $\gamma = 38°30'$. This information will be useful for relating changes in rotational strength to conformation changes.

1.9. Coupled Linear and Circular Oscillators

A second mechanism responsible for optical activity arises when a charge is constrained to move along a dissymmetric path such as a helix. If a single point charge is considered, the theory of small oscillations cannot be used, since the amplitude must be large enough for the system to display its dissymmetry through a phase difference over the region of motion.

The early investigators of the subject were able to remove the difficulty by placing a second charge on the helix, diametrically opposed to the first. If both charges can move independently under the influence of a coupling force, the problem is immediately solved in terms of the coupled oscillator model. The scalar triple product $\mathbf{b}_{12} \cdot \mathbf{b}_1 \times \mathbf{b}_2$ will be simply related to the pitch of the helix. If the two charges are rigidly joined, the system has one degree of freedom and must be treated by a new method.

Rather than solve the helical problem we will investigate three related systems which are of particular interest to actual molecules:

1. Two circularly moving charges rigidly coupled to a third constrained to move along a line perpendicular to the circle (one degree of freedom).
2. Two circularly moving charges coupled to an independently moving linear oscillator with arbitrary orientation in space (two degrees of freedom).
3. Two charges moving circularly in a plane capable of undergoing independent linear oscillations along its normal (two degrees of freedom).

The first system is shown in Figure 1.8. Charges 1 and 2 will move tangentially to the circle parallel to the vector **c**. The third charge will move along **b** perpendicular to the plane of the circle. In this rigidly coupled system the coordinates will satisfy the constraints

$$q_1 = -sq_3 \qquad (1.9.1a)$$

$$q_2 = +sq_3 \qquad (1.9.1b)$$

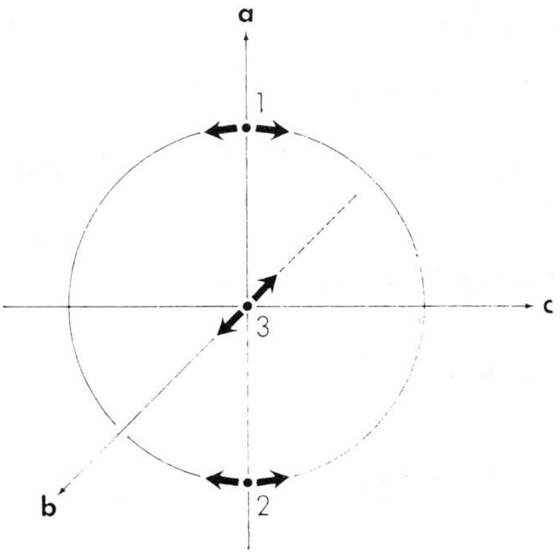

Figure 1.8. Rigidly coupled linear and circular oscillators.

for a right-handed screw motion. It will be assumed that the charges and masses are equal to e and m respectively and that each charge has a damping constant γ. A restoring force will be assumed to act independently on each charge by an amount proportional to its displacement with a constant k for all three charges.

The equation of motion may be obtained by considering the total kinetic and potential energies T and V along with the energy dissipation function W. These quantities are given by

$$T = \tfrac{1}{2}m(\dot{q}_1^2 + \dot{q}_2^2 + \dot{q}_3^2) = \tfrac{1}{2}m(2s^2 + 1)\dot{q}_3^2 \tag{1.9.2a}$$

$$V = \tfrac{1}{2}k(q_1^2 + q_2^2 + q_3^2) = \tfrac{1}{2}k(2s^2 + 1)q_3^2 \tag{1.9.2b}$$

$$W = \tfrac{1}{2}\gamma(\dot{q}_1^2 + \dot{q}_2^2 + \dot{q}_3^2) = \tfrac{1}{2}\gamma(2s^2 + 1)\dot{q}_3^2 . \tag{1.9.2c}$$

In (1.9.2c) the damping force on a charge is given by $-\gamma\dot{q}$ and the energy dissipated in time dt is $(-\gamma\dot{q})\,dq = -\gamma\dot{q}^2\,dt$. If W is defined as $\frac{1}{2}\gamma\dot{q}^2$, the power loss will equal $2W$ and the frictional force will be given by $-2W/\dot{q}$. Equations 1.9.2 indicate that in the equation of motion the quantities m, k, and γ are to be multiplied by the factor $2s^2 + 1$.

Since the coupling is rigid, a force acting on one charge is mechanically transmitted to the others. The force on the center charge is $\mathbf{b} \cdot \mathbf{E}(0)$, where $\mathbf{E}(0)$ is the field evaluated at the origin. The forces on the first two charges are $\mathbf{c} \cdot \mathbf{E}(1)$ and $\mathbf{c} \cdot \mathbf{E}(2)$, where the fields are to be evaluated at the appropriate positions. Since by (1.9.1) the first charge moves through a displacement $-sq_3$ when the third moves a distance q_3, the component of force along $\mathbf{b}$ is $-s\mathbf{c} \cdot \mathbf{E}(1)$; similarly the force on the second charge leads to $+s\mathbf{c} \cdot \mathbf{E}(2)$.

The total electric force along the motion of the third electron is given by

$$F_E = e[\mathbf{b} \cdot \mathbf{E}(0) - s\mathbf{c} \cdot \mathbf{E}(1) + s\mathbf{c} \cdot \mathbf{E}(2)]. \tag{1.9.3}$$

This is interpreted as the effective force on a single charge of mass $(2s^2 + 1)m$ and charge $(2s^2 + 1)e$.

In terms of the laboratory coordinate system **i**, **j**, **k** (**E** parallel to **i** with **k** the direction of propagation) one obtains

$$\mathbf{E}(1) = \left[E(0) + \mathbf{a} \cdot \mathbf{k} r_0 \frac{\partial E(0)}{\partial z}\right]\mathbf{i} \tag{1.9.4a}$$

$$\mathbf{E}(2) = \left[E(0) - \mathbf{a} \cdot \mathbf{k} r_0 \frac{\partial E(0)}{\partial z}\right]\mathbf{i}, \tag{1.9.4b}$$

where r_0 is the radius of the circle and $E(0) = E_0(0)e^{-i\omega t}$ is the scalar amplitude.

The subscript on q_3 may be dropped and the resulting equation of motion written as

$$\ddot{q} + \Gamma \dot{q} + \omega_0^2 q = Qe^{-i\omega t}, \tag{1.9.5}$$

where

$$\Gamma = \frac{\gamma}{m},$$

$$Q = \frac{e}{m(2s^2 + 1)}\left[\mathbf{b} \cdot \mathbf{i} E_0(0) - 2sr_0(\mathbf{a} \cdot \mathbf{k})(\mathbf{c} \cdot \mathbf{i})\frac{\partial E_0(0)}{\partial z}\right],$$

The steady state solution is obtained in the usual way by letting $q = q_0\, e^{-i\omega t}$:

$$q = \frac{Qe^{-i\omega t}}{\omega_0^2 - \omega^2 - i\omega\Gamma}. \tag{1.9.6}$$

As before, the behavior of the scattered radiation is obtained by averaging the electric and magnetic dipole moments over all orientations. This yields the relations

$$\mathbf{p} = e\langle(\mathbf{b} - s\mathbf{c} + s\mathbf{c})q\rangle_{\text{av}} = e\langle \mathbf{b} q\rangle_{\text{av}} = \frac{e^2}{m(2s^2 + 1)} \frac{e^{-i\omega t}}{\omega_0^2 - \omega^2 - i\omega\Gamma}$$

$$\times \left[\langle(\mathbf{b} \cdot \mathbf{i})\mathbf{b}\rangle_{\text{av}} E_0(0) - 2sr_0\langle(\mathbf{a} \cdot \mathbf{k})(\mathbf{c} \cdot \mathbf{i})\mathbf{b}\rangle_{\text{av}} \frac{\partial E_0(0)}{\partial z}\right]$$

$$= \frac{e^2}{m(2s^2 + 1)} \frac{1}{\omega_0^2 - \omega^2 - i\omega\Gamma}\left[\tfrac{1}{3}\mathbf{E}(0) + \tfrac{1}{3} s r_0 \frac{i\omega}{c}\mathbf{B}(0)\right] \tag{1.9.7a}$$

$$\mathbf{m} = \frac{e}{2c}\left\langle \sum_{n=1}^{3} \mathbf{r}_n \times \mathbf{v}_n \right\rangle_{\text{av}} = \frac{e}{2c}\langle 2sr_0\,\mathbf{b}\dot{q}\rangle_{\text{av}} = -sr_0\left(\frac{i\omega}{c}\right)\frac{e^2}{m(2s^2+1)}$$

$$\times \frac{1}{\omega_0^2 - \omega^2 - i\omega\Gamma}\left[\tfrac{1}{3}\mathbf{E}(0) + \tfrac{1}{3}sr_0\frac{i\omega}{c}\mathbf{B}(0)\right], \qquad (1.9.7b)$$

where the relations

$$\langle(\mathbf{a}\cdot\mathbf{k})(\mathbf{c}\cdot\mathbf{i})\mathbf{b}\rangle_{\text{av}} = \tfrac{1}{6}(\mathbf{c}\cdot\mathbf{b}\times\mathbf{a})\mathbf{j} = -\tfrac{1}{6}\mathbf{j},$$

$$\langle(\mathbf{b}\cdot\mathbf{i})\mathbf{b}\rangle_{\text{av}} = \tfrac{1}{3}\mathbf{i},$$

$$\nabla\times\mathbf{E}(0) = \mathbf{j}\frac{\partial E(0)}{\partial z} = -\frac{1}{c}\dot{\mathbf{B}} = \frac{i\omega}{c}\mathbf{B},$$

have been used.

In terms of the volume dipole moment distributions one obtains

$$\mathbf{P} = N\alpha\mathbf{E} + N\beta^{\ddagger}\mathbf{B}$$

$$\mathbf{M} = N\kappa\mathbf{B} - N\beta^{\ddagger}\mathbf{E},$$

where

$$\alpha = \frac{e^2}{3m(2s^2+1)}\frac{1}{\omega_0^2 - \omega^2 - i\omega\Gamma} \qquad (1.9.8a)$$

$$\beta^{\ddagger} = \frac{e^2}{3m(2s^2+1)}\left(\frac{i\omega sr_0}{c}\right)\frac{1}{\omega_0^2 - \omega^2 - i\omega\Gamma} \qquad (1.9.8b)$$

$$\kappa = \frac{e^2}{3m(2s^2+1)}\left(\frac{r_0^2 s^2\omega^2}{c^2}\right)\frac{1}{\omega_0^2 - \omega^2 - i\omega\Gamma}. \qquad (1.9.8c)$$

As before, the vectors **B** and **E** are interpreted to mean the effective fields. The rotation in degrees per unit path length is from (1.7.15) with $\beta = -(i/\omega)\beta^{\ddagger}$

$$\phi = \frac{4\pi NS\omega^2}{c^2}\left[\frac{e^2 sr_0}{3m(2s^2+1)}\right]\frac{\omega_0^2 - \omega^2}{(\omega_0^2 - \omega^2)^2 + \omega^2\Gamma^2}. \qquad (1.9.9)$$

Generally the conclusions from such classical models fall into two categories: those which are pertinent to actual molecules and those which are peculiar to the model. In all the examples treated in this chapter the form of the magnetic susceptibility may largely be ignored, since the complete three-dimensional degrees of freedom of an electron in orbit must be recognized to explain diamagnetism. Equation 1.9.8c does reflect the fact that $\kappa \ll \alpha$ when $r_0 \ll \lambda$ and s is not too large. The expressions for the polarizability are essentially the same as the quantum mechanical counterparts.

The equation for ϕ leads to several observations. The rotation is immediately written in terms of the polarizability, and a rough order of magnitude estimate to the expected rotations may be obtained:

$$\phi = \frac{16\pi^3 s r_0}{\lambda^2} N\alpha. \tag{1.9.10}$$

In condensed systems $\alpha \sim 1/N$; the radius r_0 will be $\sim 10^{-8}$ cm, and $\lambda \sim 3 \times 10^{-5}$ cm. This gives $\phi \sim 10^3 s$ rad/cm or $\sim 10^4 s$ deg/cm. Although a completely literal application of the model is not advisable, it may be said that the parameter s represents the ratio of the magnetic moment of a transition (in Bohr magnetons) to its electric moment (in debyes). This leads us to expect rotations of 10^4 deg/cm for solids under favorable conditions. The average values for condensed systems are not quite this high. In dilute media N is reduced by a factor of $\sim 10^3$, leading us to expect rotations of 10 deg/cm. Such high rotations are rarely observed, indicating that s is somewhat less than unity. The reason for this may be anticipated by observing that electronic motions tend to follow either circular (magnetic dipole) or linear (electric dipole) paths. In the first case $s \gg 1$ and $r_0 \sim 10^{-8}$ cm; in the second case $s < 1$ and $r_0 < 10^{-8}$ cm. In both types of transition the product $sr_0/(2s^2 + 1)$ is comparable (for a fixed value of r_0 the optimum value of s is $1/\sqrt{2}$); this again emphasizes the equivalence of electric and magnetic dipole transitions.

It follows from (1.9.9) that in the long wave region the rotation of a right-handed screw pattern is positive, a fact which seems to be recurrent in both classical and quantum theories on the subject.

It may also be observed that ϕ approaches a limiting nonzero value as $\omega \to \infty$. This is a result peculiar to a system with one degree of freedom. It is quite correct in terms of the model but only applicable to individual transitions in molecules.

A slightly more complex but highly pertinent model is provided by the coupled electric and magnetic dipole oscillators shown in Figure 1.9. The unit vectors **e** and **d** determine the position and orientation of the linear oscillator relative to the circular one. Charges 2 and 3 are rigidly confined to opposite ends of a diameter and move parallel to the **c**-axis; thus $q_3 = -q_2$. Small oscillations will again be assumed with the circular and linear motions being in general of unequal frequency but coupled by an energy term of the form $Q'_{12}q_1q_2$, as in the case of the two linear oscillators. For ordinary electrostatic coupling the dipole-quadrupole term for this system may be obtained by expanding the difference between the two dipole-dipole terms

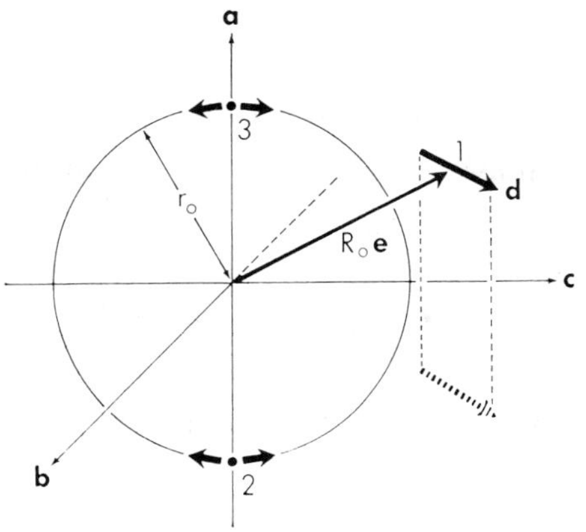

Figure 1.9. Coupled linear and circular oscillators.

as a power series in r_0 and retaining only the first term. The potential V_{12} is then given by

$$V_{12} = Q'_{12}\, q_1 q_2 = q_1 q_2\, e_1 e_2 \left\{ R_{12}^{-3} \left[(\mathbf{c} \cdot \mathbf{d}) - \frac{3(\mathbf{c} \cdot \mathbf{R}_{12})(\mathbf{d} \cdot \mathbf{R}_{12})}{R_{12}^2} \right] - R_{13}^{-3} \left[(\mathbf{c} \cdot \mathbf{d}) - \frac{3(\mathbf{c} \cdot \mathbf{R}_{13})(\mathbf{d} \cdot \mathbf{R}_{13})}{R_{13}^2} \right] \right\}$$

$$= \frac{6 r_0\, e_1 e_2}{R_0^4} [5 \gamma_a \gamma_c (\mathbf{e} \cdot \mathbf{d}) - \gamma_a (\mathbf{c} \cdot \mathbf{d}) - \gamma_c (\mathbf{a} \cdot \mathbf{d})] q_1 q_2, \tag{1.9.11}$$

where γ_a and γ_c are the direction cosines of **e** and R_{12} and R_{13} are the exact distances of separation of the indicated charges. The treatment is somewhat simplified if the mass and charge of the second two charges are one-half of the first: $m_2 = \frac{1}{2} m_1$, $e_2 = \frac{1}{2} e_1$.

In the equations of motion for the coupled system the electric field must be evaluated separately at each of the three positions of the charges. Bearing in mind that $q_3 = -q_2$, we obtain

$$m_1 \ddot{q}_1 + k_1 q_1 + \gamma_1 \dot{q}_1 + Q'_{12}\, q_2 = e_1 \mathbf{d} \cdot \mathbf{E}_0(1) e^{-i\omega t} \tag{1.9.12a}$$

$$2 m_2 \ddot{q}_2 + 2 k_2 q_2 + 2 \gamma_2 \dot{q}_2 + Q'_{12}\, q_1 = e_2 [\mathbf{c} \cdot \mathbf{E}_0(2) - \mathbf{c} \cdot \mathbf{E}_0(3)] e^{-i\omega t}. \tag{1.9.12b}$$

When the usual expansions are made for $\mathbf{E}_0(1)$, $\mathbf{E}_0(2)$, and $\mathbf{E}_0(3)$ and the substitutions $m_2 = \frac{1}{2} m_1 = \frac{1}{2} m$, $e_2 = \frac{1}{2} e_1 = \frac{1}{2} e$, there results

$$\ddot{q}_1 + \omega_1^2 q_1 + \Gamma_1 \dot{q}_1 + Q_{12}\, q_2 = Q_1\, e^{-i\omega t} \tag{1.9.13a}$$

$$\ddot{q}_2 + \omega_2^2 q_2 + \Gamma_2 \dot{q}_2 + Q_{12}\, q_1 = Q_2\, e^{-i\omega t}, \tag{1.9.13b}$$

where

$$\Gamma_1 = \frac{\gamma_1}{m_1}, \quad \Gamma_2 = \frac{\gamma_2}{m_2}, \quad Q_{12} = \frac{Q'_{12}}{m},$$

$$Q_1 = \frac{e}{m}\left[(\mathbf{d}\cdot\mathbf{i})E_0(0) + R_0(\mathbf{d}\cdot\mathbf{i})(\mathbf{e}\cdot\mathbf{k})\frac{\partial E_0(0)}{\partial z}\right],$$

$$Q_2 = -\frac{e}{2m}\left[2r_0(\mathbf{c}\cdot\mathbf{i})(\mathbf{a}\cdot\mathbf{k})\frac{\partial E_0(0)}{\partial z}\right].$$

As in Section 1.6, these equations are readily solved to give

$$q_1 = \frac{\Delta_2 Q_1 - Q_2 Q_{12}}{\Delta_1\Delta_2 - Q_{12}^2}\, e^{-i\omega t} \tag{1.9.14a}$$

$$q_2 = \frac{\Delta_1 Q_2 - Q_1 Q_{12}}{\Delta_1\Delta_2 - Q_{12}^2}\, e^{-i\omega t}, \tag{1.9.14b}$$

where

$$\Delta_1 = \omega_1^2 - \omega^2 - i\omega\Gamma_1,$$
$$\Delta_2 = \omega_2^2 - \omega^2 - i\omega\Gamma_2 .$$

The induced electric and magnetic dipole moments are found to be

$$\mathbf{p} = e\langle \mathbf{d}q_1\rangle = \frac{e^2}{m}\frac{1}{\Delta_1\Delta_2 - Q_{12}^2}\left[\tfrac{1}{3}\Delta_2\,\mathbf{E}_0(0) - \frac{Q_{12}\,r_0(\mathbf{b}\cdot\mathbf{d})}{6}\,\mathbf{j}\,\frac{\partial E_0(0)}{\partial z}\right] \tag{1.9.15a}$$

$$\begin{aligned}\mathbf{m} &= \frac{e}{2c}\left[\langle R_0\,\mathbf{e}\times\mathbf{d}\dot{q}_1\rangle_{\text{av}} + \tfrac{1}{2}\langle r_0\,\mathbf{a}\times\mathbf{c}(-\dot{q}_2)\rangle_{\text{av}} + \tfrac{1}{2}\langle -r_0\,\mathbf{a}\times\mathbf{c}\dot{q}_2\rangle_{\text{av}}\right]\\
&= \frac{e}{2c}\left(\langle \mathbf{e}\times\mathbf{d}R_0\,\dot{q}_1\rangle_{\text{av}} + \langle \mathbf{b}r_0\,\dot{q}_2\rangle_{\text{av}}\right)\\
&= -\frac{i\omega e^2}{2mc}\frac{1}{\Delta_1\Delta_2 - Q_{12}^2}\left[\tfrac{1}{6}(\mathbf{e}\times\mathbf{d})^2 R_0^2\,\mathbf{j}\,\frac{\partial E_0(0)}{\partial z}\,\Delta_2\right.\\
&\quad - \tfrac{1}{6}r_0\,R_0\,\mathbf{b}\cdot(\mathbf{e}\times\mathbf{d})Q_{12}\,\mathbf{j}\,\frac{\partial E_0(0)}{\partial z} + \tfrac{1}{6}r_0^2\,\mathbf{j}\,\frac{\partial E_0(0)}{\partial z}\,\Delta_1\\
&\quad \left. - \tfrac{1}{3}(\mathbf{b}\cdot\mathbf{d})Q_{12}\,r_0\,\mathbf{E}_0(0) - \tfrac{1}{6}r_0\,R_0\,\mathbf{b}\cdot(\mathbf{e}\times\mathbf{d})Q_{12}\,\mathbf{j}\,\frac{\partial E_0(0)}{\partial z}\right].\end{aligned} \tag{1.9.15b}$$

Once again the relation $\mathbf{j}(\partial E(0)/\partial z) = (i\omega/c)\mathbf{B}$ is used, and it will be recalled that terms of the type $\langle(\mathbf{d}\cdot\mathbf{i})(\mathbf{e}\cdot\mathbf{k})\mathbf{d}\rangle_{\text{av}} = 0$. The coefficients of **B** and **E** in the two expressions for $\mathbf{P} = N\mathbf{p}$ and $\mathbf{M} = N\mathbf{m}$ are determined to be

$$\alpha = \frac{1}{3}\frac{e^2}{m}\frac{\Delta_2}{\Delta_1\Delta_2 - Q_{12}^2} \tag{1.9.16a}$$

$$\beta^{\ddagger} = -\frac{1}{6}\frac{i\omega}{c}\frac{e^2}{m} Q_{12}\, r_0(\mathbf{b}\cdot\mathbf{d})\frac{1}{\Delta_1\Delta_2 - Q_{12}^2} \tag{1.9.16b}$$

$$\kappa = \frac{1}{12}\frac{e^2\omega^2}{mc^2}\frac{1}{\Delta_1\Delta_2 - Q_{12}^2}[(\mathbf{e}\times\mathbf{d})^2 R_0^2\Delta_2 - 2r_0 R_0\,\mathbf{b}\cdot(\mathbf{e}\times\mathbf{d})Q_{12} + r_0^2\Delta_1]. \tag{1.9.16c}$$

As can be expected, the polarizability comes from the linear oscillator; the term $\Delta_2/(\Delta_1\Delta_2 - Q_{12}^2)$ is essentially equal to $1/\Delta_1$ for weak coupling. Again the form of κ will not be taken too seriously, since it applies to restricted motion and accordingly does not provide a route to understanding diamagnetic effects.

The general behavior of the model is slightly complex; however, when $\mathbf{e}\cdot\mathbf{d} = 1$ the sign determining term, $Q_{12}(\mathbf{b}\cdot\mathbf{d})$, becomes proportional to $+\gamma_a\gamma_b\gamma_c$, since $\mathbf{a}\cdot\mathbf{d}$, $\mathbf{b}\cdot\mathbf{d}$, and $\mathbf{c}\cdot\mathbf{d}$ are now equal to γ_a, γ_b, and γ_c [cf. (1.9.11)]. When the linear oscillator is in the positive octant of the circular one, as shown in Figure 1.9, the rotation is negative. The motion conforms to a left-handed screw pattern, since when the first electron moves away from the circle the resulting dipole pulls on the top charge more strongly than on the bottom one; the motion of the central charge toward the observer is accompanied by a clockwise motion of the other two.

It may also be noted that the optical activity does not arise from the phase difference between the linear and circular oscillators as it does with two linear oscillators. Consider the two orientations shown in Figure 1.10. This is the most favorable configuration for dissymmetric scattering even though the electrostatic interaction is zero. One may assume some other type of coupling to exist and concentrate on the consequences of the coupling for the two orientations.

In the first orientation (Figure 1.10*a*), the difference in phase between the second and third charges causes a torque which is maximum when $\mathbf{E}(0) = 0$ and zero when $\mathbf{E}(0)$ is maximum. The motion of the couple is out of phase with $\mathbf{E}(0)$ and so will be the induced motion of the linear oscillator, which is not directly acted upon by the field **E**. This results in the perpendicular out of phase component of **E** required for optical activity.

In the second orientation (Figure 1.10*b*), the first charge is directly acted upon by the electric field. The circular motion of the other two charges is in phase but the magnetic moment, which is zero at the extreme positions of

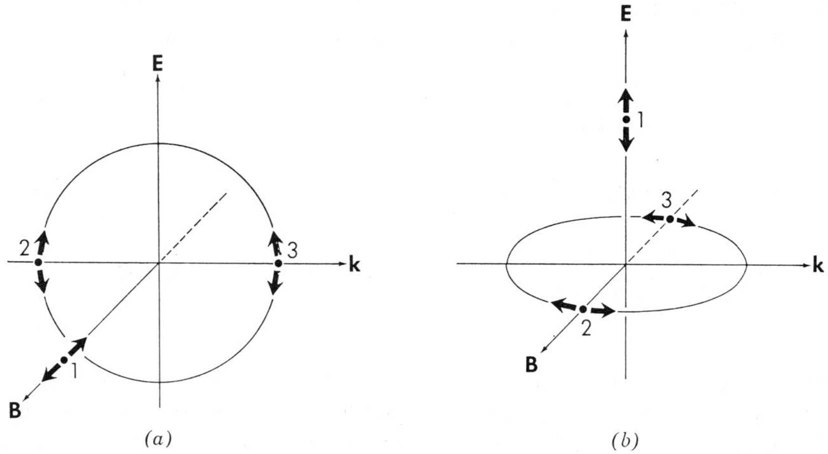

Figure 1.10. Instructive orientations for coupled linear (*a*) and circular (*b*) oscillators.

the motion of the first charge, is out of phase. There is induced a perpendicular out of phase component of **B**. It should be emphasized that in all the examples treated the scattered radiation arises from either a linear or circular motion of charge which has been induced by the motion of a charge directly driven by the radiation field. Although it was convenient to discuss the scattering of a linear oscillator in terms of its electric field and that for a circular oscillator in terms of a magnetic field, it must be remembered that the fundamental laws of electrodynamics prescribe perpendicular radiation components of magnetic or electric field. This fact would be more in evidence had we chosen to treat the problem by the direct computation of the induced radiation fields rather than solve the Maxwell equations for material media.

Comparison of (1.9.16*b*) with (1.6.13*c*) shows that the ratio of the rotatory parameters varies as $(r_0/R_0)^2$, where R_0 is the distance of separation of the two oscillators and r_0 is the radius of the circle. When R_0 is large the effect of the coupled linear oscillators would certainly predominate. This is not the whole story for molecules, as will be indicated in our last consideration.

If two charges are constrained to opposite ends of a diameter on a circle that is free to move in a perpendicular direction, a new variation results, which may be considered the classical precursor of the one-electron theory. The situation is shown in Figure 1.11. The system has two degrees of freedom and two different oscillation frequencies, a circular one ω_1 and a linear one ω_2. In addition the potential energy of each charge will depend on its distance from a fixed point *P*. In a purely mechanical model the two charges would be joined to *P* by springs. More realistically they would be acted upon by a fixed

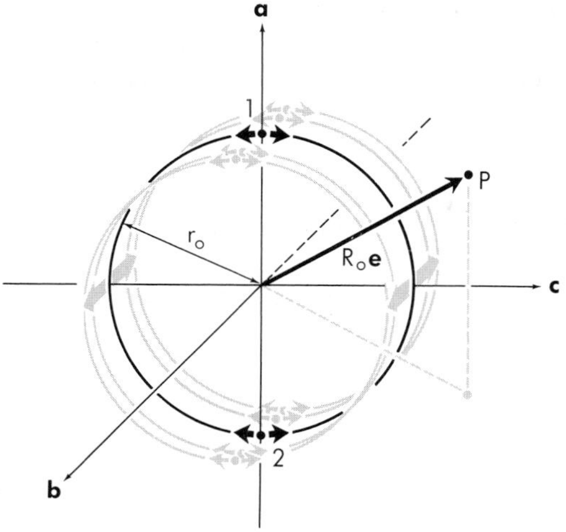

Figure 1.11. The circular oscillator with two degrees of freedom.

charge at this point. This model differs from the earlier circular oscillators in that the charges have two degrees of freedom with different frequencies of vibration. Although the magnetic component of the radiation field is now capable of altering the motion, its effect may still be neglected for frequencies in the near ultraviolet, since $v/c \ll 1$.

To determine the electrostatic coupling due to a charge at P it is convenient to define the following quantities: the position vectors of P relative to the equilibrium positions of the two charges, $\mathbf{R}_1^{(0)} = \mathbf{e}R_0 - \mathbf{a}r_0$, $\mathbf{R}_2 = \mathbf{e}R_0^{(0)} + \mathbf{a}r_0$; the position vectors of the charges relative to their own equilibrium positions, $\mathbf{r}_1 = q_1\mathbf{c} + q_2\mathbf{b}$, $\mathbf{r}_2 = -q_1\mathbf{c} + q_2\mathbf{b}$; and the vectors from the instantaneous positions of the charges to the point P, $\mathbf{R}_1 = \mathbf{R}_1^{(0)} - \mathbf{r}_1$, $\mathbf{R}_2 = \mathbf{R}_1^{(0)} - \mathbf{r}_2$. The potential of the system relative to the rest positions with a charge ρe at P is then

$$V = \rho e^2\left[\left(\frac{1}{R_1^{(0)}} - \frac{1}{R_1}\right) + \left(\frac{1}{R_2^{(0)}} - \frac{1}{R_2}\right)\right].$$

The quantities

$$\frac{1}{R_1} = \{R_1^{(0)}\sqrt{1 + [1/R_1^{(0)2}][r_1^2 - 2\mathbf{r}_1 \cdot \mathbf{R}_1^{(0)}]}\}^{-1}$$

and

$$\frac{1}{R_2} = \{R_2^{(0)}\sqrt{1 + [1/R_2^{(0)2}][r_2^2 - 2\mathbf{r}_2 \cdot \mathbf{R}_2^{(0)}]}\}^{-1}$$

may be expanded by the binomial theorem for $(1 + x)^{-1/2}$ with the retention only of the lowest order terms in $q_1 q_2$. The other terms will only involve small corrections to the zero point energy and force constants. The result is

$$V = Q'_{12} q_1 q_2 = \frac{-30\rho e^2 r_0 \gamma_a \gamma_b \gamma_c}{R_0^4} q_1 q_2, \tag{1.9.17}$$

where γ_a, γ_b, and γ_c are the direction cosines of $\mathbf{e}$ in the coordinate system **a, b, c.**

From the previous examples it should not be difficult to verify that the equations of motion for the system are

$$\ddot{q}_1 + \omega_1^2 q_1 + \Gamma_1 \dot{q}_1 + Q_{12} q_2 = Q_1 e^{-i\omega t},$$
$$\ddot{q}_2 + \omega_2^2 q_2 + \Gamma_2 \dot{q}_2 + Q_{12} q_1 = Q_2 e^{-i\omega t},$$

where

$$Q_{12} = \frac{Q'_{12}}{2m}, \quad \Gamma_1 = \frac{\gamma_1}{2m}, \quad \Gamma_2 = \frac{\gamma_2}{2m},$$

$$Q_1 = \frac{er_0}{2m}\left[2(\mathbf{a}\cdot\mathbf{k})(\mathbf{i}\cdot\mathbf{c})\frac{\partial E_0(0)}{\partial z}\right], \tag{1.9.18a}$$

$$Q_2 = \frac{e}{2m}[2E_0(0)\mathbf{i}\cdot\mathbf{b}]. \tag{1.9.18b}$$

The solutions are again

$$q_1 = \frac{\Delta_2 Q_1 - Q_2 Q_{12}}{\Delta_1 \Delta_2 - Q_{12}^2} e^{-i\omega t},$$

$$q_2 = \frac{\Delta_1 Q_2 - Q_1 Q_{12}}{\Delta_1 \Delta_2 - Q_{12}^2} e^{-i\omega t}.$$

The electric and magnetic moments are

$$\mathbf{p} = e\langle \mathbf{r}_1 + \mathbf{r}_2 \rangle_{\text{av}} = 2e\langle q_2 \mathbf{b} \rangle_{\text{av}} = \frac{2e^2}{m}\frac{e^{-i\omega t}}{\Delta_1\Delta_2 - Q_{12}^2}$$
$$\times \left\{\Delta_1(\tfrac{1}{3}\mathbf{E}_0(0)) - Q_{12} r_0 \left[-\tfrac{1}{6}\mathbf{j}\frac{\partial E_0(0)}{\partial z}\right]\right\} \tag{1.9.19a}$$

$$\mathbf{m} = \frac{er_0}{2c}\langle(\mathbf{a}\times\dot{\mathbf{r}}_1 - \mathbf{a}\times\dot{\mathbf{r}}_2)\rangle_{\text{av}} = \frac{er_0}{2c}\langle(-2\mathbf{b}\dot{q}_1)\rangle_{\text{av}}$$
$$= \frac{i\omega e^2 r_0}{mc}\frac{e^{-i\omega t}}{\Delta_1\Delta_2 - Q_{12}^2}\left\{\Delta_2\left[-\frac{r_0}{6}\mathbf{j}\frac{\partial E_0(0)}{\partial z}\right] - Q_{12}(\tfrac{1}{3})\mathbf{E}_0(0)\right\}. \tag{1.9.19b}$$

This leads to the relations

$$\alpha = \frac{2}{3}\frac{e^2}{m}\frac{\Delta_1}{\Delta_1\Delta_2 - Q_{12}^2} \tag{1.9.20a}$$

$$\beta^{\ddagger} = \frac{1}{3}\frac{e^2 r_0}{mc}\, i\omega\, \frac{Q_{12}}{\Delta_1\Delta_2 - Q_{12}^2} \tag{1.9.20b}$$

$$\kappa = \frac{e^2 r_0^2 \omega^2}{6mc^2}\frac{\Delta_2}{\Delta_1\Delta_2 - Q_{12}^2}. \tag{1.9.20c}$$

This result may be compared with the previous coupled oscillator model. From (1.9.16) and (1.9.11) and the fact that $e_2 = e_1/2 = e/2$ it follows that

$$\beta^{\ddagger}(\text{coupled}) \sim -\frac{3}{2}\frac{i\omega e^2}{m^2 c}\frac{r_0^2}{R_0^4}\gamma_a\gamma_b\gamma_c e^2,$$

where the frequency factor is omitted; and from (1.9.20) and (1.9.17) one obtains

$$\beta^{\ddagger}(\text{charge}) \sim -\frac{5 i\omega e^2}{m^2 c}\frac{r_0^2}{R_0^4}\gamma_a\gamma_b\gamma_c \rho e^2.$$

The ratio of these two quantities is

$$\frac{\beta^{\ddagger}(\text{charge})}{\beta^{\ddagger}(\text{coupled})} = \frac{10}{3}\rho,$$

which shows that the two effects may be comparable. For a positive charge ρe the scattering by this model results in left-handed or counterclockwise rotation of the plane of polarization. The motion is a left-handed screw pattern: when the circle is moved along $+\mathbf{b}$ in Figure 1.11 the first charge is pulled more strongly by the charge at P, and the accompanying circular motion is clockwise.

1.10. Octahedral Coupled Oscillator Model

Before concluding this introductory classical discussion it is worth while to explore a few of the problems of degeneracy. Two types of particular interest may be treated in one and the same model, the essential features of which are shown in Figure 1.12. Three identical linear oscillators are placed on the indicated edges of a regular octahedron. Each has one degree of freedom along its edge. In the center there is an isotropic oscillator with, in general, a different frequency. All four may be presumed coupled by electrostatic forces. The system belongs to the symmetry group D_3 with the threefold rotational axis shown in the figure.

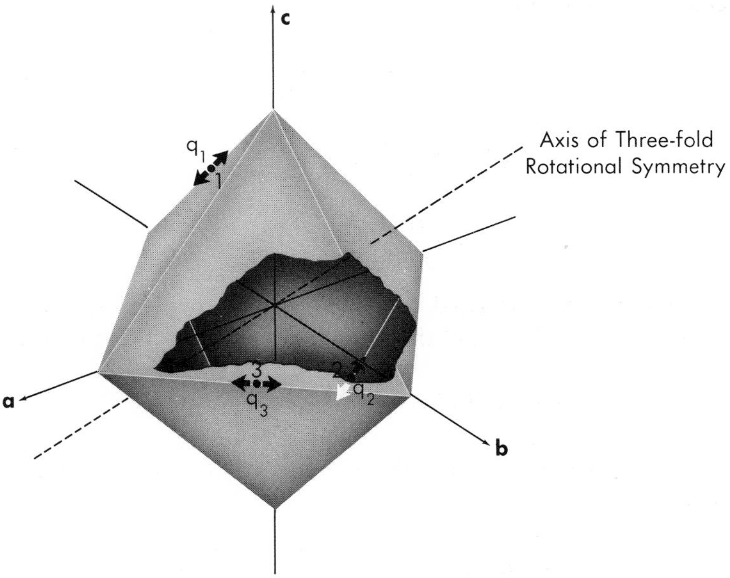

Figure 1.12. The octahedral oscillator system.

The three linear oscillators constitute a threefold group degeneracy; however, it should be noted that when the coupling is not too large they may be treated in pairs by the method already discussed. Each of the three possible pairs constitutes an identical left-handed screw pattern, and the effects of these interactions should be additive. The behavior of such a system has been displayed in Figure 1.7. The dichroism changes sign in the middle of the absorption band.

The three-dimensional oscillator exhibits intragroup degeneracy in that its three frequencies of oscillation are equal; furthermore, it will be seen that pairwise interactions between it and any of the three other oscillators will make no contribution to the dissymmetric scattering. Three-way interactions must be considered.

The following notation will be used:

$q_1\mathbf{e}_1, q_2\mathbf{e}_2, q_3\mathbf{e}_3$ = displacement vectors of the three one-dimensional oscillators;

$\mathbf{r} = u\mathbf{a} + v\mathbf{b} + w\mathbf{c}$ = displacement vector of the central oscillator;

$\mathbf{d}_1, \mathbf{d}_2, \mathbf{d}_3$ = unit vectors from the origin to the positions of the one-dimensional oscillators;

ω_0 = frequency of the isotropic oscillator;
ω_1 = frequency of the one-dimensional oscillators;
a = one-half the side of the circumscribing cube;
$R_1 = (\sqrt{3/2})a$ = distance between each pair of linear oscillators;
$R_0 = (\sqrt{2/2})a$ = distance from the origin to the linear oscillators.

The four oscillators have six possible pairings; the total dipole-dipole interaction potential is

$$V = q_1(vQ'_{v1} + wQ'_{w1}) + q_2(uQ'_{u2} + wQ'_{w2}) + q_3(uQ'_{u3} + vQ'_{v3}) + q_1q_2Q'_{12} + q_1q_3Q'_{13} + q_2q_3Q'_{23}, \quad (1.10.1)$$

where

$$Q'_{v1} = \frac{\mathbf{b} \cdot \mathbf{e}_1}{R_0^3}, \text{ etc.,}$$

$$Q'_{12} = \frac{1}{R_1^3}[(\mathbf{e}_1 \cdot \mathbf{e}_2) - 3(\mathbf{e}_1 \cdot \mathbf{d}_{12})(\mathbf{e}_2 \cdot \mathbf{d}_{12})], \text{ etc.,}$$

and $\mathbf{d}_{12}$, $\mathbf{d}_{31}$, $\mathbf{d}_{32}$ are unit vectors along the lines joining the indicated oscillators. Note that the terms Q'_{u1}, Q'_{v2}, and Q'_{w3} are zero because the vectors in all the scalar products are mutually perpendicular.

The equations of motion for this coupled system are given by

$$\ddot{u} + \omega_0^2 u + \Gamma_0 \dot{u} + q_2 Q_{u2} + q_3 Q_{u3} = Q_u e^{-i\omega t} \quad (1.10.2a)$$

$$\ddot{v} + \omega_0^2 v + \Gamma_0 \dot{v} + q_1 Q_{v1} + q_3 Q_{v3} = Q_v e^{-i\omega t} \quad (1.10.2b)$$

$$\ddot{w} + \omega_0^2 w + \Gamma_0 \dot{w} + q_1 Q_{w1} + q_2 Q_{w2} = Q_w e^{-i\omega t} \quad (1.10.2c)$$

$$\ddot{q}_1 + \omega_1^2 q_1 + \Gamma_1 \dot{q}_1 + vQ_{v1} + wQ_{w1} + q_2 Q_{12} + q_3 Q_{13} = Q_1 e^{-i\omega t} \quad (1.10.2d)$$

$$\ddot{q}_2 + \omega_1^2 q_2 + \Gamma_1 \dot{q}_2 + uQ_{u2} + wQ_{w2} + q_1 Q_{12} + q_3 Q_{23} = Q_2 e^{-i\omega t} \quad (1.10.2e)$$

$$\ddot{q}_3 + \omega_1^2 q_3 + \Gamma_1 \dot{q}_3 + uQ_{u3} + vQ_{v3} + q_1 Q_{13} + q_2 Q_{23} = Q_3 e^{-i\omega t}, \quad (1.10.2f)$$

where

$$\Gamma_0 = \frac{\gamma_0}{m}, \quad \Gamma_1 = \frac{\gamma_1}{m}, \quad Q_{12} = \frac{Q'_{12}}{m}, \text{ etc.,}$$

$$Q_u = \frac{e}{m} \mathbf{i} \cdot \mathbf{a} E_0(0),$$

$$Q_v = \frac{e}{m} \mathbf{i} \cdot \mathbf{b} E_0(0),$$

$$Q_w = \frac{e}{m} \mathbf{i} \cdot \mathbf{c} E_0(0),$$

$$Q_1 = \frac{e}{m} \left[\mathbf{i} \cdot \mathbf{e}_1 E_0(0) + (\mathbf{i} \cdot \mathbf{e}_1)(\mathbf{k} \cdot \mathbf{d}_1) R_0 \frac{\partial E_0(0)}{\partial z} \right] \tag{1.10.3a}$$

$$Q_2 = \frac{e}{m} \left[\mathbf{i} \cdot \mathbf{e}_2 E_0(0) + (\mathbf{i} \cdot \mathbf{e}_2)(\mathbf{k} \cdot \mathbf{d}_2) R_0 \frac{\partial E_0(0)}{\partial z} \right] \tag{1.10.3b}$$

$$Q_3 = \frac{e}{m} \left[\mathbf{i} \cdot \mathbf{e}_3 E_0(0) + (\mathbf{i} \cdot \mathbf{e}_3)(\mathbf{k} \cdot \mathbf{d}_3) R_0 \frac{\partial E_0(0)}{\partial z} \right], \tag{1.10.3c}$$

and **i**, **j**, **k** represent the laboratory coordinate system.

When the usual substitutions $u = u^{(0)} e^{-i\omega t}$ and $q_1 = q_1^{(0)} e^{-i\omega t}$ are made, there results the following system of linear equations written in matrix form

$$\begin{bmatrix} \Delta_0 & 0 & 0 & 0 & Q_{u2} & Q_{u3} \\ 0 & \Delta_0 & 0 & Q_{v1} & 0 & Q_{v3} \\ 0 & 0 & \Delta_0 & Q_{w1} & Q_{w2} & 0 \\ 0 & Q_{v1} & Q_{w1} & \Delta_1 & Q_{12} & Q_{13} \\ Q_{u2} & 0 & Q_{w2} & Q_{12} & \Delta_1 & Q_{23} \\ Q_{u3} & Q_{v3} & 0 & Q_{13} & Q_{23} & \Delta_1 \end{bmatrix} \begin{bmatrix} u^{(0)} \\ v^{(0)} \\ w^{(0)} \\ q_1^{(0)} \\ q_2^{(0)} \\ q_3^{(0)} \end{bmatrix} = \begin{bmatrix} Q_u \\ Q_v \\ Q_w \\ Q_1 \\ Q_2 \\ Q_3 \end{bmatrix}, \tag{1.10.4}$$

where

$$\Delta_0 = \omega_0^2 - \omega^2 - i\Gamma_0 \omega,$$
$$\Delta_1 = \omega_1^2 - \omega^2 - i\Gamma_1 \omega.$$

Even though many of the elements of the resulting determinants are zero, an exact solution to this problem would be quite tedious and unsuitable for instructional purposes; however, if only the lowest order terms are retained a great simplification results. The solutions may formally be written

$$u^{(0)} = \frac{D_u}{D} \quad (a) \qquad v^{(0)} = \frac{D_v}{D} \quad (b)$$

$$w^{(0)} = \frac{D_w}{D} \quad (c) \qquad q_1^{(0)} = \frac{D_1}{D} \quad (d) \qquad (1.10.5)$$

$$q_2^{(0)} = \frac{D_2}{D} \quad (e) \qquad q_3^{(0)} = \frac{D_3}{D} \quad (f),$$

where D is the determinant of the above matrix, and D_u, etc., is the resultant determinant obtained from D by replacing the first column with the column vector on the right of (1.10.4).

The determinant D may be approximated by its diagonal term $\Delta_0^3 \Delta_1^3$, since the rest of the terms contain higher order factors, which merely change resonance frequencies without greatly affecting the nature of the scattering. Our previous experience leads us to expect that the direct coupling of two oscillators will give a term $1/\Delta_1^2$ for the contribution to the scattering by the linear oscillators. The lowest order terms in D_1, D_2, and D_3 which contribute to the optical activity are proportional to $\Delta_0^3 \Delta_1$. Since the dissymmetric coupling of the isotropic oscillator to the linear ones is of second order, the lowest order dispersion term depending on ω_0 should be $1/\Delta_0 \Delta_1^2$; hence, we should seek out the terms in D_u, D_1, etc., proportional to $\Delta_0^2 \Delta_1$.

The average induced electric dipole moment is given by

$$\mathbf{p} = e(\langle \mathbf{a}u \rangle + \langle \mathbf{b}v \rangle + \langle \mathbf{c}w \rangle + \langle \mathbf{e}_1 q_1 \rangle + \langle \mathbf{e}_2 q_2 \rangle + \langle \mathbf{e}_3 q_3 \rangle).$$

The position and orientation vectors may be written

$$\mathbf{d}_1 = \frac{\mathbf{c} - \mathbf{b}}{\sqrt{2}} \quad (a) \qquad \mathbf{d}_2 = -\frac{\mathbf{a} + \mathbf{c}}{\sqrt{2}} \quad (b)$$

$$\mathbf{d}_3 = \frac{\mathbf{a} + \mathbf{b}}{\sqrt{2}} \quad (c) \qquad \mathbf{e}_1 = \frac{\mathbf{b} + \mathbf{c}}{\sqrt{2}} \quad (d) \qquad (1.10.6)$$

$$\mathbf{e}_2 = \frac{\mathbf{c} - \mathbf{a}}{\sqrt{2}} \quad (e) \qquad \mathbf{e}_3 = \frac{\mathbf{a} - \mathbf{b}}{\sqrt{2}}. \quad (f)$$

It happens that only terms containing Q_1, Q_2, and Q_3 will make a contribution to the ORD, since they alone contain the factor $\partial E_0(0)/\partial z$. From (1.10.6) and (1.10.3) it follows that the only nonvanishing terms of the series $\langle \mathbf{a}Q_1 \rangle$, $\langle \mathbf{b}Q_1 \rangle$, etc., are

$$\langle \mathbf{a}Q_1 \rangle = -\frac{1}{6}\frac{eR_0}{m}\frac{\partial E_0(0)}{\partial z} \qquad (1.10.7a)$$

$$\langle \mathbf{b}Q_2 \rangle = \frac{1}{6}\frac{eR_0}{m}\frac{\partial E_0(0)}{\partial z} \tag{1.10.7b}$$

$$\langle \mathbf{c}Q_3 \rangle = -\frac{1}{6}\frac{eR_0}{m}\frac{\partial E_0(0)}{\partial z}. \tag{1.10.7c}$$

The induced dipole moment is now equal to

$$e\left\{\langle \mathbf{a}u \rangle + \langle \mathbf{b}v \rangle + \langle \mathbf{c}w \rangle + \frac{1}{\sqrt{2}}[\langle(\mathbf{b}+\mathbf{c})q_1\rangle + \langle(\mathbf{c}-\mathbf{a})q_2\rangle + \langle(\mathbf{a}-\mathbf{b})q_3\rangle]\right\}. \tag{1.10.8}$$

In view of (1.10.7) only terms with the indicated factors will contribute:

$$\begin{array}{ll} u \to Q_1 & q_1 \to Q_2, Q_3 \\ v \to Q_2 & q_2 \to Q_1, Q_3 \\ w \to Q_3 & q_3 \to Q_1, Q_2. \end{array}$$

Only relatively few terms from the determinants from (1.10.4) survive the spatial averaging process.

To find $\langle \mathbf{a}u \rangle$ it is necessary to obtain those terms in D_u containing the factor $\Delta_0^2 \Delta_1 Q_1$, with the result

$$\langle \mathbf{a}u \rangle = -\frac{1}{6}\frac{eR_0}{m}\frac{Q_{12}Q_{u2} + Q_{13}Q_{u3}}{\Delta_0 \Delta_1^2}\frac{\partial E_0(0)}{\partial z} \tag{1.10.9a}$$

$$\langle \mathbf{b}v \rangle = \frac{1}{6}\frac{eR_0}{m}\frac{Q_{23}Q_{v3} + Q_{v1}Q_{12}}{\Delta_0^2 \Delta_1}\frac{\partial E_0(0)}{\partial z} \tag{1.10.9b}$$

$$\langle \mathbf{c}w \rangle = -\frac{1}{6}\frac{eR_0}{m}\frac{Q_{23}Q_{w2} + Q_{13}Q_{w1}}{\Delta_0^2 \Delta_1}\frac{\partial E_0(0)}{\partial z}. \tag{1.10.9c}$$

In the determination of $\langle(\mathbf{b}+\mathbf{c})q_1\rangle$ only terms with the factors $\Delta_0^2 \Delta_1 Q_2$ and $\Delta_0^2 \Delta_1 Q_3$ need be considered. The final results are

$$\langle(\mathbf{b}+\mathbf{c})q_1\rangle = \frac{1}{6}\frac{eR_0}{m}\frac{Q_{w1}Q_{w2} - Q_{v1}Q_{v3}}{\Delta_0 \Delta_1^2}\frac{\partial E_0(0)}{\partial z} \tag{1.10.10a}$$

$$\langle(\mathbf{c}-\mathbf{a})q_2\rangle = \frac{1}{6}\frac{eR_0}{m}\frac{Q_{w1}Q_{w2} - Q_{u2}Q_{u3}}{\Delta_0 \Delta_1^2}\frac{\partial E_0(0)}{\partial z} \tag{1.10.10b}$$

$$\langle(\mathbf{a}-\mathbf{b})q_3\rangle = -\frac{1}{6}\frac{eR_0}{m}\frac{Q_{v1}Q_{v3} + Q_{u2}Q_{u3}}{\Delta_0 \Delta_1^2}\frac{\partial E_0(0)}{\partial z}. \tag{1.10.10c}$$

The second order coupling constants in these equations may be interpreted in terms of the physical process taking place. In $\langle \mathbf{a}u \rangle$ the factor $Q_{12}Q_{u2}$

arises from the motion of #2 induced by a displacement u along the **a**-axis. (The electric field **E** can be presumed to be along this axis.) This in turn through the coupling constant Q_{12} induces the motion of #1, which is not directly affected by **E** or motion along **a**. A similar interpretation may be put upon each of the products in (1.10.9).

The terms of (1.10.10) are actually second order modifications to the coupled motion of the linear oscillators; for example, $Q_{w1}Q_{w2}$ describes the motion of #2 induced by #1 through the intermediate influence of the isotropic oscillator moving along **c**. This coupling will exhibit a maximum at the frequency ω_0 as well as at ω_1, where it makes a small addition to the direct coupling. The result is that all the terms of (1.10.8) will be of equal importance.

From (1.10.6) the coupling constants are found to be

$$Q_{v1} = Q_{w1} = Q_{w2} = Q_{u3} = -Q_{u2} = -Q_{v3} = \frac{e^2}{\sqrt{2}\, mR_0^3} \tag{1.10.11a}$$

$$Q_{12} = -Q_{13} = -Q_{23} = \frac{e^2}{4mR_1^3}. \tag{1.10.11b}$$

The combination of (1.10.8), (1.10.9), and (1.10.10) leads to the result

$$\mathbf{p}' = \frac{i\omega}{c}\frac{1}{6}\frac{e^6}{m^3R_0^2}\frac{1}{\Delta_0\,\Delta_1^2}\frac{3}{2}\sqrt{2}\left(\frac{1}{2R_1^3}+\frac{1}{R_0^3}\right)\mathbf{B}, \tag{1.10.12}$$

where only the part $\mathbf{p}'$ of the dipole moment leading to dissymmetric scattering has been considered. The configuration in Figure 1.12 is dextrorotatory on the low frequency side of the spectrum; furthermore, the ORD and CD behave normally in the absorption region $\omega = \omega_0$, as can be seen by writing

$$\frac{1}{\Delta_0\,\Delta_1^2} \sim \frac{1}{\Delta_0(\omega_1^2 - \omega_0^2)^2}, \tag{1.10.13}$$

which is valid when $\omega \sim \omega_0$. The dispersion now exhibits normal behavior. It also follows that the dichroism will not change sign within the absorption band as it does for the frequency ω_1. The overall behavior of the system is shown in Figure 1.13.

The motion may be seen to follow a right-handed screw pattern so far as the role of the isotropic oscillator is concerned. In Figure 1.14 the electric field along **c** causes a displacement of charge along the position **c**-direction. The dipole-dipole interaction formula indicates that charge #1 moves in the manner shown; this motion in turn causes #3 to move in a counterclockwise manner as viewed along the (−) **c**-axis. The net result of the motion of the isotropic oscillator and the third linear oscillator is a right-handed screw pattern, again which identifies this form of motion with positive

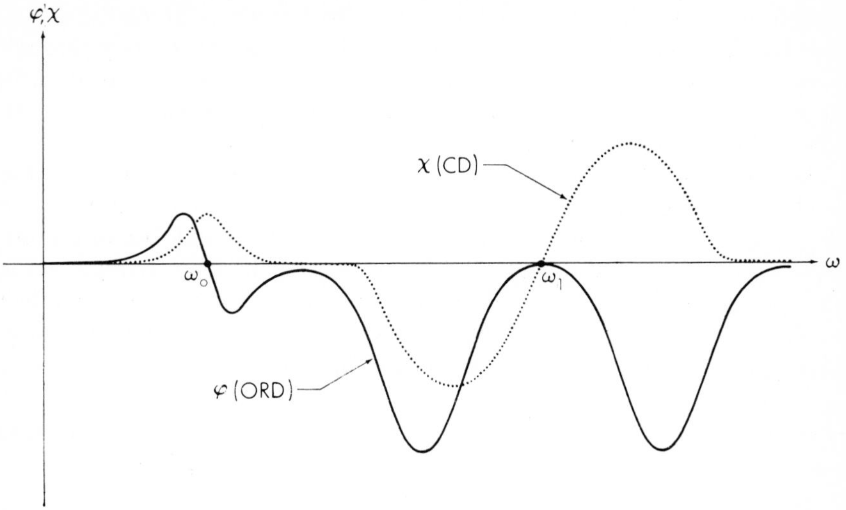

Figure 1.13. The ORD and CD behavior of the octahedral coupled oscillator system.

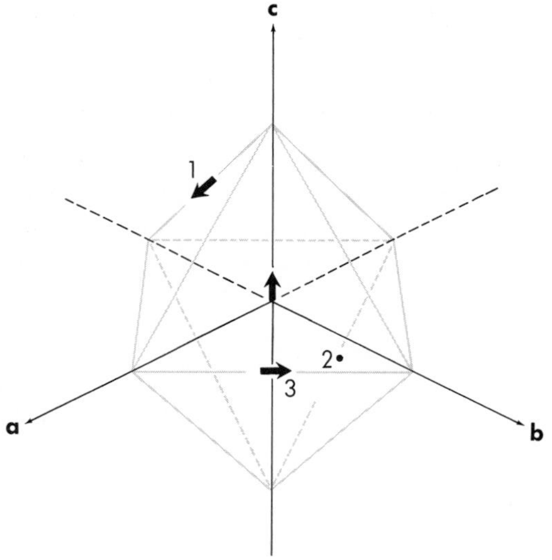

Figure 1.14. The resolution of second order coupling into a right-handed screw pattern.

rotation. An analysis of the central oscillator's motion along the other two axes **a** and **b** also leads to a right-handed screw pattern; thus, all three directions of the degenerate motion have identical scattering properties, and there is no tendency for cancellation. A more general discussion of degeneracy will be presented after the quantum mechanical development of the subject.

CHAPTER 2

The Quantum Theory

2.1. The Lagrangian and Hamiltonian Formulations

It will now be necessary to undertake the quantum mechanical formulation of the subject. This chapter will be devoted to the derivation of the Rosenfeld equation for optical activity in nonabsorbing regions of the spectrum followed by an exposition of the Kronig-Kramers relations and their application to absorbing regions. The development of this difficult subject cannot follow the simple classical treatment using the Newtonian equations of motion, since quantum theory is cast in the Hamiltonian formulation. The problems involved will become clearer as we briefly review the rudiments of the Lagrangian and Hamiltonian theories and their application to quantum mechanics.

The Newtonian equation of motion for the Cartesian coordinate x_i of particle i is

$$F_i = m\ddot{x}_i = \dot{p}_i. \tag{2.1.1}$$

This system of equations may be inconvenient particularly if the coordinates are not all independent. In this case it would be desirable to formulate a principle which directly leads to the minimum number of equations required to describe the system's motion. If the forces are derived from a potential $V(x_i)$, then $F_i = -(\partial V/\partial x_i)$. The relations 2.1.1 may be multiplied by $\dot{x}_i$ and added; when all the derivatives are expressed in terms of the independent coordinates q_j the standard reductions give*

$$\sum_j \left[\frac{d}{dt}\left(\frac{\partial T}{\partial \dot{q}_j}\right) - \frac{\partial T}{\partial q_j} + \frac{\partial V}{\partial q_j}\right]\dot{q}_j = 0. \tag{2.1.2}$$

Since the q_j are now independent, the individual coefficients of $\dot{q}_j$ may each be set equal to zero with the resulting Lagrangian equations of motion. If V is independent of $\dot{q}_j$ the equations may be written

$$\frac{d}{dt}\left(\frac{\partial L}{\partial \dot{q}_j}\right) - \frac{\partial L}{\partial q_j} = 0, \tag{2.1.3}$$

where $L = T - V$.

* See H. Goldstein, *Classical Mechanics*, Addison-Wesley, Reading, Mass., 1956.

Comparison of this equation with (2.1.1) shows that $\partial L/\partial \dot{q}_j$ now plays the role of a generalized momentum. When V is independent of velocity, $p_j = \partial L/\partial \dot{q}_j = \partial T/\partial \dot{q}_j$. If q_j is the Cartesian coordinate x_j, then $\partial T/\partial \dot{x}_j = m\dot{x}_j$, which corresponds to the original Newtonian definition of momentum. In other coordinate systems the conventional forms of angular momentum as well as various types of composite momenta will be involved. The relation $p_j = \partial L/\partial \dot{q}_j$ is strictly a definition of the momentum p_j *conjugate* to the coordinate q_j. Only when V is independent of velocity will the conjugate momentum p_j of a Cartesian coordinate x_j be equal to the Newtonian linear momentum $m\dot{x}_j$.

The Lagrangian function $L = T - V$ has the often undesirable feature that it is not a constant of motion for conservative systems. It is therefore prudent to search for variables other than q_j and $\dot{q}_j$. A logical path leads to the selection of q_j and $p_j = \partial L/\partial \dot{q}_j$ as the independent variables, and a straightforward manipulation of partial derivatives gives the Hamilton equations of motion:

$$\dot{q}_j = \frac{\partial H}{\partial p_j} \tag{2.1.4a}$$

$$\dot{p}_j = -\frac{\partial H}{\partial q_j} \tag{2.1.4b}$$

$$\frac{\partial L}{\partial t} = -\frac{\partial H}{\partial t}, \tag{2.1.4c}$$

where $H = \sum_i \dot{q}_i p_i - L$. For a single linear degree of freedom x this reduces to $H = m\dot{x}^2 - (\frac{1}{2}m\dot{x}^2 - V(x)) = T + V$. For conservative systems H will be equal to the constant value of the total energy.

The crux of the damping problem can be seen by observing that (2.1.3) cannot be used to describe a frictional force $-\gamma\dot{x}$ without some modification. A second function F, the dissipation function encountered in Chapter 1, is defined for a single particle as $F = \frac{1}{2}(\gamma_1 \dot{x}_1^2 + \gamma_2 \dot{x}_2^2 + \gamma_3 \dot{x}_3^2)$. The equation

$$\frac{d}{dt}\left(\frac{\partial L}{\partial \dot{x}_i}\right) - \frac{\partial L}{\partial x_i} + \frac{\partial F}{\partial \dot{x}_i} = 0,$$

immediately leads to the correct Newtonian equations of motion in Cartesian coordinates with the generalization

$$\frac{d}{dt}\left(\frac{\partial L}{\partial \dot{q}_i}\right) - \frac{\partial L}{\partial q_i} + \frac{\partial F}{\partial \dot{q}_i} = 0. \tag{2.1.5}$$

Two functions must be used to describe damped motion in the Lagrangian method and the transformation to Hamilton's equations 2.1.4 is not possible.

In the Hamilton method the energy lost per unit time is an explicit function of the velocities, which may only be obtained in terms of the instantaneous values of p_i and q_i after the problem has been solved.

It will next be necessary to express the total electromagnetic force on a charge in a form suitable for Lagrange's equations. The Lorentz force on a charge e with velocity $\mathbf{v}$ in an electromagnetic field described by the vectors $\mathbf{E}$ and $\mathbf{B}$ is

$$\mathbf{F} = e\left[\mathbf{E} + \left(\frac{\mathbf{v}}{c}\right) \times \mathbf{B}\right]. \tag{2.1.6}$$

In this brief review of classical mechanics it will suffice to verify that the desired Lagrangian function is

$$L = T - e\phi + \frac{e}{c}\mathbf{A} \cdot \mathbf{v}, \tag{2.1.7}$$

where $\mathbf{E}$ and $\mathbf{B}$ are related to the scalar and vector potentials ϕ and $\mathbf{A}$ by the relations

$$\mathbf{E} = -\nabla\phi - \frac{1}{c}\dot{\mathbf{A}},$$

$$\mathbf{B} = \nabla \times \mathbf{A}.$$

For a single particle the Lagrangian equations may be written in vector form as

$$\frac{d}{dt}\left(\frac{\partial L}{\partial \mathbf{v}}\right) - \nabla L = 0, \tag{2.1.8}$$

where

$$\frac{\partial L}{\partial \mathbf{v}} = \mathbf{i}\frac{\partial L}{\partial v_x} + \mathbf{j}\frac{\partial L}{\partial v_y} + \mathbf{k}\frac{\partial L}{\partial v_z}.$$

The necessary derivatives are

$$\frac{d}{dt}\frac{\partial L}{\partial \mathbf{v}} = m\dot{\mathbf{v}} + \frac{e}{c}[\dot{\mathbf{A}} + (\mathbf{v} \cdot \nabla)\mathbf{A}] \tag{2.1.9a}$$

$$\nabla L = -e\nabla\phi + \frac{e}{c}[\mathbf{v} \times \nabla \times \mathbf{A} + (\mathbf{v} \cdot \nabla)\mathbf{A}], \tag{2.1.9b}$$

where the total derivative of $\partial L/\partial \mathbf{v}$ must be separated into a partial time derivative and a velocity dependent term to take into account those changes in time due to the motion of the particle. In the expression for ∇L the vector identity $\nabla(\mathbf{V}_1 \cdot \mathbf{V}_2) = \mathbf{V}_1 \times \nabla \times \mathbf{V}_2 + \mathbf{V}_2 \times \nabla \times \mathbf{V}_1 + (\mathbf{V}_1 \cdot \nabla)\mathbf{V}_2 + (\mathbf{V}_2 \cdot \nabla)\mathbf{V}_1$ has been used.

From (2.1.7) the generalized momentum of a single particle in an electromagnetic field is seen to be

$$\mathbf{p} = \frac{\partial L}{\partial \mathbf{v}} = m\mathbf{v} + \frac{e}{c}\,\mathbf{A}. \tag{2.1.10}$$

Reference to (2.1.4) and (2.1.7) shows the Hamiltonian to be given by

$$H = \mathbf{p} \cdot \mathbf{v} - L = \tfrac{1}{2}mv^2 + e\phi. \tag{2.1.11}$$

This result is independent of the magnetic field, which is not surprising, since **B** always acts at right angles to the velocity and does not directly change the energy of the system.

In general H is only a constant when **A** and ϕ are independent of time. Equation 2.1.11 is unsuitable for further calculation, since it is expressed in terms of **v** and **r** rather than **p** and **r**. The substitution of (2.1.10) into (2.1.11) gives

$$H = \tfrac{1}{2}m\left(\frac{\mathbf{p}}{m} - \frac{e}{mc}\,\mathbf{A}\right)^2 + e\phi, \tag{2.1.12}$$

where the explicit dependence of H on **p** and **r** is displayed.

2.2. The Quantum Mechanical Perturbation Operator

In the transition from classical to quantum mechanics it must be remembered that the operator $-i\hbar\nabla$ corresponds to the *generalized* momentum **p** and not the Newtonian momentum $m\mathbf{v}$. The quantum mechanical electromagnetic Hamiltonian may be written

$$H = \frac{1}{2m}\left(-i\hbar\nabla - \frac{e}{c}\,\mathbf{A}\right) \cdot \left(-i\hbar\nabla - \frac{e}{c}\,\mathbf{A}\right) + e\phi, \tag{2.2.1}$$

where due regard must be paid to the order of the terms. The term $(i\hbar e/c)\nabla \cdot \mathbf{A}$ may be transformed by determining its effect when H operates on a function ψ:

$$\nabla \cdot (\mathbf{A}\psi) = \psi\nabla \cdot \mathbf{A} + \mathbf{A} \cdot \nabla\psi. \tag{2.2.2}$$

In most problems of interest, particularly those dealing with radiation, $\nabla \cdot \mathbf{A} = 0$. This assumes that the charge density is constant throughout the interaction time.

Equation 2.2.1 then becomes

$$H = -\frac{\hbar^2\nabla^2}{2m} + \frac{e}{mc}\,i\hbar\mathbf{A} \cdot \nabla + \frac{e^2}{2mc^2}\,\mathbf{A}^2 + e\phi. \tag{2.2.3}$$

In the succeeding development we will only be interested in off-diagonal terms of the perturbing Hamilton function; and, therefore, the second term will in general lead to nonvanishing matrix elements. The ratio of the third term to the second can be shown to be governed by the ratio of the electrical work done on the system to the differences in energy between the states, which is presumed small at low radiation intensities.

The Hamiltonian for a molecular system in an electromagnetic field is then $H = H_0 + H'$, where

$$H' = -\frac{e}{mc}\sum_i \mathbf{A}(\mathbf{r}_i)\cdot\mathbf{p}_i\,. \tag{2.2.4}$$

The summation is over all electrons (the effect on the nuclei will be neglected in this discussion), and the vector potential is to be evaluated separately at the position of each electron. It must now be borne in mind that the matrix elements of H' involve an integration of $\mathbf{A}(\mathbf{r}_i)\cdot\mathbf{p}_i$ over all space and thereby describe the average effects of an oscillating electron cloud.

As in the classical treatment of dissymmetric scattering by point charges, it will be necessary to distinguish among the phases of the charge cloud at different points. The potentials $\mathbf{A}(\mathbf{r}_i)$ may not be approximated by their values at a common origin but must be expanded in the form

$$\mathbf{A}(\mathbf{r}) = \mathbf{A}(0) + (\mathbf{r}\cdot\nabla_0)\mathbf{A}(0), \tag{2.2.5}$$

where ∇_0 operates only on $\mathbf{A}$, and the result is to be evaluated at the origin. Equation 2.2.4 then requires the evaluation of terms like

$$\mathbf{A}\cdot\mathbf{p} + (\mathbf{r}\cdot\nabla_0)(\mathbf{A}\cdot\mathbf{p}),$$

where it is understood that $\mathbf{A}$ and its derivatives are to be evaluated at the origin and $\mathbf{r}$ is the coordinate of an electron with conjugate momentum $\mathbf{p} = -i\hbar\nabla$.

The above expression may formally be transformed by means of the vector identity

$$(\mathbf{V}_1\cdot\mathbf{V}_2)(\mathbf{V}_3\cdot\mathbf{V}_4) = \tfrac{1}{2}(\mathbf{V}_2\times\mathbf{V}_3)\cdot(\mathbf{V}_1\times\mathbf{V}_4) + \tfrac{1}{2}[(\mathbf{V}_1\cdot\mathbf{V}_2)(\mathbf{V}_3\cdot\mathbf{V}_4) + (\mathbf{V}_1\cdot\mathbf{V}_3)(\mathbf{V}_2\cdot\mathbf{V})_4]$$

into

$$(\mathbf{r}\cdot\nabla_0)(\mathbf{A}\cdot\mathbf{p}) = \tfrac{1}{2}(\nabla_0\times\mathbf{A})\cdot(\mathbf{r}\times\mathbf{p}) + \tfrac{1}{2}[(\mathbf{r}\cdot\nabla_0)(\mathbf{A}\cdot\mathbf{p}) + (\mathbf{r}\cdot\mathbf{A})(\nabla_0\cdot\mathbf{p})] \tag{2.2.6}$$

where ∇_0 is considered as operating to the left on $\mathbf{A}$ in the last term.

In the last term it will be convenient to reverse the order of the terms when matrix elements of (2.2.6) are taken. When attention is paid to noncommuting terms one obtains

$$\begin{aligned}(\mathbf{r}\cdot\mathbf{A})(\mathbf{\nabla}_0\cdot\mathbf{p}) - (\mathbf{\nabla}_0\cdot\mathbf{p})(\mathbf{r}\cdot\mathbf{A}) \\ = (xp_x - p_x x)\left(\frac{\partial A_x}{\partial x}\right)_0 + (yp_y - p_y y)\left(\frac{\partial A_y}{\partial y}\right)_0 + (zp_z - p_z z)\left(\frac{\partial A_z}{\partial z}\right)_0 \\ = i\hbar\mathbf{\nabla}_0\cdot\mathbf{A} = 0. \qquad (2.2.7)\end{aligned}$$

By use of the quantum mechanical Poisson bracket relation

$$\mathbf{p} = \left(\frac{im}{\hbar}\right)(H\mathbf{r} - \mathbf{r}H),$$

the matrix element of the second term in (2.2.6) between states m and n may be written

$$\begin{aligned}\tfrac{1}{2}\langle m|\,(\mathbf{r}\cdot\mathbf{\nabla}_0)(\mathbf{A}\cdot\mathbf{p}) + (\mathbf{\nabla}_0\cdot\mathbf{p})(\mathbf{r}\cdot\mathbf{A})\,|n\rangle \\ = \frac{im}{2\hbar}\{\langle m|\,(\mathbf{r}\cdot\mathbf{\nabla}_0)H(\mathbf{r}\cdot\mathbf{A}) - (\mathbf{r}\cdot\mathbf{\nabla}_0)H(\mathbf{r}\cdot\mathbf{A})\,|n\rangle \\ + \langle m|\,H(\mathbf{r}\cdot\mathbf{\nabla}_0)(\mathbf{A}\cdot\mathbf{r}) - (\mathbf{r}\cdot\mathbf{\nabla}_0)(\mathbf{r}\cdot\mathbf{A})H\,|n\rangle\} \\ = \frac{im}{2\hbar}(E_m - E_n)\langle m|\,(\mathbf{r}\cdot\mathbf{\nabla}_0)\,(\mathbf{A}\cdot\mathbf{r})\,|n\rangle, \qquad (2.2.8)\end{aligned}$$

where H does not operate on $\mathbf{A}$.

The complete spin neglected interaction Hamiltonian to first order is

$$\begin{aligned}H' = -\frac{e}{mc}\Big\{\sum_i \mathbf{A}(0)\cdot\mathbf{p}_i + \tfrac{1}{2}(\mathbf{\nabla}_0\times\mathbf{A}(0))\cdot(\mathbf{r}_i\times\mathbf{p}_i) \\ + \frac{im}{2\hbar}[H(\mathbf{r}\cdot\mathbf{\nabla}_0)(\mathbf{A}(0)\cdot\mathbf{r}) - (\mathbf{r}\cdot\mathbf{\nabla}_0)(\mathbf{A}(0)\cdot\mathbf{r})H]\Big\}. \qquad (2.2.9)\end{aligned}$$

The last term is related to the quadrupole moment tensor and will be shown to make no contribution to the optical activity of isotropic media. Its role in anisotropic media such as crystals has not been thoroughly investigated. There appears to be no reason why its contribution should be neglected in general, for it is of the same order of magnitude as the magnetic dipole term.

2.3. The Time Dependent Schrödinger Equation

Before solving the quantum mechanical equations of motion via perturbation theory, it will be worthwhile to review the consequences of the time dependent Schrödinger equation and its solutions for a time independent Hamiltonian. The general equation for wave mechanics is

$$H\Psi = i\hbar \frac{\partial \Psi}{\partial t}. \tag{2.3.1}$$

This equation differs markedly from the classical wave equation in that it must be expressed in complex form and is first order in time. This fact is a consequence of the requirement that the energy should be proportional to the first, not the second, power of the frequency. The classical wave equation and its solution in complex form is given by

$$\nabla^2 \chi = \frac{1}{c^2} \frac{\partial^2 \chi}{\partial t^2} \tag{2.3.2a}$$

$$\chi = e^{-i(\omega t - 2\pi \mathbf{k} \cdot \mathbf{r}/\lambda)}. \tag{2.3.2b}$$

If a moving particle is to be described by a wavelength $\lambda = 2\pi\hbar/p$ and a frequency $\omega = E/\hbar$, one should anticipate a wave of the form

$$\Psi = e^{i(\mathbf{p} \cdot \mathbf{r}/\hbar - Et/\hbar)}. \tag{2.3.3}$$

Since $E = p^2/2m$ for a free particle, it is not possible for such a function to satisfy a wave equation that is second order in both space and time coordinates; for

$$\nabla^2 \Psi = -\frac{p^2}{\hbar^2} \Psi \tag{2.3.4a}$$

$$\frac{\partial \Psi}{\partial t} = -\frac{iE}{\hbar}\Psi = -\frac{ip^2}{2m\hbar}\Psi. \tag{2.3.4b}$$

If an equation is sought in which the operators have the dimensions of energy, the simplest relation is

$$-\frac{\hbar^2}{2m}\nabla^2 \Psi = i\hbar \frac{\partial \Psi}{\partial t}, \tag{2.3.5}$$

which leads to the correspondences

$$-i\hbar \nabla \rightarrow \mathbf{p} \tag{2.3.6a}$$

$$i\hbar \frac{\partial}{\partial t} \rightarrow E. \tag{2.3.6b}$$

The minus sign appears in (2.3.6*a*) in order that $-i\hbar \nabla \Psi = +\mathbf{p}\Psi$.

In the more general case where $\mathbf{p}$ is not constant the operator $-(\hbar^2/2m)\nabla^2$ must be replaced by the Hamiltonian operator for the total energy: $H = -(\hbar^2 \nabla^2/2m) + V$. The interpretation of the quantum wave function differs markedly from the classical. In the latter case only the real part of the wave function is used, which is seen to satisfy the equation also. By contrast the real part of (2.3.3) does not satisfy (2.3.5), nor will any linear combinations of sine and cosine terms with real coefficients. Furthermore, it is not possible to formulate a *real* equation that is second order in space and first order in time which is satisfied by terms of the form $A\cos(\mathbf{p}\cdot\mathbf{r}/\hbar - Et/\hbar) + B\sin(\mathbf{p}\cdot\mathbf{r}/\hbar - Et/\hbar)$, even with complex coefficients.

The square of the classical wave function is a measure of the intensity of the disturbance. For material waves it is proportional to the kinetic energy and for electromagnetic waves proportional to the energy density. A similar interpretation cannot be put upon the quantum wave function, since the energy is determined by the factors appearing in the phase.

A revealing relation which points toward the proper interpretation of Ψ is obtained by writing the general time dependent Schrödinger equation and its complex conjugate:

$$-\frac{\hbar^2}{2m}\nabla^2\Psi + V\Psi = i\hbar\frac{\partial\Psi}{\partial t} \tag{2.3.7a}$$

$$-\frac{\hbar^2}{2m}\nabla^2\Psi^* + V\Psi^* = -i\hbar\frac{\partial\Psi^*}{\partial t}. \tag{2.3.7b}$$

The complex conjugate is introduced because it will now be possible to write a relation for Ψ and its derivatives which does not include the potential energy. Multiplication of (2.3.7*a*) by Ψ^* and (2.3.7*b*) by Ψ gives upon subtraction

$$-\frac{\hbar_2}{2m}(\Psi^*\nabla^2\Psi - \Psi\nabla^2\Psi^*) = i\hbar\frac{\partial(\Psi^*\Psi)}{\partial t}. \tag{2.3.8}$$

The left-hand side may be rewritten as $-(\hbar^2/2m)\nabla\cdot(\Psi^*\nabla\Psi - \Psi\nabla\Psi^*)$. This result immediately brings to mind the conservation equation for fluid motion

$$\nabla\cdot\mathbf{J} + \frac{\partial\rho}{\partial t} = 0, \tag{2.3.9}$$

where $\mathbf{J}$ is the vector rate of flow of material per unit area per unit time and ρ is the density. This equation states that if there is a net flow of material out from a given volume there must be a corresponding reduction in density. Equation 2.3.8 may then be interpreted as a conservation equation with

$$\rho = \Psi^*\Psi \tag{2.3.10a}$$

$$\mathbf{J} = \frac{\hbar}{2im}(\Psi^*\nabla\Psi + \Psi\nabla\Psi^*). \tag{2.3.10b}$$

It will be noted that in order for ρ to have the dimension of $(\text{volume})^{-1}$ and $\mathbf{J}$ of $(\text{area} \times \text{time})^{-1}$, Ψ must be proportional to $(\text{volume})^{-1/2}$. This is readily accomplished in a bound state problem for which $\int \Psi^*\Psi \, d\tau$ over all space is finite. The product $\Psi^*\Psi \, d\tau$ is accordingly to be interpreted as the probability of finding the particle in a volume element $d\tau$ with $e\Psi^*\Psi$ as the charge density. Since the total probability of finding it somewhere must be unity, it must be true that

$$\int \Psi^*\Psi \, d\tau = 1. \tag{2.3.11}$$

Equation 2.3.3 may not be so normalized, but the integral of $\Psi^*\Psi$ over any finite volume V equals V. In any problem involving freely traveling waves within a volume V, where boundary effects can be neglected (2.3.3) may be written $\Psi = (1/\sqrt{V})e^{i(\mathbf{p}\cdot\mathbf{r}/\hbar - Et/\hbar)}$. There is an equal probability of finding the particle anywhere in the volume. When there are no restrictions on the free particle there is an equal probability of finding it anywhere in space. If this is so, one might ask the question: How is the presence of such a thinly spread entity detected at all? The answer lies in the initial and boundary conditions. In general a free particle will have originated from a bound state and would appear as a diffusing cloud; as $t \to \infty$ this cloud will completely pervade all space only if it does not come under the influence of any other force fields.

If now the particle is confined to a specified volume with the requirement that Ψ be zero outside the bounding surfaces, no single exponential function will satisfy both (2.3.5) and the boundary conditions. The function (2.3.3) represents a wave traveling along the positive $\mathbf{r}$-direction and a reversal in sign $\mathbf{p}$ will give a wave in the opposite direction. The difference between these two functions gives a standing wave

$$\Psi' = e^{i(\mathbf{p}\cdot\mathbf{r}/\hbar - Et/\hbar)} - e^{-i(\mathbf{p}\cdot\mathbf{r}/\hbar + Et/\hbar)} = 2i \sin \frac{\mathbf{p}\cdot\mathbf{r}}{\hbar} e^{-iEt/\hbar}, \tag{2.3.12}$$

since the product, $\Psi'^*\Psi' = 4\sin^2(\mathbf{p}\cdot\mathbf{r}/\hbar)$, is independent of time.

In the one-dimensional case the function $\sin(2\pi px/h)$ will have nodes for $px/h = n/2$, $n = 1, 2, 3, \ldots$. If the length of the box is adjusted to correspond with the values $L = nh/2p$, a series of one-dimensional boxes will result, all of which can contain a particle whose momentum is p with a zero probability of finding it at the boundaries $x = 0$ and $x = L$. The requirement that the entire charge distribution be confined to the box is satisfied by the normalization condition

$$N^2 \int_0^L \sin^2 \frac{2\pi px}{h} \, dx = N^2 \int_0^{nh/2p} \sin^2 \frac{2\pi px}{h} \, dx = \tfrac{1}{2} N^2 \frac{nh}{2p} = 1. \tag{2.3.13}$$

The functions $2\sqrt{p/nh}\,\sin(2\pi px/h)$ describe a particle with momentum p in a one-dimensional box of length $L = nh/2p$.

Conversely, if the length of the box is fixed, standing waves will occur only for certain values of the momentum according to the requirement

$$\sin \frac{2\pi pL}{h} = 0, \tag{2.3.14}$$

which leads to the result

$$p = \frac{hn}{2L} \qquad \text{and} \qquad E = \frac{p^2}{2m} = \frac{h^2h^2}{8mL^2}, \qquad n = 1, 2, 3, \ldots .$$

The probability distribution of these states is constant in time but non-uniform in the spatial coordinate. Were it possible to observe the state without perturbing it, one would see a periodic distribution of charge clouds with nodes at the boundaries and evenly spaced nodes intervening.

A particle with any energy above the ground state and any initial charge distribution consistent with that energy which vanishes at the boundaries may be confined within a box; but in general the probability distribution $\Psi^*\Psi$ will no longer be independent of time. If for simplicity we confine ourselves to odd functions, a function $\phi_0(x)$ may be expanded in terms of the complete set of stationary states for a box of length L:

$$\phi(x, t) = \sum_{n=1}^{\infty} c_n \sin \frac{n\pi x}{L}\, e^{-iE_nt/\hbar}, \tag{2.3.15}$$

where

$$c_n = \left(\frac{2}{L}\right)^{1/2} \int_0^L \sin \frac{n\pi x}{L}\, \phi(x)\, dx,$$

$$\phi(x, 0) = \phi_0(x),$$

$$E_n = \frac{n^2h^2}{8mL^2}.$$

When $t = 0$ this corresponds to the Fourier expansion of the initial charge distribution. Equation 2.3.15 accordingly describes the motion of a particle whose initial distribution is $\phi_0(x)$; (2.3.5) is satisfied for any c_n.

From (2.3.6) and the orthogonality of the sine functions the energy of the particle is

$$E = \sum_{n=1}^{\infty} c_n^* c_n E_n \tag{2.3.16}$$

with $\sum_{n=1}^{\infty} c_n^* c_n = 1$. The energy is thus unambiguously specified by the charge distribution in view of the uniqueness of the Fourier expansion.

In (2.3.15) let $c_1 = c_2 = \sqrt{1/L}$, $c_3 = c_4 = \cdots = 0$. The time dependent charge or probability density will be

$$\phi^*(x, t)\phi(x, t) = \frac{1}{L}\left(\sin^2 \frac{\pi x}{L} + \sin^2 \frac{2\pi x}{L}\right) + \frac{2}{L} \sin \frac{\pi x}{L} \sin \frac{2\pi x}{L} \cos \omega_{12} t, \tag{2.3.17}$$

where $\omega_{12} = (E_2 - E_1)/\hbar$. The extremes of the motion will occur when $\omega_{12} t = n\pi$ and they are shown by the solid and dotted lines in Figure 2.1.

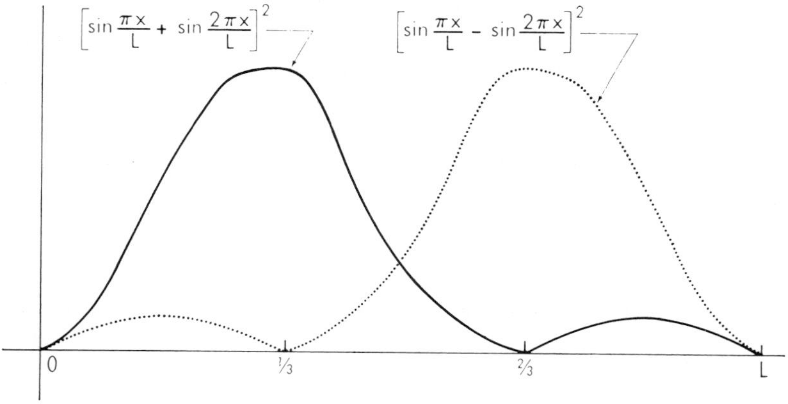

Figure 2.1. The charge density of the time dependent particle in a box problem.

This example shows how the energy differences between the stationary states of a system determine the natural frequencies of oscillation for non-stationary states. In summary, it may be said that any closed or bound system will have a series of stationary states $\Psi_n = \psi_n e^{-iE_n t/\hbar}$ for which $\Psi_n^* \Psi$ is independent of time. These states are characterized by stationary charge cloud distributions which do not appear to exhibit any motion in the same way that the standing waves of vibrating strings appear to minimize the effect of motion. When the system finds itself in any other than these "pure" states, it will undergo composite oscillations at the natural frequencies $\omega_{mn} = (E_m - E_n)/\hbar$. The neglect of $e^{-iE_n t/\hbar}$ factors in any time dependent problem is analgous to the neglect of the restoring forces $-k_n q_n$ in a classical problem. It is hoped that this digression will help the quantum equations of dissymmetric scattering to take on more physical meaning.

2.4. Derivation of the Optical Rotatory Parameter

When the Hamiltonian does not explicitly contain the time, (2.3.1) is separable with solutions

$$\Psi_n^{(0)} = \psi_n^{(0)} \exp\left(\frac{-iE_n^{(0)}t}{\hbar}\right), \tag{2.4.1}$$

where $H_0\Psi_n^{(0)} = E_n^{(0)}\Psi_n^{(0)}$. As the preceding section has shown, individually these functions determine the stationary states and collectively they describe the natural oscillations of the nonstationary states.

The introduction of a time dependent term H' into the Hamiltonian will cause the system to undergo forced oscillations. If H' changes very slowly in time compared to the natural frequencies, that is, $|(\partial H'/\partial t)/H'| \ll \omega_{nm}$, the methods of time independent perturbation theory under the so-called adiabatic hypothesis may be used. The system will continuously pass from one series of stationary states to the next without the absorption or emission of radiation.

When the perturbation consists of a rapidly fluctuating field with $\omega \sim \omega_{mn}$ the time dependent Schrödinger equation must be used. The equation to be solved is

$$(H_0 + H')\Psi = i\hbar \frac{\partial \Psi}{\partial t}. \tag{2.4.2}$$

If $\Psi_n^{(0)} = \psi_n^{(0)} \exp(-iE_n^{(0)}\,t/\hbar)$ are the stationary states satisfying the equations

$$H_0\Psi_n^{(0)} = i\hbar \frac{\partial \Psi_n^{(0)}}{\partial t} \tag{2.4.3}$$

for the time independent Hamiltonian H_0, any state function describing the perturbed system may be expanded in terms of them.

In classical mechanics the initial state of the system is described by specifying the magnitudes of all the coordinates and momenta at $t = 0$. In quantum theory this is not possible; instead one may specify the initial state of the system, which may be pure or composite. In general

$$\Psi^{(0)} = \sum_n c_n(0)\Psi_n^{(0)}, \tag{2.4.4}$$

where the $c_n^{(0)}$ are arbitrary. Under the influence of the perturbation the coefficients are changed. The time dependent state function may formally be written

$$\Psi = \sum_n c_n(t)\Psi_n^{(0)}, \tag{2.4.5}$$

where the $c_n(t)$ are the time dependent coefficients for the spatial expansion of Ψ in terms of the $\Psi_n^{(0)}$.

When (2.4.5) is substituted into (2.4.2) there results

$$\sum_n [c_n(t)H_0\Psi_n^{(0)} + c_n(t)H'\Psi_n^{(0)}] = i\hbar \sum_n \left[\frac{dc_n(t)}{dt} + c_n \frac{\partial \Psi_n^{(0)}}{\partial t}\right]. \tag{2.4.6}$$

In view of (2.4.3) this becomes

$$\sum_n c_n(t)H'\Psi_n^{(0)} = i\hbar \sum_n \frac{dc_n(t)}{dt} \Psi_n^{(0)}. \tag{2.4.7}$$

The orthogonality of the $\Psi_n^{(0)}$ may be used to eliminate the summation on the right. Multiplication of both sides by $\Psi_m^{(0)*}$ and integration over space gives

$$i\hbar \frac{dc_m(t)}{dt} = \sum_n c_n(t) \int \Psi_m^{(0)*}H'\Psi_n^{(0)}\, d\tau. \tag{2.4.8}$$

At this stage (2.4.8) is exact and applies to any perturbation, no matter how large. For small oscillations where the wave function at any time differs little from $\Psi^{(0)}$ the first approximation to the solution of (2.4.8) will be sufficient. This is obtained by setting $c_n(t) = c_n(0)$ on the right-hand side of (2.4.8). Since the explicit form of $\Psi_n^{(0)}$ and H' is known, the $c_m(t)$ may be found by elementary integration. In the actual molecular system there are damping mechanisms, which have not been included in this treatment. After a certain time solutions to the classical equation for damped motion

$$\ddot{q} + \omega_0^2 q + \Gamma\dot{q} = F(t) \tag{2.4.9}$$

will no longer contain terms proportional to $\sin \omega_0 t$ and $\cos \omega_0 t$, since the particular solutions to this equation decay exponentially with time. When the solutions to (2.4.8) are used to evaluate matrix elements, terms proportional to $e^{i(E_m - E_n)t/\hbar}$ are to be rejected, since these natural oscillations of the system will have decayed to zero amplitude. In general the $c_m(0)$ will not be zero.

In the problems to be discussed the system will be initially in one of the stationary states $\Psi_n^{(0)}$ with $c_n(0) = 1$ and all the $c_m(0)$ small. (They are not zero in order that the transients may be eliminated.) It will be assumed that at all times during the motion $c_n(t) \sim 1$ and $c_m(t) \sim 0$; otherwise the first approximation to the solution of (2.4.8) is not valid. Under these assumptions (2.4.8) becomes to first order

$$i\hbar \frac{dc_m(t)}{dt} = \int \Psi_m^{(0)*}H'\Psi_n^{(0)}\, d\tau, \tag{2.4.10}$$

$(m \neq n)$ with $c_n(t) = 1$. The general solution is

$$c_m(t) = c_m^{(0)} - \frac{i}{\hbar} \int \left(\int \Psi_m^{(0)*}H'\Psi_n^{(0)}\, d\tau \right) dt, \tag{2.4.11}$$

where the indefinite integral with respect to time is used and the volume integral is over all space.

The behavior of an observable quantity Q such as the electric or magnetic dipole moment of a molecule is governed by its expectation value, which may be written

$$\langle Q\rangle_{nn} = \int \Psi_n'^* Q \Psi_n' \, d\tau, \tag{2.4.12}$$

where $\Psi_n' = \Psi_n^{(0)} + \sum_m c_m(t)\Psi_m^{(0)}$. When the time dependence of the $\Psi_m^{(0)}$ is explicitly displayed, this becomes to first order

$$\langle Q\rangle_{nn} = \langle n|\, Q\,|n\rangle + 2\,\mathrm{Re}\left[\sum_m \langle n|\, Q\,|m\rangle e^{-i\omega_{nm}t} c_m(t)\right], \tag{2.4.13}$$

where

$$\langle n|\, Q\,|m\rangle = \int \psi_n^{(0)*} Q \psi_m^{(0)} \, d\tau,$$

$$\omega_{nm} = \frac{E_m^{(0)} - E_n^{(0)}}{\hbar}.$$

For a monochromatic wave the operator H' will have the form $H' = \overline{H}' \cos \omega t$, where $\overline{H}'$ is independent of time. Equation 2.4.11 then becomes

$$\begin{aligned} c_m(t) &= c_m^{(0)} - \frac{i}{\hbar} \langle m|\, \overline{H}'\,|n\rangle \int \cos \omega t e^{i\omega_{nm}t} \, dt \\ &= c_m^{(0)} + i \frac{\langle m|\, \overline{H}'\,|n\rangle e^{i\omega_{nm}t}}{\hbar(\omega_{nm}^2 - \omega^2)} (i\omega_{nm} \cos \omega t + \omega \sin \omega t). \end{aligned} \tag{2.4.14}$$

The substitution of this into (2.4.13) gives

$$\begin{aligned} \langle Q\rangle_{nn} = \langle n|\, Q\,|n\rangle + 2\,\mathrm{Re}\Bigg\{\sum_m \Bigg[c_m^{(0)}\langle n|\, Q\,|m\rangle e^{-i\omega_{mn}t} + \frac{\langle n|\, Q\,|m\rangle\langle m|\, \overline{H}'\,|n\rangle}{\hbar(\omega_{nm}^2 - \omega^2)} \\ \times (-\omega_{nm} \cos \omega t + i\omega \sin \omega t)\Bigg]\Bigg\}. \end{aligned} \tag{2.4.15}$$

The transient terms will be eliminated if $c_m^{(0)} = 0$, which does *not* correspond to $c_m(0) = 0$. Under this condition (2.4.15) becomes

$$\begin{aligned} \langle Q\rangle_{nn} &= \langle n|\, Q\,|n\rangle - \sum_{m\neq n} \frac{2}{\hbar(\omega_{nm}^2 - \omega^2)} \{\mathrm{Re}(\langle n|\, Q\,|m\rangle\langle m|\, \overline{H}'\,|n\rangle)\omega_{nm} \cos \omega t \\ &\qquad + \mathrm{Im}(\langle n|\, Q\,|m\rangle\langle m|\, \overline{H}'\,|n\rangle)\, \omega \sin \omega t\} \\ &= \langle n|\, Q\,|n\rangle - \sum_{m\neq n} \frac{2}{\hbar(\omega_{nm}^2 - \omega^2)} \Bigg[\omega_{nm}\, \mathrm{Re}(\langle n|\, Q\,|m\rangle\langle m|\, H'\,|n\rangle) \\ &\qquad - \mathrm{Im}\left(\langle n|\, Q\,|m\rangle\left\langle m\left|\frac{\partial H'}{\partial t}\right|n\right\rangle\right)\Bigg], \end{aligned} \tag{2.4.16}$$

where $\langle m|\, H' \,|n\rangle = \int \psi_m^{(0)*} H' \psi_n^{(0)}\, d\tau$ and $H' = \bar{H}' \cos \omega t$ is the only time dependent quantity in the integral.

The vector potential for an electromagnetic wave evaluated at the origin will be designated $\mathbf{A}(0) = \mathbf{A}_0^{(0)} \cos \omega t$. From the first two terms of (2.2.9) and the relation $\mathbf{p} = (im/\hbar)(H\mathbf{r} - \mathbf{r}H)$ one obtains

$$\langle m|\, H' \,|n\rangle = -\frac{e}{mc}\sum_i \left[\frac{im}{\hbar}(E_m - E_n)\langle m|\, \mathbf{r}_i \,|n\rangle \cdot \mathbf{A}(0) + \tfrac{1}{2}(\nabla \times \mathbf{A}(0)) \cdot \langle m|\, \mathbf{r}_i \times \mathbf{p}_i \,|n\rangle\right]$$

$$= -\frac{i}{c}\,\omega_{nm}\langle m|\, \boldsymbol{\mu} \,|n\rangle \cdot \mathbf{A}(0) - (\nabla \times \mathbf{A}(0)) \cdot \langle m|\, \mathbf{m} \,|n\rangle \qquad (2.4.17a)$$

$$\left\langle m \left| \frac{\partial H'}{\partial t} \right| n \right\rangle = -\frac{i}{c}\,\omega_{nm}\langle m|\, \boldsymbol{\mu} \,|n\rangle \cdot \frac{\partial \mathbf{A}(0)}{\partial t} - \left(\nabla \times \frac{\partial \mathbf{A}(0)}{\partial t}\right) \cdot \langle m|\, \mathbf{m} \,|n\rangle, \qquad (2.4.17b)$$

where the electric and magnetic moment operators are given by

$$\boldsymbol{\mu} = e \sum_i \mathbf{r},$$

$$\mathbf{m} = \frac{e}{2mc}\sum_i \mathbf{r}_i \times \mathbf{p}_i .$$

The field vectors **E** and **B** are related to **A** through the equations

$$\mathbf{E} = -\frac{1}{c}\frac{\partial \mathbf{A}}{\partial t} \quad (a) \qquad \frac{\partial \mathbf{E}}{\partial t} = -\frac{1}{c}\frac{\partial^2 \mathbf{A}}{\partial t^2} = \frac{\omega^2}{c}\mathbf{A} \quad (b)$$

$$\mathbf{B} = \nabla \times \mathbf{A} \quad (c) \qquad \frac{\partial \mathbf{B}}{\partial t} = \nabla \times \frac{\partial \mathbf{A}}{\partial t}, \quad (d) \qquad (2.4.18)$$

where the quantities are understood to be evaluated at the origin. Substitution of (2.4.17) and (2.4.18) into (2.4.16) gives

$$\langle Q\rangle_{nn} = \langle n|\, Q \,|n\rangle + \sum_{m\neq n} \frac{2}{\hbar(\omega_{nm}^2 - \omega^2)}\left[\frac{\omega_{nm}^2}{\omega^2}\,\mathrm{Re}(i\langle n|\, Q \,|m\rangle\langle m|\, \boldsymbol{\mu} \,|n\rangle) \cdot \frac{\partial \mathbf{E}}{\partial t} + \omega_{nm}\,\mathrm{Re}(\langle n|\, Q \,|m\rangle\langle m|\, \mathbf{m} \,|n\rangle) \cdot \mathbf{B} + \omega_{nm}\,\mathrm{Im}(i\langle n|\, Q \,|m\rangle\langle m|\, \boldsymbol{\mu} \,|n\rangle) \cdot \mathbf{E} - \mathrm{Im}(\langle n|\, Q \,|m\rangle\langle m|\, \mathbf{m} \,|n\rangle) \cdot \frac{\partial \mathbf{B}}{\partial t}\right]. \qquad (2.4.19)$$

This expression gives the expectation value of an observable Q in a state n with a fixed orientation of the molecular coordinate system in the laboratory frame determined by the vectors **E** and **B**. The observables $\langle Q\rangle_{nn}$ must next be averaged over all orientations. In order to determine the scattering properties of a medium it is necessary to find the quantities $\overline{\langle \boldsymbol{\mu}\rangle}_{nn}$ and $\overline{\langle \mathbf{m}\rangle}_{nn}$, where the bar denotes averaging over orientations. This will require the averaging of quantities like $\langle n|\,\mathbf{Q}\,|m\rangle\langle m|\,\mathbf{m}\,|n\rangle\cdot\partial\mathbf{B}/\partial t$. From the methods outlined in Chapter 1 this is equal to $\frac{1}{3}(\langle n|\,\mathbf{Q}\,|m\rangle\cdot\langle m|\,\mathbf{m}\,|n\rangle)(\partial\mathbf{B}/\partial t)$.

The term

$$\sum_{m\neq n}\frac{\omega_{mn}^2}{(\omega_{nm}^2-\omega^2)\omega^2}\,\mathrm{Re}(i\langle n|\,Q\,|m\rangle\langle m|\,\boldsymbol{\mu}\,|n\rangle)$$

is equal to

$$\sum_{m\neq n}\frac{-\mathrm{Im}(\langle n|\,Q\,|m\rangle\langle m|\,\boldsymbol{\mu}\,|n\rangle)}{\omega_{nm}^2-\omega^2}-\omega^{-2}\sum_{m}\mathrm{Im}\langle n|\,Q\,|m\rangle\langle m|\,\boldsymbol{\mu}\,|n\rangle)$$
$$+\,\omega^{-2}\,\mathrm{Im}(\langle n|\,Q\,|n\rangle\langle n|\,\boldsymbol{\mu}\,|n\rangle),\quad (2.4.19a)$$

where the second summation is over all states including n. Since the diagonal matrix elements of observables are real, the last term is zero. By the sum rule for matrix elements the second term is $-(1/\omega^2)\mathrm{Im}(\langle n|\,Q\mu\,|n\rangle)$, which is also zero.

From the above discussion the orientation averaged vector observables may finally be written:

$$\overline{\langle\mathbf{Q}\rangle}_{nn}=\frac{2}{3\hbar}\sum_{m\neq n}\frac{1}{\omega_{nm}^2-\omega^2}\Bigg[-\mathrm{Im}(\langle n|\,\mathbf{Q}\,|m\rangle\cdot\langle m\,|\,\boldsymbol{\mu}\,|n\rangle)\frac{\partial\mathbf{E}}{\partial t}$$
$$+\,\omega_{nm}\,\mathrm{Re}(\langle n|\,\mathbf{Q}\,|m\rangle\cdot\langle m|\,\mathbf{m}\,|n\rangle)\mathbf{B}$$
$$+\,\omega_{nm}\,\mathrm{Re}(\langle n|\,\mathbf{Q}\,|m\rangle\cdot\langle m|\,\boldsymbol{\mu}\,|n\rangle)\,\mathbf{E}$$
$$-\,\mathrm{Im}(\langle n|\,\mathbf{Q}\,|m\rangle\cdot\langle m|\,\mathbf{m}\,|n\rangle)\frac{\partial\mathbf{B}}{\partial t}\Bigg].\quad (2.4.20)$$

The vanishing of the quadrupole moment terms may now be demonstrated. If the averaging process used to obtain (2.4.20) from (2.4.16) is applied to the last term of (2.2.9), one will be led to consider terms like

$$\overline{\langle n|\,\mathbf{Q}\,|m\rangle\langle m|\,(\mathbf{r}\cdot\boldsymbol{\nabla}_0)(\mathbf{A}(0)\cdot\mathbf{r})\,|n\rangle},$$

where **Q** is either **μ** or **m**. By the matrix sum rule this may be written

$$\overline{\langle n|\,\mathbf{Q}\,|m\rangle\sum_s\langle m|\,\mathbf{r}\cdot\boldsymbol{\nabla}_0\,|s\rangle\langle s|\,\mathbf{A}(0)\cdot\mathbf{r}\,|n\rangle}$$
$$=\tfrac{1}{6}\Big(\langle n|\,\mathbf{Q}\,|m\rangle\cdot\sum_s\langle m|\,\mathbf{r}\,|s\rangle\times\langle s|\,\mathbf{r}\,|n\rangle\Big)(\boldsymbol{\nabla}_0\times\mathbf{A}(0))$$
$$=\tfrac{1}{6}(\langle n|\,\mathbf{Q}\,|m\rangle\cdot\langle m|\,\mathbf{r}\times\mathbf{r}\,|n\rangle)(\boldsymbol{\nabla}_0\times\mathbf{A}(0))=0,\quad (2.4.21)$$

where the relation

$$\overline{(\mathbf{A}_1 \cdot \mathbf{B}_1)(\mathbf{A}_2 \cdot \mathbf{B}_2)(\mathbf{A}_3 \cdot \mathbf{B}_3)} = \tfrac{1}{6}(\mathbf{A}_1 \cdot \mathbf{A}_2 \times \mathbf{A}_3)(\mathbf{B}_1 \cdot \mathbf{B}_2 \times \mathbf{B}_3)$$

has been used.

When $\mathbf{Q}$ is equal to $\boldsymbol{\mu}$ in (2.4.20) the first term is zero, since

$$\langle n|\,\boldsymbol{\mu}\,|m\rangle \cdot \langle m|\,\boldsymbol{\mu}\,|n\rangle$$

is real; and when $\mathbf{Q}$ is equal to $\mathbf{m}$ the fourth term vanishes. The required average dipole moments are found to be

$$\overline{\langle \boldsymbol{\mu} \rangle}_{nn} = \alpha_n \mathbf{E} - \gamma_n \mathbf{B} + \frac{\beta_n}{c}\frac{\partial \mathbf{B}}{\partial t} \tag{2.4.22a}$$

$$\overline{\langle \mathbf{m} \rangle}_{nn} = \kappa_n \mathbf{B} + \gamma_n \mathbf{E} + \frac{\beta_n}{c}\frac{\partial \mathbf{E}}{\partial t} \tag{2.4.22b}$$

where

$$\alpha_n = \frac{2}{3h}\sum_{m \neq n} \frac{\nu_{nm}|\langle n|\,\boldsymbol{\mu}\,|m\rangle|^2}{\nu_{nm}^2 - \nu^2}$$

$$\kappa_n = \frac{2}{3h}\sum_{m \neq n} \frac{\nu_{nm}|\langle n|\,\mathbf{m}\,|m\rangle|^2}{\nu_{nm}^2 - \nu^2}$$

$$\gamma_n = \frac{2}{3h}\sum_{m \neq n} \frac{\nu_{nm}\,\mathrm{Re}\,(\langle n|\,\boldsymbol{\mu}\,|m\rangle \cdot \langle m|\,\mathbf{m}\,|n\rangle)}{\nu_{nm}^2 - \nu^2}$$

$$\beta_n = \frac{c}{3\pi h}\sum_{m \neq n} \frac{\mathrm{Im}\,(\langle n|\,\boldsymbol{\mu}\,|m\rangle \cdot \langle m|\,\mathbf{m}\,|n\rangle)}{\nu_{nm}^2 - \nu^2}.$$

The coefficients of $\partial\mathbf{B}/\partial t$ and $\partial\mathbf{E}/\partial t$ have been written in the form β_n/c to conform with convention in the quantum mechanical formulation.

Since the wave function for an unperturbed molecule may always be written in the form $e^{i\lambda}\psi$, where ψ is real, the parameter γ_n may be set equal to zero. When force fields other than the radiation field are present, this will not always be true; however, it can be shown that the term can make at most only a higher order contribution to the rotatory dispersion.

The consequences of (2.4.22) with $\gamma_n = 0$ have already been discussed in Chapter 1. The rotation in radians per unit length is accordingly given by

$$\phi = \frac{16\pi^2}{3ch} N \sum_{m \neq n} \frac{\nu^2 R_{nm}}{\nu_{nm}^2 - \nu^2}, \tag{2.4.23}$$

where $R_{nm} = \mathrm{Im}(\langle n|\,\boldsymbol{\mu}\,|m\rangle \cdot \langle m|\,\mathbf{m}\,|n\rangle)$ is the rotational strength of the transition and N is the number density of the molecules. In most cases n is the ground state; when higher states are appreciably populated the terms in (2.4.23) will have to be statistically weighted.

The quantity R_{nm} is to be compared with the analogous quantity S_{nm} in the expression for the polarizability, which may be written

$$\alpha_n = \frac{2}{3h} \sum_m \frac{\nu_{nm} S_{nm}}{\nu_{nm}^2 - \nu^2},$$

where $S_{nm} = |\langle n| \boldsymbol{\mu} |m\rangle|^2$. This quantity is called the *line strength* of the transition from n to m.

A useful parameter in the study of a given transition is Kuhn's anisotropy factor

$$g_{nm} = R_{nm}/S_{nm}. \tag{2.4.24}$$

If the angle between the electric dipole moment and the magnetic dipole moment of a transition is θ_{nm}, the anisotropy factor may be written

$$g_{nm} = \frac{|\langle n| \mathbf{m} |m\rangle|}{|\langle n| \boldsymbol{\mu} |m\rangle|} \cos \theta_{nm}. \tag{2.4.25}$$

In the extreme case of a transition with large electric and magnetic dipole moments parallel to each other g_{nm} is $\sim 10^{-3}$, where $|\langle n| \mathbf{m} |m\rangle|$ has been assumed to be one Bohr magneton, $e\hbar/2mc \sim 10^{-20}$ cgs and $|\langle n| \boldsymbol{\mu} |m\rangle|$ has been given the typical value of one debye unit, 5×10^{-18} cgs.

For most transitions large magnetic moments will be accompanied by small electric moments and vice versa. The reason for this is that most transitions are largely confined to localized groups of atoms which themselves are not dissymmetric. It is the function of small perturbations by the rest of the molecule to provide the necessary moment parallel to the electric or magnetic dipole moment of the particular group responsible for the transition.

It may be expected that such components of electric or magnetic moment caused by dissymmetric perturbations will be at least an order of magnitude lower than their maximum values used above. A typical value of g_{nm} for a strong electric dipole transition (octyl alcohol) is $\sim 10^{-6}$. Strong magnetic dipole transitions with small electric dipole moments, such as occur in the ethylene diamine and oxalate complexes of chromium and cobalt, will exhibit values of $g_{nm} \sim 10^{-2}$.

The Kuhn-Thomas sum rule states that

$$\sum_m f_{nm} = n_e, \tag{2.4.26}$$

where n_e is the total number of electrons in the molecule and

$$f_{nm} = \frac{8\pi^2 m}{3e^2 h} \nu_{nm} S_{nm}.$$

The quantity f_{nm} is called the oscillator strength of the transition from n to m; the polarizability α_n may be written

$$\alpha_n = \frac{e^2}{4\pi^2 m} \sum_m \frac{f_{nm}}{\nu_{nm}^2 - \nu^2}.$$

An analogous rule exists for the rotational strengths, R_{nm}:

$$\sum_m R_{nm} = 0. \qquad (2.4.27)$$

The proof follows from the matrix sum rule:

$$\sum_m R_{nm} = \mathrm{Im}\left(\sum_m \langle n| \boldsymbol{\mu} |m\rangle \cdot \langle m| \mathbf{m} |n\rangle\right)$$
$$= \mathrm{Im}(\langle n| \boldsymbol{\mu}\mathbf{m} |n\rangle - \langle n| \boldsymbol{\mu} |n\rangle \cdot \langle n| \mathbf{m} |n\rangle) = 0,$$

since the diagonal elements are real. From (2.4.23) and (2.4.27) it follows that $\phi \to 0$ as $\nu \to 0$ or ∞, for

$$\sum_m \frac{\nu^2 R_{nm}}{\nu_{nm}^2 - \nu^2} \to 0 \text{ as } \nu \to 0 \qquad \text{and} \qquad \sum_m \frac{\nu^2 R_{nm}}{\nu_{nm}^2 - \nu^2} \to -\sum_m R_{nm} = 0 \text{ as } \nu \to \infty.$$

2.5. The Kronig-Kramers Transforms

The form of the parameters appearing in (2.4.22) applies only outside of absorption regions, where $|\nu_{nm} - \nu| \gg 0$. A special theory of line shapes is required to predict the correct form of the resonance expressions. The formalism of ordinary dispersion and absorption is fairly well understood, but the detailed application to particular systems has not often given impressive agreement with experiment. For molecules the greatest success has been attained with empirical methods.

The classical treatment of line widths in the absorption of monatomic gases divided the contributions into essentially three groups:

1. Natural line width or radiation damping.
2. Doppler effect caused by the motion of the atoms.
3. Interactions or collisions.

In classical language radiation damping is caused by reradiation from the accelerated electrons resulting in a broader band and the absorption of energy from the electromagnetic field. This effect has been treated by the models in Chapter 1; the absorption and dispersion curves exhibit the so-called Lorentzian behavior. In quantum theory this natural line width is presented in terms of the lifetime of excited states and their natural tendency to decay to the ground. Simple calculations indicate that this makes a small contribution to the line width of even atomic systems.

The Doppler effect is well understood and easily calculated from the Boltzmann distribution of molecular velocities. It arises from a change in the wavelength of the radiation emitted by an atom or molecule in motion relative to the observer. This same effect is used to estimate the motion of celestial bodies relative to the earth. Since the distribution of velocities is Gaussian, it will happen that this contribution to the line shape will also be Gaussian. This effect appears to be quite small compared to observed molecular line widths.

Most theories of atomic line shape have centered around atomic interactions. The results have yielded both exponential and Lorentzian expressions, none of which appear to be applicable to complex molecules. The observed molecular bands are much broader than atomic spectra and often may be empirically fitted to a Gaussian curve. It has been possible to make an impressive correlation of fine structure with vibrations. It appears that molecular line shapes cannot even be estimated by the fixed nuclei approximation.

Despite this difficult situation there is one approach which will allow the correlation of absorption and circular dichroism data with calculated dispersion expressions outside the absorption band. The optical parameters in (2.4.22) are in general complex. This may be seen from the classical models in Chapter 1, where the dispersion was governed by the real part of the optical rotatory parameter and the circular dichroism by its imaginary part; both the ORD and the CD are obtained from the same complex function. The general methods of complex variable theory may be employed to relate the real part of a function to its imaginary part.

In order to do this it will be necessary to derive some simple properties of the optical constants. In Chapter 1 it was found that a periodic force $F = F_0 e^{-i\omega t}$, where F_0 is real, gave rise to a response $X = X_0 e^{-i\omega t}$, where X_0 is complex. This may also be written

$$X = \alpha F_0 e^{-i\omega t}. \tag{2.5.1}$$

If one writes $\alpha = \alpha' + i\alpha''$, the real part of (2.5.1) is

$$\operatorname{Re} X = \operatorname{Re}[(\alpha' + i\alpha'')F_0(\cos \omega t - i \sin \omega t)] = (\alpha' \cos \omega t + \alpha'' \sin \omega t)F_0. \tag{2.5.2}$$

The energy absorbed per cycle is given by

$$\int_0^{2\pi/\omega} (\operatorname{Re} \dot{X})(\operatorname{Re} F)\, dt$$

$$= \omega F_0^2 \int_0^{2\pi/\omega} (-\alpha' \sin \omega t + \alpha'' \cos \omega t)\cos \omega t\, dt = \pi\alpha'' F_0^2. \tag{2.5.3}$$

In the most general case the response of a system depends on the values of the driving force at all previous instants. This fact may be expressed mathematically in the form

$$X(t) = \int_0^\infty K(\tau)F(t-\tau)\,d\tau, \tag{2.5.4}$$

where $K(\tau)$ is real. This states that the current value of X at time t has a linear dependence on the values of F at all prior times but not on subsequent ones. As τ varies from 0 to ∞, the argument of F varies from t to $-\infty$. This is an expression of the principle of causality.

The dispersion law is obtained by making a Fourier analysis of the driving force F and the response X:

$$F(t) = \int_{-\infty}^\infty e^{-i\omega t} f(\omega)\,d\omega \tag{2.5.5a}$$

$$X(t) = \int_{-\infty}^\infty e^{-i\omega t} x(\omega)\,d\omega, \tag{2.5.5b}$$

where $f(\omega)$ and $x(\omega)$ are amplitude factors which govern the frequency distribution. If f and x are even functions of ω, F and X will be real; but this is not necessary in the theory. Both f and x will be considered as complex; for the moment ω is a real variable with the integration taken along the real axis.

Substitution of these relations into (2.5.4) gives

$$\int_{-\infty}^\infty e^{-i\omega t} x(\omega)\,d\omega = \int_{-\infty}^\infty e^{-i\omega t}\left[\int_0^\infty e^{i\omega\tau}K(\tau)\,d\tau\right] f(\omega)\,d\omega. \tag{2.5.6}$$

From this it follows that

$$x(\omega) = \alpha(\omega)f(\omega), \tag{2.5.7}$$

where $\alpha(\omega) = \int_0^\infty e^{i\omega\tau}K(\tau)\,d\tau$. This is now the most general form for a linear response parameter $\alpha(\omega)$.

This expression implies that $\alpha(-\omega) = \alpha^*(\omega)$, from which one obtains $\alpha'(-\omega) = \alpha'(\omega)$, $\alpha''(-\omega) = -\alpha''(\omega)$; that is, $\alpha'(\omega)$ is an even function and $\alpha''(\omega)$ is odd. The examples in Chapter 1 all conform to this rule.

In the ensuing development it is well to emphasize that initially $\alpha(\omega)$ is a complex function of a real variable. The real and imaginary parts of this function will respectively describe dispersion and absorption phenomena. In order to relate these two functions it will be necessary to extend the domain of ω to complex numbers. First, for real values of ω it may be argued that on physical grounds $\alpha(\omega)$ approaches a finite limiting value as $\omega \to 0$, which may be taken as zero with no loss in generality. In the event $\alpha(0) \neq 0$ one may replace $\alpha(\omega)$ by $\alpha(\omega) - \alpha(0)$ in all the resulting formulas. Second, it will happen that $\alpha(\infty) = 0$, since the inertia of a system prevents it from following infinitely rapid fluctuations. These two facts are also reflected in the models of Chapter 1.

If one seeks to extend the values of ω into the complex domain, $\omega = \omega' + i\omega''$, the exponential factor $e^{i\omega\tau}$, in the integral expression for $\alpha(\omega)$ will insure that this function decreases exponentially for large positive imaginary components, since $e^{i\omega\tau} = e^{i\omega'\tau}e^{-\omega''\tau}$. All real systems of interest will be absorbing and ω'' will be positive. The complex function $\alpha(\omega)$, when regarded from a strictly mathematical point of view as a function of a complex variable ω, will be analytic in the upper half plane and will approach zero as $e^{-\omega''\tau}$.

A few central results of complex variable theory will now be reviewed:

1. The line integral $\oint_C f(z)\,dz$ around a closed loop C of an analytic function $f(z)$ is zero.

2. The line integral of any function around a closed loop is independent of the path provided the same singularities are enclosed.

From these facts it follows that $\oint_{n\neq -1} z^n\,dz = 0$ for positive and negative integers and all contours circumscribing the origin; for all such contours may be deformed to circles of radius R centered on the origin. In this case $z = \mathrm{Re}^{i\theta}$, $dz = i\,\mathrm{Re}^{i\theta}$, and

$$\oint z^n\,dz = iR^{n+1}\int_0^{2\pi} e^{(n+1)i\theta}\,d\theta. \tag{2.5.8}$$

This is zero except when $n = -1$, where it has the value $2\pi i$.

This argument may be readily extended to show that

$$\oint (z-a)^n\,dz = \begin{cases} 0, & n \neq -1 \\ 2\pi i, & n = -1 \end{cases} \tag{2.5.9}$$

for any complex constant a. The special role of the reciprocal of $z - a$ is used throughout the entire field of complex variable analysis. In particular the Cauchy integral theorem follows from the above considerations:

$$f(z) = \frac{1}{2\pi i}\int_C \frac{f(z')}{z'-z}\,dz', \tag{2.5.10}$$

where $f(z)$ is analytic over the region of the loop. It may be proved by expanding $f(z')$ as a power series in $(z'-z)$, $f(z') = f(z) + (z'-z)f'(z) + \cdots$. Integration over all powers of $z'-z$ gives zero except for $n = -1$, and the result immediately follows.

A corollary to (2.5.10) is

$$\lim_{r\to 0}\int_{C(r,\Omega)} \frac{f(z')}{z'-z}\,dz' = i\Omega f(z), \tag{2.5.11}$$

where $C(r, \Omega)$ is an arc of angle Ω on a circle with radius r and center z. The proof again follows by expanding $f(z')$ in terms of $(z' - z)$. This gives

$$\lim_{r\to 0} \int_{C(r,\Omega)} \sum_{n=0}^{\infty} \frac{f^{(n)}(z)}{n!} (z' - z)^n \frac{dz'}{z' - z}$$

$$= \lim_{r\to 0} \sum_{n=0}^{\infty} \frac{f^{(n)}(z) i r^n}{n!} \int_0^{\Omega} e^{ni\theta}\, d\theta = i\Omega f(z). \quad (2.5.12)$$

It is important to remember that this result only holds in the limit as $r \to 0$. Only when $\Omega = 2\pi$ may the radius be arbitrary.

We are now in a position to derive a relation between the real and imaginary parts of a complex function of a real variable. Toward this end the result of (2.5.11) will be kept in mind. Consider the loop in Figure 2.2. The function

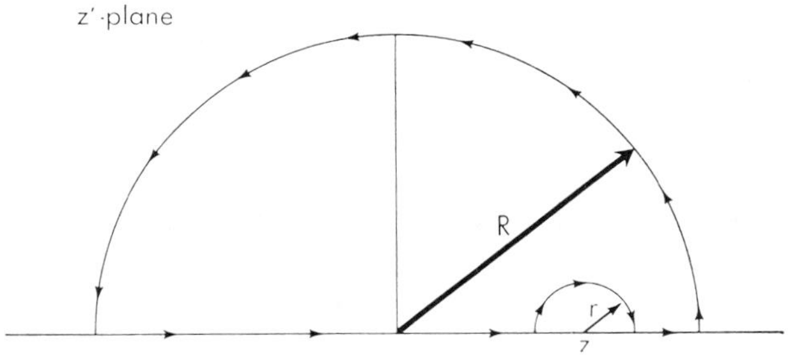

Figure 2.2. Contour of integration for Kronig-Kramers transformation.

$f(z')/(z' - z)$ is analytic inside this region, since the point $z' = z$ has been excluded. One may therefore write

$$\oint \frac{f(z')}{z' - z} dz' = \int_{C_R} \frac{f(z')}{z' - z} dz' + \int_{C_r} \frac{f(z')}{z' - z} dz'$$

$$+ \int_{-R}^{-r+z} \frac{f(z')}{z' - z} dz' + \int_{r+z}^{R} \frac{f(z')}{z' - z} dz' = 0, \quad (2.5.13)$$

where C_R is the large semicircle centered on the origin and C_r is the small one around z.

If $f(z)$ is now identified with $\alpha(\omega)$ in (2.5.7), it will be seen that $\alpha(z')/(z' - z)$ goes to zero faster than $1/R$ on the semicircle because the real part of the exponent in the factor $e^{iz\tau}$ is negative in the upper half plane. Accordingly, as $R \to \infty$, the integral over C_R vanishes. From (2.5.11) the integral over C_r as $r \to 0$ is $-\pi i f(z)$; the minus sign appears because the integral is taken in the clockwise rather than counterclockwise sense. The remaining two integrals are evaluated for real values of z', but $f(z)$ is still complex. The sum as $r \to 0$ and $R \to \infty$ is the definition of the Cauchy principal value of the integral from $-\infty$ to $+\infty$, which is denoted by the symbol $⨍$. Equation 2.5.13 becomes

$$⨍_{-\infty}^{\infty} \frac{f(z')}{z' - z}\, dz' = \pi i f(z), \tag{2.5.14}$$

where it is emphasized that both z' and z are real.

The analytic function $f(z)$ may now be identified with $\alpha(\omega) = \alpha'(\omega) + i\alpha''(\omega)$. When z', z are replaced by ω, ω_0, (2.5.14) becomes

$$⨍_{-\infty}^{\infty} \frac{\alpha'(\omega) + i\alpha''(\omega)}{\omega - \omega_0}\, d\omega = \pi i \alpha'(\omega_0) - \pi\alpha''(\omega_0). \tag{2.5.15}$$

Equating real and imaginary parts leads to the Kronig-Kramers transforms

$$\alpha'(\omega_0) = \frac{1}{\pi} ⨍_{-\infty}^{\infty} \frac{\alpha''(\omega)}{\omega - \omega_0}\, d\omega \tag{2.5.16a}$$

$$\alpha''(\omega_0) = -\frac{1}{\pi} ⨍_{-\infty}^{\infty} \frac{\alpha'(\omega)}{\omega - \omega_0}\, d\omega. \tag{2.5.16b}$$

In (2.5.16a) $\alpha''(\omega)$ is an odd function, and we may write

$$\begin{aligned}
\alpha'(\omega_0) &= \frac{1}{\pi}\left[⨍_{-\infty}^{0} \frac{\alpha''(\omega)}{\omega - \omega_0}\, d\omega + ⨍_{0}^{\infty} \frac{\alpha''(\omega)}{\omega - \omega_0}\, d\omega\right] \\
&= \frac{1}{\pi}\left[⨍_{0}^{\infty} \frac{\alpha''(\omega)}{\omega + \omega_0}\, d\omega + ⨍_{0}^{\infty} \frac{\alpha''(\omega)}{\omega - \omega_0}\, d\omega\right] \\
&= \frac{2}{\pi} ⨍_{0}^{\infty} \frac{\omega\alpha''(\omega)}{\omega^2 - \omega_0^2}\, d\omega.
\end{aligned}$$

Similarly one may make use of the evenness of $\alpha'(\omega)$ to obtain

$$\alpha''(\omega_0) = -\frac{2}{\pi}\omega_0 ⨍_{0}^{\infty} \frac{\alpha'(\omega)}{\omega^2 - \omega_0^2}\, d\omega.$$

This alternative mode of expression is given by

$$\alpha'(\omega_0) = \frac{2}{\pi} ⨍_{0}^{\infty} \frac{\omega\alpha''(\omega)}{\omega^2 - \omega_0^2}\, d\omega \tag{2.5.16a$'$}$$

$$\alpha''(\omega_0) = -\frac{2}{\pi}\omega_0 ⨍_{0}^{\infty} \frac{\alpha'(\omega)}{\omega^2 - \omega_0^2}\, d\omega. \tag{2.5.16b$'$}$$

In Chapter 1 it was demonstrated that the average index of refraction and absorption coefficient were determined by the complex polarizability α, and the difference between these quantities for left and right circularly polarized light was determined by the complex optical rotatory parameter β. Both α and β are response parameters, and their real and imaginary parts are related by the above transformations. The appropriate indices of refraction are connected by the relation

$$(n'_- - n'_+) + i(n''_- - n''_+) = 8\pi NS \frac{\omega}{c} \beta = 8\pi NS \frac{\omega}{c} (\beta' + i\beta''). \tag{2.5.17}$$

The rotation ϕ and the circular dichroism θ are given by

$$\phi = 4\pi NS \frac{\omega^2}{c^2} \beta' \tag{2.5.18a}$$

$$\theta = 16\pi NS \frac{\omega^2}{c^2} \beta''. \tag{2.5.18b}$$

The substitution of (2.5.18) into (2.5.16)′ gives

$$\phi(\omega_0) = \frac{\omega_0^2}{2\pi} \int_0^\infty \frac{\theta(\omega)\, d\omega}{\omega(\omega^2 - \omega_0^2)}. \tag{2.5.19}$$

The simplest way of portraying a spectrum of nonoverlapping absorption bands is to write

$$\theta(\omega) = \sum_n \theta_n \delta(\omega - \omega_n), \tag{2.5.20}$$

where $\delta(\omega - \omega_n)$ is a function which is infinite at ω_n and zero elsewhere in such a way that $\int \delta(\omega - \omega_n)\, d\omega = 1$. In addition it is supposed to have the property that $\int f(\omega)\delta(\omega - \omega_n)\, d\omega = f(\omega_n)$. Although this function is not of the soundest mathematical vintage, its unfailing success in avoiding tedious proofs in physical problems has greatly enhanced its pragmatic stature.

The integrand in (2.5.19) will have no singularities if $\omega_0 \neq \omega_n$. From (2.5.19) and (2.5.20) it follows that

$$\phi(\omega_0) = \frac{\omega_0^2}{2\pi} \sum_n \frac{\theta_n}{\omega_n(\omega_n^2 - \omega_0^2)} \tag{2.5.21}$$

Comparison of this result with (2.4.23) gives for a transition $0 \to n$

$$R_{0n} = \text{Im}(\boldsymbol{\mu}_{0n} \cdot \mathbf{m}_{n0}) = \frac{3ch}{32\pi^3} \frac{\theta_n}{NS\omega_n}. \tag{2.5.22}$$

This furnishes a direct comparison of the calculated rotational strength R_{0n} with the experimentally determined area under the dichroism band θ_n. This result indicates that the limiting form of the dispersion is independent of line shape, as is implicit in the derivation of (2.4.23).

The above result will be accurate only so long as the bands do not overlap.

It will also suffer inaccuracies for broad bands, which may be considered a special case of overlapping bands, if for no other reason than the ambiguity in ω_n. For the present it seems that the error in (2.5.22) is considerably less than the precision of current methods for calculating R_{0n}.

The two most widely used empirical forms of absorption curves have been the Lorentzian $\Gamma\omega/[(\omega_n^2 - \omega^2)^2 + \Gamma^2\omega^2]$ and the Gaussian $e^{-a^2(\omega-\omega_n)^2}$. The theoretical aspects of the former have been presented in Chapter 1, where it was found that the dispersion and absorption were derived from a single complex response parameter of the form $A/[(\omega_n^2 - \omega^2) - i\Gamma\omega]$. It is an instructive exercise in integration to verify that the real and imaginary parts of this function are connected by the relations 2.5.16. It is worth noting that this function satisfies the conditions under which the Kronig-Kramers transforms were derived in that its two poles, $\omega_\pm = (-i\Gamma \pm \sqrt{4\omega_n^2 - \Gamma^2})/2$, are in the lower half plane, not the upper.

An important question to be answered is the mathematical form of the dispersion for a Gaussian absorption. It will be recalled that the imaginary part of the complex response parameter must be an odd function of ω. The simplest Gaussian which satisfies this requirement is

$$\alpha''(\omega) = A(e^{-a^2(\omega-\omega_n)^2} - e^{-a^2(\omega+\omega_n)^2}). \tag{2.5.23}$$

In the ensuing discussion it will be necessary to evaluate integrals of the form $⨍_{-\infty}^{\infty} e^{-x^2}/(x+a)\,dx$; this is a common type and there are various techniques described in mathematical texts. In one of the general methods use is made of the fact that

$$\int_0^R e^{\pm i(x\pm a)\theta}\,d\theta = \frac{1}{\pm i(x\pm a)}(e^{\pm i(x\pm a)R} - 1)$$

and

$$\lim_{R\to\infty}\int_{x_1}^{x_2} f(x)e^{ixR}\,dx = 0$$

to deduce the result

$$⨍_{-\infty}^{\infty}\frac{e^{-x^2}}{x+a}\,dx = 2\sqrt{\pi}\,e^{-a^2}\int_0^a e^{x^2}dx. \tag{2.5.24}$$

When (2.5.23) is substituted into (2.5.16*a*) this equation leads to the dispersion term

$$\alpha'(\omega) = \frac{2\sqrt{\pi}}{\pi}A\left[e^{-a^2(\omega_n-\omega)^2}\left(\int_0^{a(\omega_n-\omega)} e^{x^2}\,dx\right) + e^{-a^2(\omega_n+\omega)^2}\left(\int_0^{a(\omega_n+\omega)} e^{x^2}\,dx\right)\right]. \tag{2.5.25}$$

This is an even function of ω, as it should be. Inside the absorption region the second term may be neglected and the first approximation to the dispersion becomes

$$\alpha'(\omega) = \frac{2}{\sqrt{\pi}} A e^{-a^2(\omega_n-\omega)^2} a(\omega_n - \omega), \tag{2.6.26}$$

where only the first term has been retained in the expansion of the integral.

This will not be an accurate estimate throughout the entire absorption region, but it does indicate Gaussian, rather than Lorentzian, behavior near the center of the band. This should put one on his guard not to expect a Lorentzian dispersion to be associated with a Gaussian absorption curve. The asymptotic behavior as $\omega \to \infty$ is of particular interest. The asymptotic behavior of the function

$$e^{-a^2}\int_0^a e^{x^2}\,dx = \int_0^a e^{x^2-a^2}\,dx$$

was investigated by Stokes. It may be determined by making the substitution $y = x^2 - a^2$, from which it follows that

$$\int_0^a e^{x^2-a^2}\,dx = \frac{1}{2}\int_{-a^2}^0 \frac{e^y}{\sqrt{a^2+y}}\,dy = \frac{1}{2a}\int_{-a^2}^0 e^y\left(1 - \frac{1}{2}\frac{y}{a^2} + \frac{3}{8}\frac{y^2}{a^4} - \cdots\right) dy$$
$$= \frac{1}{2a}\left\{(1 - e^{-a^2}) - \frac{1}{2a^2}\left[-1 + (a^2+1)e^{-a^2}\right] + \cdots\right\} \sim \frac{1}{2a} + \frac{1}{4a^3}, \tag{2.5.27}$$

where only the first two inverse powers of a have been retained. The limiting form of (2.5.25) is found to be

$$\alpha'(\omega) \to \frac{2}{\sqrt{\pi}} A\left[\frac{1}{2a(\omega_n - \omega)} + \frac{1}{2a(\omega_n + \omega)}\right] = \frac{2A}{a\sqrt{\pi}}\frac{\omega_n}{\omega_n^2 - \omega^2}. \tag{2.5.28}$$

This result assures us that a Gaussian absorption curve is consistent with the required limiting form of the dispersion.

A second instructive example will demonstrate that not all forms of absorption curve will lead to an acceptable dispersion. We seek the absorption associated with a Gaussian dispersion curve. It will be realized that according to classical and quantum theories such a function is not possible, because it does not have the proper limiting form. It is nonetheless interesting to display the corresponding absorption required by (2.5.16*b*) in order to illustrate the general principle that an investigator is not displaying his data to best advantage by using empirical absorption expressions which do not lead to the correct limiting form for the dispersion.

Consider the even function

$$\alpha'(\omega) = B[(\omega_n - \omega)e^{-a^2(\omega_n-\omega)^2} + (\omega_n + \omega)e^{-a^2(\omega_n+\omega)^2}]. \qquad (2.5.29)$$

In the absorbing region centered around $\omega = \omega_n$ the first term dominates and gives rise to the typical S-shaped dispersion form. The reciprocally related absorption curve is given by

$$\alpha''(\omega_0) = -\frac{1}{\pi}⨍_{-\infty}^{\infty} \frac{\alpha'(\omega)}{\omega - \omega_0}\, d\omega$$

$$= \frac{B}{\pi}\int_{-\infty}^{\infty} \left[\left(1 - \frac{\omega_n - \omega_0}{\omega - \omega_0}\right)e^{-a^2(\omega_n-\omega)^2} - \left(1 + \frac{\omega_n + \omega_0}{\omega - \omega_0}\right)e^{-a^2(\omega_n+\omega)^2}\right] d\omega$$

$$= \frac{B}{\pi}\left[\frac{\sqrt{\pi}}{a} - (\omega_n - \omega_0)2\sqrt{\pi}\, e^{-a^2(\omega_n-\omega_0)^2}\int_0^{a(\omega_n-\omega_0)} e^{x^2}\, dx\right.$$

$$\left. - \frac{\sqrt{\pi}}{a} + (\omega_n + \omega_0)2\sqrt{\pi}\, e^{-a^2(\omega_n+\omega_0)^2}\int_0^{a(\omega_n+\omega_0)} e^{x^2}\, dx\right]. \qquad (2.5.30)$$

Near the center of the band this function is Gaussian with an $(\omega_n - \omega_0)^2 e^{-a^2(\omega_n-\omega_0)^2}$ dependence. It is interesting to note that if this represented the entire absorption curve the corresponding dispersion would not be pure Gaussian and would reduce to the correct $1/(\omega_n^2 - \omega_0^2)$ limiting form outside the band. The asymptotic behavior of (2.5.30) can be found from (2.5.26), which leads to the limiting form

$$\alpha''(\omega) \to \frac{B}{2a^3\sqrt{\pi}}\left[-\frac{1}{(\omega_n - \omega)^2} + \frac{1}{(\omega_n + \omega)^2}\right] = -\frac{2B}{a^3\sqrt{\pi}}\frac{\omega\omega_n}{(\omega_n^2 - \omega^2)^2}, \qquad (2.5.31)$$

which parallels the limiting behavior of Lorentzian absorption.

In summary it may be said that the Kronig-Kramers transforms impose a requirement of self-consistency on the absorption and dispersion curves both for the average and differential quantities of optical activity. This all follows from the opportunity the physical situation provides in writing the dispersion and absorption response parameters as the real and imaginary parts of a single complex function. In the course of the analysis it followed that the dispersion parameters had to be even functions of the frequency and the absorption parameters odd functions. These transformations in conjunction with the quantum mechanical limiting form $A/(\omega_n^2 - \omega^2)$ will greatly facilitate the interpretation of dispersion and absorption curves in a self-consistent manner as well as point the way toward feasible methods of correlating calculated and observed quantities.

2.6. General Symmetry Considerations

There are certain general conclusions which can be made by studying the symmetry properties of the rotational strength $R_{0n} = \mathrm{Im}(\boldsymbol{\mu}_{0n} \cdot \mathbf{m}_{n0})$. If Ω is a linear operator corresponding to one of the molecule's group operations, then for nondegenerate states $\psi_n(\Omega\mathbf{r}) = \sigma_\Omega \psi_n(\mathbf{r})$, where $\sigma_\Omega = \pm 1$. The integrals associated with matrix elements may be evaluated in any coordinate system. In particular an integral may first be evaluated in an arbitrary system and then in the system obtained from one of the group operations; the two results must be identical. If $\mathbf{T}(\mathbf{r}, \boldsymbol{\nabla})$ is a quantum mechanical operator, this procedure gives

$$T_{0n} = \int \psi_0(\mathbf{r})\mathbf{T}(\mathbf{r}, \boldsymbol{\nabla})\psi_n(\mathbf{r})\, d\tau = \int \psi_0(\Omega\mathbf{r})\mathbf{T}(\Omega\mathbf{r}, \Omega\boldsymbol{\nabla})\psi_n(\Omega\mathbf{r})\, d\tau, \qquad (2.6.1)$$

where use has been made of the length preserving nature of Ω. Improper rotations can only cause changes of sign in the integrand; the change in sign of $d\tau$ is compensated by a reversal in the limits of integration over all space. In one dimension one may write

$$\int_{-\infty}^{\infty} f(x)\, dx = \int_{\infty}^{-\infty} f(-x)(-dx) = \int_{-\infty}^{\infty} f(-x)\, dx.$$

The operators $\boldsymbol{\mu}$ and $\mathbf{m}$ have the form

$$\boldsymbol{\mu} = e \sum_a (\mathbf{i}x_a + \mathbf{j}y_a + \mathbf{k}z_a) \qquad (2.6.2a)$$

$$\mathbf{m} = \left(\frac{e\hbar}{2mc}\right) i \sum_a \left[\mathbf{i}\left(z_a \frac{\partial}{\partial y_a} - y_a \frac{\partial}{\partial z_a}\right) + \mathbf{j}\left(x_a \frac{\partial}{\partial z_a} - z_a \frac{\partial}{\partial x_a}\right) + \mathbf{k}\left(y_a \frac{\partial}{\partial x_a} - x_a \frac{\partial}{\partial y_a}\right)\right]. \qquad (2.6.2b)$$

Both transform contragrediently for proper rotations through an angle θ about the z-axis:

$$\begin{Bmatrix} \mu_x' \\ m_x' \end{Bmatrix} = \begin{Bmatrix} \mu_x \\ m_x \end{Bmatrix} \cos\theta - \begin{Bmatrix} \mu_y \\ m_y \end{Bmatrix} \sin\theta \qquad (2.6.3a)$$

$$\begin{Bmatrix} \mu_y' \\ m_y' \end{Bmatrix} = \begin{Bmatrix} \mu_x \\ m_x \end{Bmatrix} \sin\theta + \begin{Bmatrix} \mu_y \\ m_y \end{Bmatrix} \cos\theta \qquad (2.6.3b)$$

$$\begin{Bmatrix} \mu_z' \\ m_z' \end{Bmatrix} = \begin{Bmatrix} \mu_z \\ m_z \end{Bmatrix}. \qquad (2.6.3c)$$

For improper rotations the transformation properties are

$$\begin{Bmatrix} \mu'_x \\ m'_x \end{Bmatrix} = \begin{Bmatrix} \mu_x \\ -m_x \end{Bmatrix} \cos\theta - \begin{Bmatrix} \mu_y \\ -m_y \end{Bmatrix} \sin\theta \tag{2.6.4a}$$

$$\begin{Bmatrix} \mu'_y \\ m'_y \end{Bmatrix} = \begin{Bmatrix} \mu_x \\ -m_x \end{Bmatrix} \sin\theta + \begin{Bmatrix} \mu_y \\ -m_y \end{Bmatrix} \cos\theta \tag{2.6.4b}$$

$$\begin{Bmatrix} \mu'_z \\ m'_z \end{Bmatrix} = \begin{Bmatrix} -\mu_z \\ m_z \end{Bmatrix}. \tag{2.6.4c}$$

If the symmetry group of the molecule contains an improper rotation, (2.6.1) and (2.6.4) give the result

$$\boldsymbol{\mu}_{0n} \cdot \mathbf{m}_{n0} = (\mu_x)_{0n}(m_x)_{n0} + \cdots = -(\mu_x)_{0n}(m_x)_{n0} - \cdots = -\boldsymbol{\mu}_{on} \cdot \mathbf{m}_{n0}, \tag{2.6.5}$$

from which it follows that $\boldsymbol{\mu}_{0n} \cdot \mathbf{m}_{n0} = 0$. For a center of inversion $\boldsymbol{\mu}' = -\boldsymbol{\mu}$, $\mathbf{m}' = m$; and (2.6.1) again leads to the vanishing of the rotational strength.

For a group operation Ω degenerate states have the transformation property

$$\psi_s(\Omega\mathbf{r}) = \sum_t c_t^{(s)} \psi_t(\mathbf{r}). \tag{2.6.6}$$

The coefficients $c_t^{(s)}$ are the elements of a matrix whose rows and columns are required by group theory to be orthogonal; that is, $\sum_s c_t^{(s)} c_{t'}^{(s)} = \delta_{tt'}$. This fact, along with (2.6.1), (2.6.4), and (2.6.6), leads to the result $\sum_s \boldsymbol{\mu}_{0s} \cdot \mathbf{m}_{s0} = -\sum_s \boldsymbol{\mu}_{0s} \cdot \mathbf{m}_{s0} = 0$ and the conclusion that the total contribution from the degenerate band is zero.

The above arguments serve to establish as a necessary condition for optical activity the requirement that the symmetry group of a molecule contain no improper rotations, that is, a reflection plane, center of inversion, or rotation-reflection axis. Traditionally attention has been focused on the first two; however, the symmetry groups S_4, S_8, S_{12}, ... are Abelian groups of order 4, 8, 12, ... with their generating elements consisting of rotation-reflections through 90°, 45°, 22.5°, ... Molecules with these symmetry properties have no reflection planes or centers of inversion, yet they are inactive. Molecules with none of the improper rotations described above all have the property of being nonsuperimposable on their mirror images. This fact has traditionally served as the criterion for optical activity.

If a molecule is optically active, the above methods may be used to show that its mirror image molecule has an equal and opposite signed rotational strength. Now it will happen that for a reflection $\psi(\Omega_R \mathbf{r}) \neq \pm\psi(\mathbf{r})$, but $\int \psi_0(\Omega_R \mathbf{r})\mathbf{T}(\mathbf{r}, \nabla)\psi_n(\Omega_R \mathbf{r})\, d\tau = \int \psi_0(\mathbf{r})\mathbf{T}(\Omega_R \mathbf{r}, \Omega_R \nabla)\psi_n(\mathbf{r})\, d\tau$, from which it follows that $\boldsymbol{\mu}_{0n}^{(R)} \cdot \mathbf{m}_{n0}^{(R)} = -\boldsymbol{\mu}_{0n} \cdot \mathbf{m}_{n0}$. In this argument a transformation $\Omega_R \mathbf{r}$ has been made on the original function to produce the corresponding one for the mirror image molecule; and a variable change $\Omega_R \mathbf{r}$ has been made in the evaluation of the matrix elements along with the use of the relation $\Omega_R^2 = 1$ for a reflection.

Most optically active molecules, particularly those of biochemical interest, belong to groups of quite low symmetry. Quite often these will contain chromophores of high symmetry such as a benzene ring. The question then arises as to the rule of exact and near degeneracy in dissymmetric molecules. A preliminary answer may be obtained by first considering an optically active molecule with exact degeneracy such as in the groups C_n, $D_n (n > 2)$, T, or $\mathcal{O}$. While it is true that the Jahn-Teller effect will remove any such degeneracy for excited states, it is believed that the small alteration in nuclear conformation will leave the following arguments substantially unaltered.

If $\psi_1, \ldots, \psi_N$ are a linearly independent set of N degenerate wave functions, the total contribution of the band will be

$$R = \text{Im}\left\{\sum_{i=1}^{N} \boldsymbol{\mu}_{0i} \cdot \mathbf{m}_{i0}\right\}. \tag{2.6.7}$$

Any linearly independent combination of the ψ_i's will serve equally well in determining R. In particular one may choose the set

$$\psi_i' = C_1^{(i)}\psi_1 + \sum_{j=2}^{N} c_j^{(i)}\psi_j, \qquad i = 1, \ldots, N, \tag{2.6.8}$$

where $C_1^{(i)} \sim 1$ and the $c_j^{(i)}$ are vanishingly small but adjusted to make the ψ_i' functions linearly independent. The total rotational strength becomes

$$R = \text{Im}\left\{\sum_{i=1}^{N} C_1^{(i)^2} \boldsymbol{\mu}_{01} \cdot \mathbf{m}_{10} + \text{vanishingly small terms}\right\}$$

$$\sim \text{Im}\{N\boldsymbol{\mu}_{01} \cdot \mathbf{m}_{10}\}. \tag{2.6.9}$$

Thus all functions or linear combinations of functions corresponding to a particular degenerate eigenvalue give $1/N$ of the total rotational strength of the band. This result applies strictly to exact degeneracy, but it has important consequences for near degeneracy; for example, starting from an inactive chromophore such as the D_{3h} benzene derivative (**I**), one may substitute the molecule in such a way as to introduce C_3(**II**) or D_3(**III**) symmetry. The degeneracy is retained and the molecule is optically active. In the fixed nuclei approximation a simple dichroism curve would be observed; in the actual case complex vibronic fine structure is often found. The above rule expressed in (2.6.9) will apply, and the contributions from both components of the doubly degenerate bands will be equal and of the same sign.

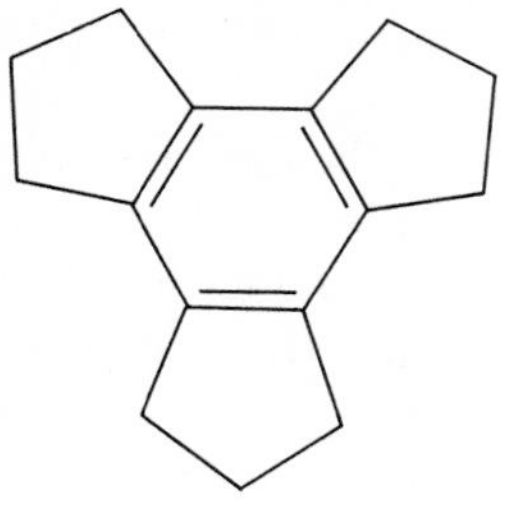

I

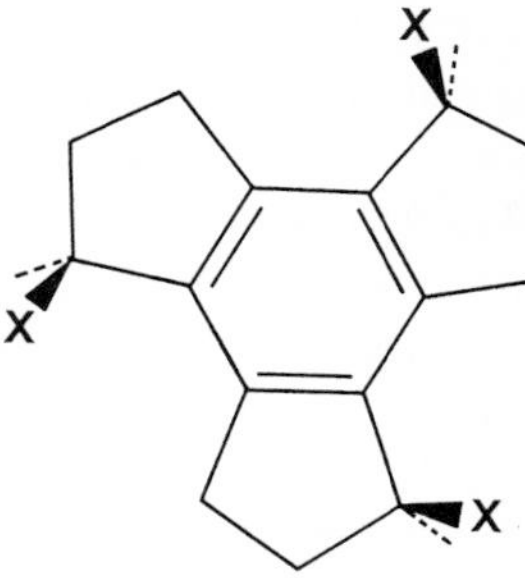

II

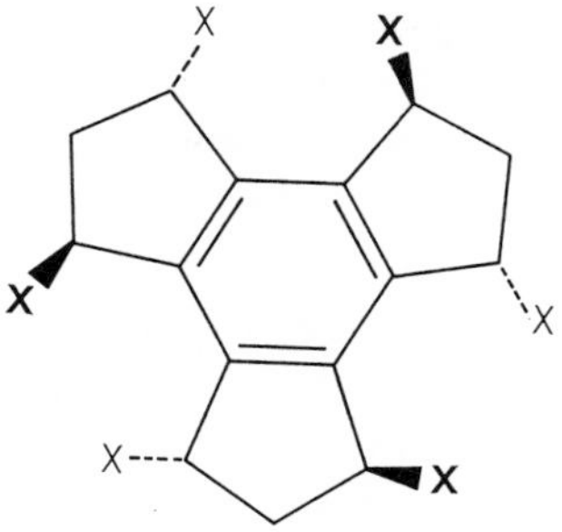

III

If now the molecules, II and III, are further substituted in such a way as to destroy the degeneracy, the individual contributions will no longer be equal (II′, III′). It appears that when an inactive molecule of high symmetry is

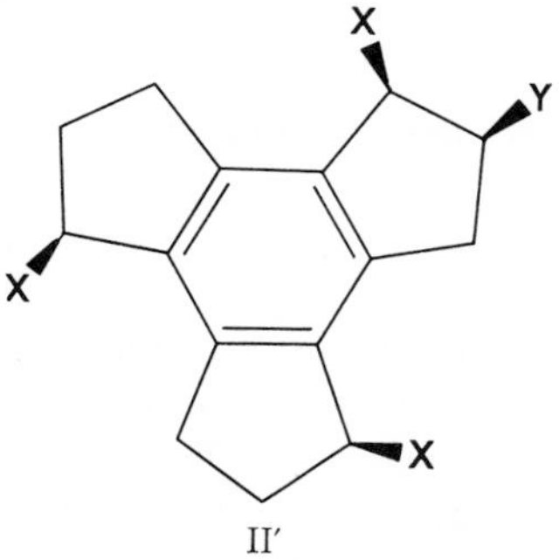

II′

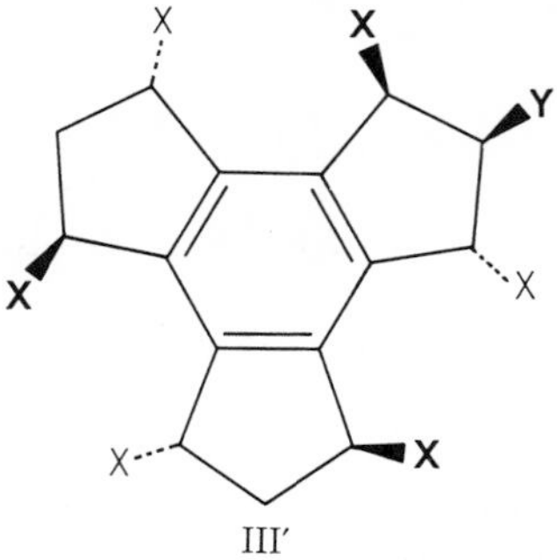

III′

dissymmetrically substituted two extremes may be observed. When a degree of latent symmetry persists with a small splitting of the level, a nearly symmetrical bell-shaped dichroism curve is observed similar to that expected for the completely degenerate case. For large perturbations one often observes an S-shaped dichroism with nearly equal extrema.

Since the only requirement for optical activity is the absence of improper rotation elements the complete absence of symmetry will not be a necessary condition for optical activity. Since three points determine a plane, the prototype of a dissymmetric molecule should be four point scatterers at the corners of an irregular tetrahedron having no center or plane of symmetry. In addition to the optically active tetrahedral carbon atom surrounded by four different groups there are the spiro-compounds, which have a screw pattern of symmetry such as (**IV**). As with the asymmetric carbon atom the four groups may be considered to lie at the corners of an irregular tetrahedron.

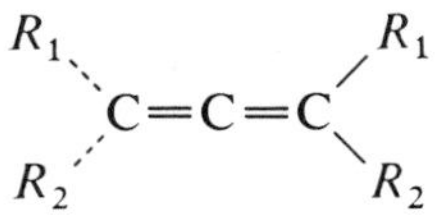

IV

In the compound hexahelicene (**V**) an overall molecular dissymmetry is displayed because of steric interference between the pairs of atoms (a, c) and (b, d). It has been pointed out that the various bands responsible for optical rotation are primarily electric or magnetic dipole transitions which acquire parallel magnetic or electric moments from other transitions by means of dissymmetric perturbations.

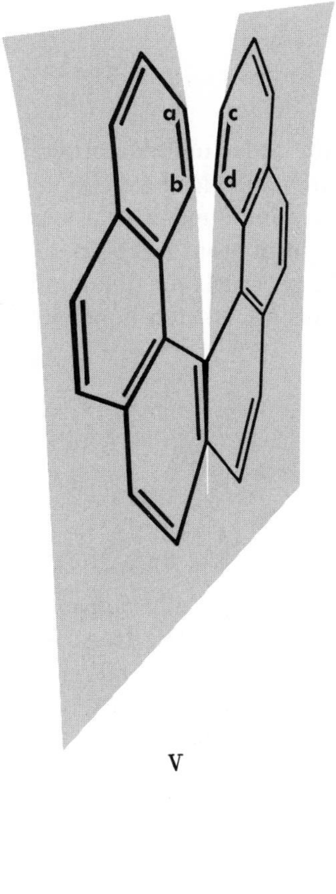

V

Owing to the complete conjugation in hexahelicene, the entire molecule must be regarded as a single chromophore and all its transitions are both electric and magnetic dipole allowed.

This compound falls in the category of skewed or inherently dissymmetric chromophores, which commonly exhibit large rotations because of appreciable parallel electric and magnetic moments for any given transition. A simple quantum mechanical model for such compounds is discussed in the next chapter.

Although most of the optically active compounds that have been investigated have carbon as the primary atom involved in the dissymmetry of the molecule, there are numerous examples where other elements play a leading role. Quaternary salts (**VI**) of nitrogen, phosphorus, and arsenic may be resolved and closely resemble the quadrivalent carbon compounds in structure. One might expect the neutral compounds (**VII**) to exist in active forms as well; however, the inversion barrier appears to be too low and no activity has even been observed.

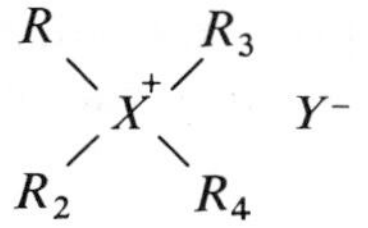

VI

$X =$ N, P, As
$Y =$ Br, Cl^-, etc.

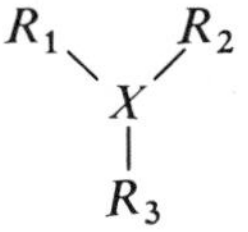

VII

$X =$ N, P, As

In principle the optically active unit comprised of the minimum number of four tangent spheres is embodied in the compounds of sulfur, selenium, and telurium (**VIII**). In all the compounds so far synthesized at least one of the groups attached to the central atom has been complex, consisting of several atoms, and at present the prospects for obtaining compounds where R_1, R_2, and R_3 are all single atoms are not too hopeful.

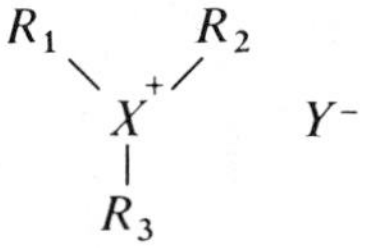

VIII

$X =$ S, Se, Te
$Y = Br^-$, Cl^-, etc.

In the carbon family itself optically active analogues of silicon and tin have been prepared and resolved. The transition metal complexes provide a fertile field for the study of optical rotation. For example the octahedral complexes (**IX**) and (**X**) are dissymmetric (only **X** is asymmetric) and will be optically active. The cobalt complex **XI** has both a plane and a center of symmetry and is inactive. These compounds have transitions in the visible spectral region, and their Cotton effect curves may be observed over their entire absorption regions provided the absorption is not prohibitively high for the measurement of rotations.

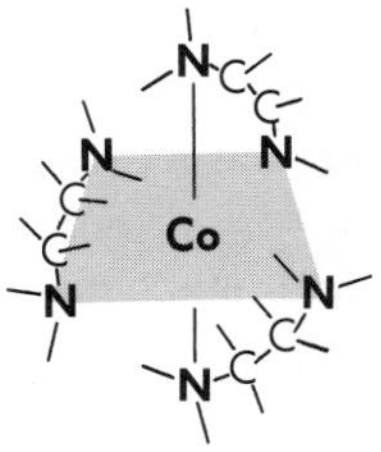

IX

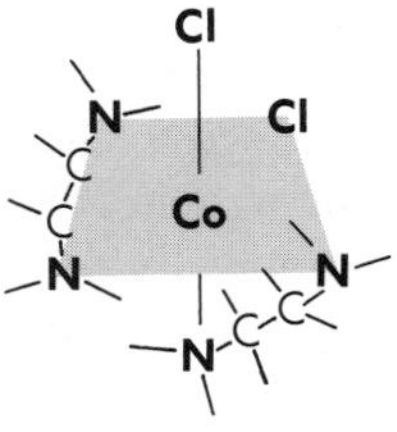

X

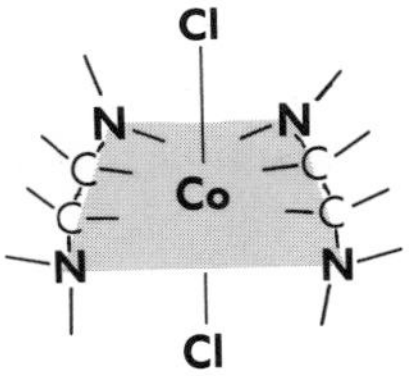

XI

Since almost all the current methods for evaluating the terms in the Rosenfeld equation are pairwise interaction theories, it is well to consider the experimental and theoretical justification for this. In a pairwise interaction theory it is assumed that each pair of groups makes a contribution to the total rotation which is independent of the nature and disposition of the other groups in the molecule. In a molecule like H_2O_2

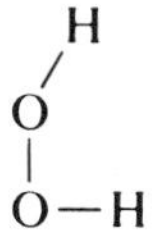

XII

the total contribution to the rotation would come from the interaction of just two identical groups with no further interactions.

In order for this approach to be at all valid it is necessary that there exist at least one moiety comprised of two groups which has no plane or center of symmetry; otherwise all the pairwise interactions would vanish as in $CHCH_3ClBr$. In fact, all pairwise interactions are zero in molecules containing axially symmetric groups joined to a central carbon along their axes of symmetry.

It may be expected that if the pairwise interactions are not zero they will account for the major portion of the rotation. In an attempt to delineate the boundaries for the validity of pairwise interactions Kauzmann et al. (1940) have concluded that higher order interactions may make contributions as high as 20° to the molecular rotation. This means that the simultaneous interaction of 3, 4, or more groups does not necessarily play a negligible role in optical rotation. The compound $CH_3CHBrCN$, which has four axially symmetric groups attached to a central atom, has a molecular rotation of 21°. In this compound the transitions of the $-C{\equiv}N$ group will be considered to acquire parallel components of electric and magnetic moment under the joint influence of two of the other three groups, since the central carbon and any two of the groups attached to it have a plane of symmetry.

In the theory of optical rotation the division of the molecule into groups is largely arbitrary and it is desirable to retain the simplicity of the pairwise interaction approach. This may often be done by combining two groups into one and considering their combined effect on a third. Here what would normally be called a three-way interaction is treated like a pairwise interaction.

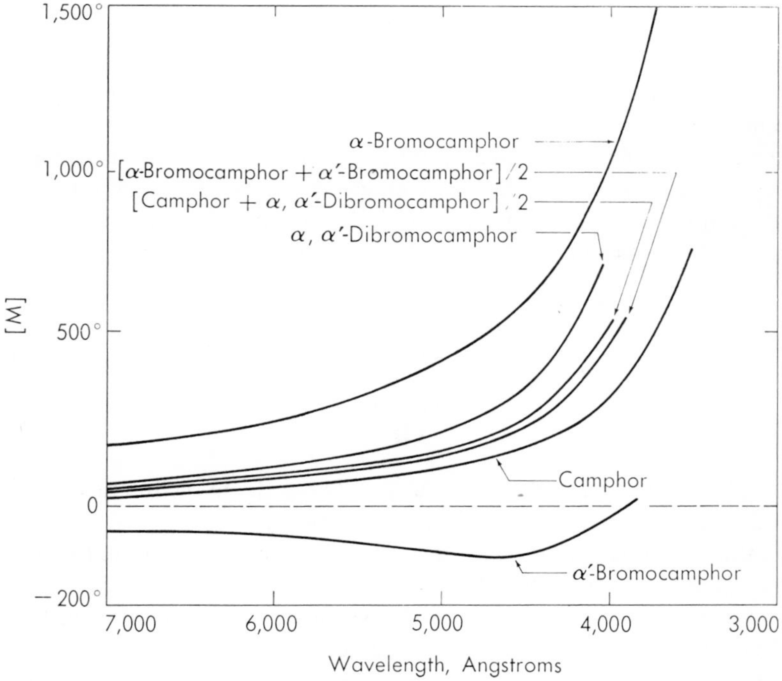

Figure 2.3. The rotations of camphor derivatives. (After Lowry, 1935.)

Although much of the data necessary for a complete analysis of the subject is lacking, Kauzmann et al. have derived relationships based on pairwise interactions among several classes of compounds. For this purpose it was advantageous to consider only rigid molecules where orientation effects are minimized. A certain degree of regularity was observed in the rotations of cyclopropane, cyclobutane, cyclopentane, cyclohexane, camphor, sugar, and steroid derivatives when analyzed by the pairwise interaction theory; for example, $[M]_{5461}$ of camphor is 79.7°, of 3α-bromocamphor 324.2, and of 3β-bromocamphor −101.1. The pairwise interaction theory would predict the rotation of 3,3-dibromocamphor to be the sum of the rotations of the monobromo derivatives less that of camphor. This sum is 143.4°, which compares favorably with the observed rotation of 147.6°. The composite dispersion curve obtained by adding the camphor and dibromocamphor curves is nearly coincident with the curve obtained from the addition of the α- and β-monobromocamphor dispersion curves (Figure 2.3). In many other instances the results are not so encouraging and more data are needed to separate true deviations from apparent ones caused by solvent effects.

CHAPTER 3

Quantum Mechanical Models

3.1. Group Theory

As with all optical phenomena one is ultimately faced with the task of evaluating matrix elements. Before undertaking the task of optical activity and $\boldsymbol{\mu}_{0n} \cdot \mathbf{m}_{n0}$, it is worthwhile to summarize the situation for ordinary dispersion and absorption as governed by the quantity $\boldsymbol{\mu}_{0n} \cdot \boldsymbol{\mu}_{n0}$. In the fixed nuclei approximation transitions are divided into electric dipole allowed and forbidden. The status of a transition originating from the totally symmetrical ground state is determined by the representation spanned by the excited state. For a fixed nuclear conformation all states must transform under the group operations of the molecule according to definite patterns.

A group operation R effects a coordinate transformation described by the matrix $\mathbf{A}^{(R)}$ such that

$$\begin{bmatrix} x' \\ y' \\ z' \end{bmatrix} = \begin{bmatrix} A_{11}^{(R)} & A_{12}^{(R)} & A_{13}^{(R)} \\ A_{21}^{(R)} & A_{22}^{(R)} & A_{23}^{(R)} \\ A_{31}^{(R)} & A_{32}^{(R)} & A_{33}^{(R)} \end{bmatrix} \begin{bmatrix} x \\ y \\ z \end{bmatrix}. \tag{3.1.1}$$

In general a wave function $\psi_i(\mathbf{r})$ belonging to a degenerate set $\psi_1(\mathbf{r}), \ldots, \psi_N(\mathbf{r})$ will be transformed by $\mathbf{A}^{(R)}$ into a linear combination of these functions:

$$\psi_i(\mathbf{A}^{(R)}\mathbf{r}) = \sum_{j=1}^{N} B_{ij}^{(R)} \psi_j(\mathbf{r}) \qquad i = 1, \ldots, N. \tag{3.1.2}$$

This defines a matrix $\mathbf{B}^{(R)}$ such that

$$\begin{bmatrix} \psi_1(\mathbf{A}^{(R)}\mathbf{r}) \\ \psi_2(\mathbf{A}^{(R)}\mathbf{r}) \\ \vdots \\ \psi_N(\mathbf{A}^{(R)}\mathbf{r}) \end{bmatrix} = \begin{bmatrix} B_{11}^{(R)} & B_{12}^{(R)} & \cdots & B_{1N}^{(R)} \\ B_{21}^{(R)} & B_{22}^{(R)} & \cdots & B_{2N}^{(R)} \\ \vdots & \vdots & \vdots\vdots\vdots & \vdots \\ B_{N1}^{(R)} & B_{N2}^{(R)} & \cdots & B_{NN}^{(R)} \end{bmatrix} \begin{bmatrix} \psi_1(\mathbf{r}) \\ \psi_2(\mathbf{r}) \\ \vdots \\ \psi_N(\mathbf{r}) \end{bmatrix}. \tag{3.1.3}$$

The spherical symmetry group consists of the complete set of all proper and improper rotations about the origin; these bring a sphere into coincidence with itself. The number of linearly independent functions transformed according to (3.1.2) or (3.1.3) is the dimension of the representation. For the spherical group there are an infinite number of distinct representations with dimensions 1, 2, ... Corresponding to each one there is an infinite set of transformation matrices with the property that

$$\mathbf{B}^{(R)\dagger} = \mathbf{B}^{(R)-1}$$

and

$$\mathrm{Tr}\,\mathbf{B}^{(R)} = \sum_{i=1}^{N} B_{ii}^{(R)} = \mathrm{Tr}\,\mathbf{C} = \sum_{i=1}^{N} C_{ii}^{(R)} \tag{3.1.4}$$

for all matrices $\mathbf{B}^{(R)}$, $\mathbf{C}^{(R)}$, etc., belonging to the particular representation. This particular sum is called the character. Each group operation has a different character for every representation. The spherical group is of infinite order and any operation is described by three parameters, which specify the axis and angle of rotation. The three Cartesian coordinates x, y, z span a three dimensional representation and their matrices may be found from simple geometrical considerations. For a rotation θ about the z-axis one obtains

$$\begin{bmatrix} x' \\ y' \\ z' \end{bmatrix} = \begin{bmatrix} \cos\theta & -\sin\theta & 0 \\ \sin\theta & \cos\theta & 0 \\ 0 & 0 & 1 \end{bmatrix} \begin{bmatrix} x \\ y \\ z \end{bmatrix}. \tag{3.1.5}$$

The trace of this matrix is $1 + 2\cos\theta$; it so happens that the trace of a rotation about an arbitrary axis depends only on the angle of rotation and not the orientation of the axis. The character of all such rotations is then $1 + 2\cos\theta$; for improper rotations consisting of a rotation followed by a reflection in the plane perpendicular to the axis the character is $-1 + 2\cos\theta$. The identity element $\begin{bmatrix} 1 & 0 & 0 \\ 0 & 1 & 0 \\ 0 & 0 & 1 \end{bmatrix}$ and the inversion matrix $\begin{bmatrix} -1 & 0 & 0 \\ 0 & -1 & 0 \\ 0 & 0 & -1 \end{bmatrix}$ are seen to have characters of 3 and -3.

Any function of $r = \sqrt{x^2 + y^2 + z^2}$ is invariant under all rotations and reflections and belongs to the totally symmetrical one dimensional representation for which all the matrices are one dimensional and equal to the number 1. General polynomials of the form $x^a y^b z^c$ transform according to representations of higher dimension; for example, the functions xy, yz, $x^2 - y^2$, $x^2 + y^2 - 2z^2$ span a five dimensional representation with characters $3 + 2\cos 2\theta$. In the hydrogen atom s-functions belong to the totally symmetrical representation, p-functions to the same three dimensional one as (x, y, z), and d-functions to the above-mentioned five dimensional representation. The f-functions are based on certain third order polynomials and belong to a seven dimensional representation.

All space groups of lower symmetry are subgroups of the spherical group. The operations which leave a cone invariant belong to the $C_{\infty v}$ group and include all rotations about the z-axis along with reflections in all planes containing this axis; the $D_{\infty h}$ group consists of all the operations which bring a right circular cylinder into coincidence with itself, which includes all rotations about the z-axis, all rotations perpendicular to this axis, and the corresponding reflections. Homonuclear diatomic and nonpolar linear molecules such as CO_2 belong to the $D_{\infty h}$ group; whereas heteronuclear diatomic and polar linear molecules such as HCN belong to the $C_{\infty v}$ group.

Groups of finite order consist of those operations which bring certain classes of geometrical figures without cylindrical or spherical symmetry into coincidence with themselves. A figure for which there exist no reflections or rotations which bring it into coincidence with itself is called asymmetric and belongs to the group C_1 consisting of only the identity element. Most optically active molecules are asymmetric; a substantial number particularly among the transition metal complexes are merely dissymmetric. This means that certain rotations will bring the molecule into coincidence with itself, as illustrated by the example of multibladed propellers.

Subgroups of $C_{\infty v}$ and $D_{\infty h}$ may be formed by considering an infinite series of regular polygons beginning with the equilateral triangle. If a solid figure is now formed by connecting the vertices to two arbitrary points above and below the plane on the axis of symmetry, a figure of D_{nh} symmetry is obtained if the points are equidistant; otherwise C_{nv} symmetry results. As n increases the number of representations increases but their dimensions never exceed two. For example, C_{3v} and C_{4v} have a single two dimensional representation; C_{5v} and C_{6v} have two such representations; and C_{7v} and C_{8v} have three, etc. If the plane figure is a rectangle, the above procedure leads to D_{2h} and C_{2v} symmetry, all of whose representations are one dimensional. Any function belonging to a one dimensional representation will always be transformed into itself or its negative under any of the group operations. It is important to emphasize that if an arbitrary rotation is performed which does not bring the nuclei into coincidence, the resulting wave functions will not be eigenfunctions of the Hamiltonian for the prescribed nuclear conformation.

A further set of symmetry groups is obtained by forming regular polyhedrons from equilateral triangles. The simplest is the tetrahedron with four faces and four vertices belonging to the group T_h; each vertex is common to three faces. The figure has four three-fold rotation axes passing through the center and the four vertices. The next step is to consider figures with four faces common to a vertex; this leads to the octahedron with six vertices and eight faces belonging to the symmetry group $\mathcal{O}_h$. Like the tetrahedron it also has a set of four three-fold rotation axes. If one seeks to construct a polyhedron with five triangular faces common to a vertex, the result is the regular icosahedron of the group $\mathscr{I}_h$. This figure has 20 sides and 12 vertices. It has 10 threefold and 6 fivefold rotation axes, and contains representations with dimensions up to five.

Such regular polyhedrons with more than five sides common to a vertex are not possible, since six equilateral triangles with a common vertex must lie in a plane and the figure could not be closed. There is then an upper limit to the number of regular polyhedrons which are geometrically possible. Contrary to expectation one cannot approach the symmetry of the sphere through a series of polyhedrons with progressively higher symmetry.

If regular polygons of more than three sides are considered, it follows that any closed figure must have at least three faces common to a vertex. The square may have only three, since four squares common to a vertex are coplanar; the resulting polyhedron is, of course, the cube, which also has $\mathscr{O}_h$ symmetry. It is possible for three regular pentagons to be common to a vertex but not coplanar, since $3 \times 108° = 324° < 360°$. The resulting figure is the regular dodecahedron with 12 faces and 20 vertices; this is to be compared with the icosahedron with 20 faces and 12 vertices. Both these figures have 10 threefold and 6 fivefold rotation axes and belong to the $\mathscr{I}_h$ symmetry group. It is not possible to construct a regular polyhedron with hexagonal faces, because three regular hexagons with a common vertex are coplanar.

This exhausts the search for regular polyhedrons and confines the list to five geometrical shapes: the tetrahedron (T_h), octahedron ($\mathscr{O}_h$), cube ($\mathscr{O}_h$), dodecahedron ($\mathscr{I}_h$), and icosahedron ($\mathscr{I}_h$) (Figure 3.1). In certain mystical philosophies these figures are given a special significance, such as Plato's association of them with the fundamental elements, earth, air, fire, water, and ether. The icosahedron is not just a geometrical curiosity for chemists; for it is known that certain virus molecules are arranged in icosahedral patterns in an attempt to attain spherical symmetry.

Beginning with the space groups C_{nv}, D_{nh}, T_h, $\mathscr{O}_h$, and $\mathscr{I}_h$, it is possible to derive subgroups of lower symmetry by excluding all improper rotations; this leads to the optically active groups C_n, D_n, T, $\mathscr{O}$, and $\mathscr{I}$, whose symmetry operations consist exclusively of the rotation elements in the parent group without the reflections. The geometrical prototypes may be obtained by placing an irregular protrusion anywhere on one of the faces of the original figure except on a plane or axis of symmetry. Additional identical protrusions at the positions attained by the first under all combinations of the original group's proper rotations will lead to the desired lower symmetry. The procedure is straightforward for the groups C_n and D_n, but is somewhat harder to visualize for the T, $\mathscr{O}$, and $\mathscr{I}$ groups; no optically active molecules with T, $\mathscr{O}$, or $\mathscr{I}$ symmetry have ever been studied.

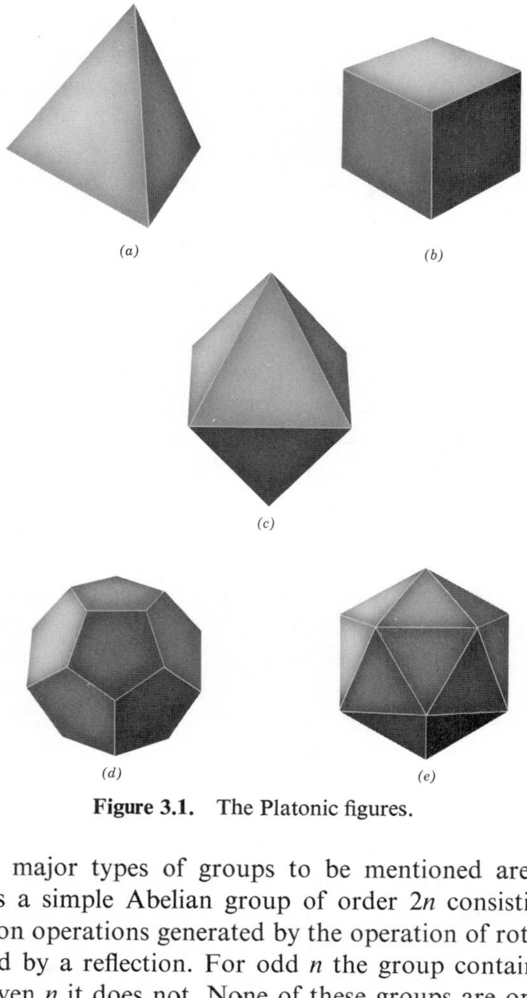

Figure 3.1. The Platonic figures.

The last two major types of groups to be mentioned are the S_{2n} and C_{nh}. The first is a simple Abelian group of order $2n$ consisting of $2n$-fold rotation-reflection operations generated by the operation of rotation through $360°/2n$ followed by a reflection. For odd n the group contains a center of inversion; for even n it does not. None of these groups are optically active. The groups S_3, S_5, etc., do not exist because an even number of successive reflections are required to return the figure to its original configuration. The C_{nh} groups consist of the rotation operations of the C_n groups along with the additional improper rotations accompanying a plane of symmetry. They may also be formed from the D_{nh} groups by placing an element in the horizontal plane of symmetry away from any of the dihedral reflection planes and generating $n - 1$ identically oriented elements by the rotations about the n-fold axis; Hero's boiler is an example of C_{4h} symmetry.

At a large distance an object may appear to have a high degree of symmetry, but as one approaches, certain imperfections and appendages appear which more often than not render the structure devoid of any symmetry; yet the greatest single impression made by the object is its approximate symmetry. The same is true of molecules where the properties of a transition are not so much governed by the exact symmetry of the molecule as by the local symmetry of the group itself.

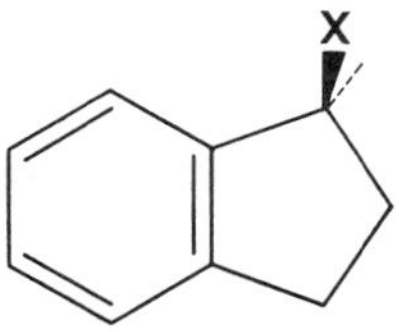

I

Associated with most transitions will be two or sometimes three levels of symmetry, the overall molecular symmetry, the group or chromophore symmetry, and often the symmetry of the distorted chromophore, which may not be identical with the molecular symmetry. For example, the indan derivative (I) is asymmetric (C_1); the undistorted π-electron system has D_{6h} symmetry; and the distorted chromophore system of the unsubstituted indan has C_{2v} symmetry. The spectra of benzene, indan, and the substituted compounds (I) are qualitatively similar. A great enhancement of the forbidden B_{1u} and B_{2u} transitions in benzene is found for indan, which has been attributed to the destruction of D_{6h} symmetry by hyperconjugation. In benzene these transitions become allowed by departures from the fixed nuclei approximation. For the time being the discussion will be confined to those aspects of optical activity governed by the fixed nuclei approximation; although it is unquestionably true that circular dichroism curves often display a rich vibronic secondary structure with even sign changes. It will be best to postpone the theory of these effects until more has been said about the simpler and better known mechanisms.

If an efficient direct method of approximating the exact solutions to molecular wave functions were available, effective symmetry of the chromophore would take care of itself; this would also be true for a complete self-consistent field calculation. Most theories of optical activity can be reduced to perturbative techniques, where a judicious choice of zeroth order wave functions is crucial. Once the appropriate symmetry of a group has been determined, transitions will fall into the following categories:

1. (*a*) Electric allowed—magnetic forbidden.
   (*b*) Magnetic allowed—electric forbidden.
   Groups
   C_i, C_{nh}, D_{nh}, D_{nd} $(n \neq 2)$, S_{2n} (n odd), $\mathcal{O}_h$, T_d, $\mathcal{I}_h$.

2. Electric and magnetic allowed, but perpendicular.
   Groups
   C_s, C_{nv}, D_{2d}, S_{2n} (n even).
3. Electric and magnetic allowed, parallel.
   Groups
   C_n, D_n, T, $\mathcal{O}$, $\mathcal{I}$.

To date the great majority of optical activity theory has centered around the first class, in which zeroth order functions describing allowed transitions of either an electric or magnetic character are used. Two methods may be used to obtain the desired dissymmetric functions of the third group: perturbation theory and molecular orbital theory. We shall next occupy ourselves with a discussion of three simple models based on these approaches; the details of the general theory of optically active molecules will be presented in Chapter 4.

3.2. The Harmonic Oscillator

The simplest model for the perturbation technique is the harmonic oscillator with potential

$$V_0 = \tfrac{1}{2}(k_1 x_1^2 + k_2 x_2^2 + k_3 x_3^2). \tag{3.2.1}$$

A rotation of the coordinate system about a given axis converts this into the general bilinear form

$$V_0 = k_{11}x_1'^2 + k_{22}x_2'^2 + k_{33}x_3'^2 + k_{12}x_1'x_2' + k_{13}x_1'x_3' + k_{23}x_2'x_3'. \tag{3.2.2}$$

Conversely any such form as (3.2.2) can be brought into the diagonal form (3.2.1) by rotation about a suitably chosen axis. It happens that all quadratic potentials can be expressed in the form of (3.2.1); a potential field with this form has D_{2h} symmetry consisting of three mutually perpendicular reflection planes, a center of inversion, and three perpendicular twofold rotation axes (Figure 3.2).

The product $x_1x_2x_3$ is the only cubic term which changes sign on inversion and all reflections; its addition to (3.2.1) produces a dissymmetric field

$$V = V_0 + V' = \tfrac{1}{2}(k_1 x_1^2 + k_2 x_2^2 + k_3 x_3^2) + Ax_1x_2x_3. \tag{3.2.3}$$

This field actually has D_2 symmetry, since it is unchanged by reversing the sign of any pair of coordinates as a result of a 180° rotation about one of the axes.

The unperturbed wave functions are

$$\psi(n_1, n_2, n_3) = \phi_{n1}(X_1)\phi_{n2}(X_2)\phi_{n3}(X_3), \tag{3.2.4}$$

where

$$\phi_n(X_i) = (2^n n! \sqrt{\pi})^{-1/2} H_n(X_i) e^{-X_i^2/2},$$

$$H_n(X_i) = \frac{1}{2^n n!} e^{X_i^2} \frac{d^n}{dX_i^n} e^{-X_i^2},$$

$$X_i = x_i / a_i,$$

$$a_i = \frac{1}{2\pi} \sqrt{\frac{h}{m\nu_i}}.$$

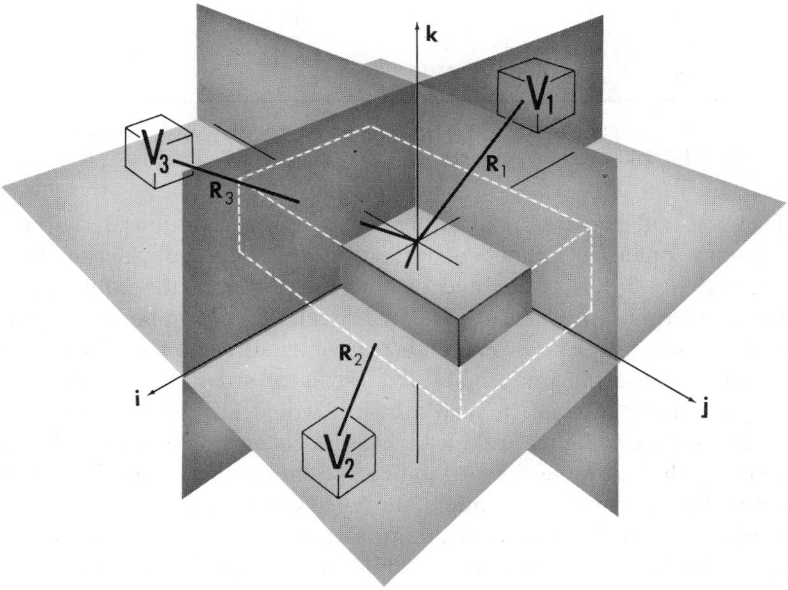

Figure 3.2. D_{2h} symmetry.

There are three different frequencies of oscillation along the mutually perpendicular axes of symmetry ν_1, ν_2, ν_3. If one considers the general excited state with the $n_i \geqslant 1$, there will be a total of 18 allowed transitions of the electric or magnetic type, 9 absorptions and 9 emissions. These are summarized in Table 3.1. It will be assumed that $\nu_1 > \nu_2 > \nu_3$. Only the 9 absorption transitions are listed; the emission transitions are obtained by reversing the appropriate signs. For example, a strong magnetic emission transition along the *i*-axis would be to the state $(n_1, n_2 - 1, n_3 + 1)$ with the frequency $|\nu_3 - \nu_2|$.

TABLE 3.1

Absorption Transitions

Designation	Type[a]	Frequency	Polarization[b]
(n_1+1, n_2, n_3)	E	ν_1	**i**
(n_1, n_2+1, n_3)	E	ν_2	**j**
(n_1, n_2, n_3+1)	E	ν_3	**k**
(n_1, n_2+1, n_3-1)	SM	$\nu_2-\nu_3$	**i**
(n_1+1, n_2, n_3-1)	SM	$\nu_1-\nu_3$	**j**
(n_1+1, n_2-1, n_3)	SM	$\nu_1-\nu_2$	**k**
(n_1, n_2+1, n_3+1)	WM	$\nu_2+\nu_3$	**i**
(n_1+1, n_2, n_3+1)	WM	$\nu_1+\nu_3$	**j**
(n_1+1, n_2+1, n_3)	WM	$\nu_1+\nu_2$	**k**

[a] E = strong electric; SM = strong magnetic; WM = weak magnetic.
[b] **i, j, k** are vectors along the x_1, x_2, x_3 directions.

The role of emission transitions requires special consideration. The elementary quantum theory of radiation makes no distinction between the probability of absorption and of emission so far as the influence of the radiation field is concerned. An isolated oscillator with none of its quantum numbers equal to zero will make no net contribution to the absorption coefficients, because the frequencies and oscillator strengths are identical for absorption and emission. In such a case it would happen that one form of circularly polarized light would lead to a net absorption and the other to an emission with the average absorption coefficient equal to zero. This situation is not realistic because of the interaction of systems with each other and with the radiation field. The simple assumption of complete Boltzmann equilibrium leads to the Einstein transition probabilities for spontaneous emission.

It is best to avoid the emission question altogether by concentrating on ground states. For a one electron oscillator this eliminates the strong magnetic transitions and greatly reduces the instructional value of the model. The alternative is to consider the excited state in a system of noninteracting electrons with all lower states occupied. The simplest situation which illustrates the equivalent role of electric and magnetic dipole transitions is a ground state represented by the function,

$$\psi_0 = (000)^2(001)^2, \tag{3.2.5}$$

where the superscript has the usual role of designating the number of electrons in the orbital.

We will next develop an abbreviated form of one electron perturbation theory. The familiar expressions for perturbed wave functions are

$$\psi'_0 = \psi_0 - \sum_t \frac{V_{t0}\psi_t}{E_t - E_0} \tag{3.2.6a}$$

$$\psi'_n = \psi_n - \sum_s \frac{V_{sn}\psi_s}{E_s - E_n}. \tag{3.2.6b}$$

To first order the electric dipole moment is

$$\boldsymbol{\mu}'_{0n} = \langle\psi'_0|\,\boldsymbol{\mu}\,|\psi'_n\rangle = \boldsymbol{\mu}_{0n} - \frac{V_{0n}}{h\nu_{0n}}(\boldsymbol{\mu}_{nn} - \boldsymbol{\mu}_{00})$$

$$- \sum_{s\neq 0,n} \frac{V_{sn}\boldsymbol{\mu}_{0s}}{E_s - E_n} - \sum_{t\neq 0,n} \frac{V_{0t}\boldsymbol{\mu}_{tn}}{E_t - E_0} \tag{3.2.7a}$$

$$\mathbf{m}'_{n0} = \langle\psi'_n|\,\mathbf{m}\,|\psi'_0\rangle = \mathbf{m}_{n0} - \frac{V_{n0}}{h\nu_{0n}}(\mathbf{m}_{nn} - \mathbf{m}_{00})$$

$$- \sum_{s\neq 0,n} \frac{V_{ns}\,\mathbf{m}_{s0}}{E_s - E_n} - \sum_{t\neq 0,n} \frac{V_{t0}\,\mathbf{m}_{nt}}{E_t - E_0}. \tag{3.2.7b}$$

The mixing of ground and excited state functions has been explicitly displayed. To first order the rotational strength becomes

$$\boldsymbol{\mu}'_{0n}\cdot\mathbf{m}'_{n0} = \boldsymbol{\mu}_{0n}\cdot\mathbf{m}_{n0} - \frac{V_{0n}}{h\nu_{0n}}(\boldsymbol{\mu}_{nn} - \boldsymbol{\mu}_{00})\cdot\mathbf{m}_{n0}$$

$$- \sum_{s\neq 0,n} \frac{V_{sn}}{E_s - E_n}(\boldsymbol{\mu}_{0s}\cdot\mathbf{m}_{n0} + \boldsymbol{\mu}_{0n}\cdot\mathbf{m}_{s0})$$

$$- \sum_{t\neq 0,n} \frac{V_{t0}}{E_t - E_0}(\boldsymbol{\mu}_{tn}\cdot\mathbf{m}_{n0} + \boldsymbol{\mu}_{0n}\cdot\mathbf{m}_{nt}). \tag{3.2.8}$$

Real wave functions have been assumed with no degeneracy; the term in the permanent magnetic moments has been dropped. For the unperturbed chromophore $\boldsymbol{\mu}_{0n}\cdot\mathbf{m}_{n0}$ is zero; the second term is often called a charge transfer term, which is zero for groups with D_{nh} symmetry. The third and fourth terms arise from the perturbation of the excited and ground states, respectively.

Consider the general case of a many electron system. The states (000), (001), (010), etc., will be filled with a maximum of two electrons in the order of increasing energy. Even when the relative magnitudes of ν_1, ν_2, ν_3 are specified, a separate ordering of the frequencies $\nu_1 - \nu_2$, $\nu_2 - \nu_3$, $\nu_1 - \nu_2$ must also be specified. An exhaustive treatment of all possibilities would be quite tedious and misleading, since the only purpose of the model is to indicate overall trends in chromophores of D_{2h} symmetry.

Of particular interest will be magnetic dipole transitions. Without loss of generality it may be assumed that the x_3-axis is the direction of polarization. Let the transition be represented by $(n_1 n_2 n_3) \rightarrow (n_1 + 1, n_2 - 1, n_3)$; this tacitly assumes that $\nu_1 > \nu_2$. It will next be necessary to consider all those parallel electric transitions which involve either one of these orbitals. The others will make no contribution, because V, $\boldsymbol{\mu}$, and $\mathbf{m}$ are one electron operators and matrix elements vanish unless the two functions differ in no more than one orbital.

The electric and magnetic moments between individual orbitals can be found from the recursion relation

$$X_i \phi_{n_i} = (n_i + \tfrac{1}{2})^{1/2} \phi_{n_i+1} + (n_i/2)^{1/2} \phi_{n_i-1} \tag{3.2.9}$$

and the familiar quantum relations

$$m_1 = \frac{e}{2mc}(x_2 p_3 - x_3 p_2), \text{ etc.} \tag{3.2.10a}$$

$$\langle n_i' | p_i | n_i \rangle = 2\pi i m a_i (n_i' - n_i) \nu_i \langle n_i' | X_i | n_i \rangle. \tag{3.2.10b}$$

The results are

$$\langle n_1 n_2 n_3 | \mu_1 | n_1 \pm 1, n_2 n_3 \rangle = e a_1 \langle n_1 n_2 n_3 | X_1 | n_1 \pm 1, n_2 n_3 \rangle = e a_1 \left(\frac{\bar{n}_1}{2} \right)^{1/2} \tag{3.2.11a}$$

$$\langle n_1, n_2 \pm 1, n_3 \pm 1 | m_1 | n_1 n_2 n_3 \rangle = i \left(\frac{e\hbar}{2mc} \right) \frac{a_2 a_3}{2} \left(\pm \frac{1}{a_3^2} \pm \frac{1}{a_2^2} \right) (\bar{n}_2 \bar{n}_3)^{1/2}, \tag{3.2.11b}$$

where $\bar{n}_i$ is the larger of n_i and $n_i + 1$ or $n_i - 1$, and the relation $\nu_i = h/[m(2\pi a_i)^2]$ has been used. The moments along the x_2 and x_3 directions are obtained by cyclic permutation.

It will be observed that there are 6 electric dipole and 12 magnetic dipole transitions:

Electric

$$(n_1 n_2 n_3) \rightarrow (n_1 \pm 1, n_2, n_3)$$
$$(n_1 n_2 n_3) \rightarrow (n_1, n_2 \pm 1, n_3)$$
$$(n_1 n_2 n_3) \rightarrow (n_1, n_2, n_3 \pm 1)$$

Magnetic

$$(n_1 n_2 n_3) \rightarrow (n_1, n_2 \pm 1, n_3 \pm 1)$$
$$(n_1 n_2 n_3) \rightarrow (n_1 \pm 1, n_2, n_3 \pm 1)$$
$$(n_1 n_2 n_3) \rightarrow (n_1 \pm 1, n_2 \pm 1, n_3).$$

The moments of the weak magnetic transitions will be proportional to $(1/a_i^2 - 1/a_j^2)$; these may be neglected in the perturbation treatment.

$$(n_1 + 1, n_2 - 1, n_3 + 1)\text{—}$$
$$(n_1, n_2, n_3, +1)\text{—}$$
$$(n_1 + 1, n_2 - 1, n_3)\text{—}$$
$$(n_1 n_2 n_3)\#$$
$$(n_1 + 1, n_2 - 1, n_3 - 1)\#$$
$$(n_1, n_2, n_3 - 1)\#$$

II

One will in the course of considering the transition $(n_1 n_2 n_3) \rightarrow (n_1 + 1, n_2 - 1, n_3)$ require a knowledge of all electric dipole transitions along the x_3-axis between both these states. The four required states will be $(n_1 n_2 n_3 \pm 1)$ and $(n_1 + 1, n_2 - 1, n_3 \pm 1)$. The rotational strength will depend on the relative order of these six states. It has already been assumed that $\nu_1 > \nu_2$ in order to insure that $(n_1 n_2 n_3)$ is lower in energy than $(n_1 + 1, n_2 - 1, n_3)$. To insure that the transition is low lying one will assume that $\nu_1 - \nu_2$ is lower than ν_1, ν_2, and ν_3. In the course of the development it will become evident that the result is unaffected by the relative magnitude of ν_3 so long as $\nu_3 > \nu_1 - \nu_2$. The order of energies is shown in II, where all orbitals below $(n_1 n_2 n_3)$ are occupied.

The appropriate electric transitions which originate from the ground state are $(n_1 n_2 n_3) \rightarrow (n_1, n_2, n_3 + 1)$ $(n_1 + 1, n_2 - 1, n_3 - 1) \rightarrow (n_1 + 1, n_2 - 1, n_3)$; only one transition is connected with the excited state $(n_1 + 1, n_2 - 1, n_3) \rightarrow (n_1 + 1, n_2 - 1, n_3 + 1)$. The $(n_1 n_2 n_3 - 1) \rightarrow (n_1 n_2 n_3)$ is not included because both these orbitals are filled. The appropriate states will be given by

$$\psi_0 = |\cdots (n_1 n_2 n_3)\overline{(n_1 n_2 n_3)} \cdots| \tag{3.2.12a}$$

$$\psi_n = |\cdots (n_1 n_2 n_3)\overline{(n_1 + 1, n_2 - 1, n_3)} \cdots| \tag{3.2.12b}$$

$$\psi_A = |\cdots (n_1 n_2 n_3)\overline{(n_1 n_2 n_3 + 1)} \cdots| \tag{3.2.12c}$$

$$\psi_B = |\cdots (n_1 + 1, n_2 - 1, n_3 - 1)\overline{(n_1 + 1, n_2 - 1, n_3)} \cdots| \tag{3.2.12d}$$

$$\psi_C = |\cdots (n_1 n_2 n_3)\overline{(n_1 + 1, n_2 - 1, n_3 + 1)} \cdots|, \tag{3.2.12e}$$

where the bar indicates antiparallel spin and only singly excited states are considered as indicated. The normalization has been omitted; in the course of evaluating matrix elements of such determinental functions for one electron operators one may proceed as though there were only a single term, since $N!$ identical terms are obtained.

Equation 3.2.8 gives

$$R_{0n} = \mathrm{Im}\, \boldsymbol{\mu}'_{0n} \cdot \mathbf{m}'_{n0} = -\mathrm{Im}\left[\left(\frac{\boldsymbol{\mu}_{0A} V_{An}}{E_A - E_n} + \frac{\boldsymbol{\mu}_{0B} V_{Bn}}{E_B - E_n} + \frac{\boldsymbol{\mu}_{Cn} V_{0C}}{E_C - E_0}\right) \cdot \mathbf{m}_{n0}\right]. \tag{3.2.13}$$

From (3.2.11) and (3.2.12) one obtains

$$\mathbf{m}_{n0} = -i\,\frac{a_1 a_2}{2}\left(\frac{1}{a_1^2} + \frac{1}{a_2^2}\right)\sqrt{(n_1+1)n_2}\left(\frac{e\hbar}{2mc}\right) \tag{3.2.14a}$$

$$\boldsymbol{\mu}_{0A} = e a_3 \left(\frac{n_3+1}{2}\right)^{1/2} \tag{3.2.14b}$$

$$\boldsymbol{\mu}_{0B} = e a_3 \left(\frac{n_3}{2}\right)^{1/2} \tag{3.2.14c}$$

$$\boldsymbol{\mu}_{Cn} = e a_3 \left(\frac{n_3+1}{2}\right)^{1/2} \tag{3.2.14d}$$

$$(xyz)_{An} = a_1 a_2 a_3 \left[\frac{(n_1+1)n_2(n_3+1)}{8}\right]^{1/2} \tag{3.2.14e}$$

$$(xyz)_{Bn} = a_1 a_2 a_3 \left[\frac{(n_1+1)n_2 n_3}{8}\right]^{1/2} \tag{3.2.14f}$$

$$(xyz)_{0C} = a_1 a_2 a_3 \left[\frac{(n_1+1)n_2(n_3+1)}{8}\right]^{1/2} \tag{3.2.14g}$$

$$E_A - E_n = h[\nu_3 - (\nu_1 - \nu_2)] \tag{3.2.14h}$$

$$E_B - E_n = h[\nu_3 - (\nu_1 - \nu_2)] \tag{3.2.14i}$$

$$E_C - E_0 = h[\nu_3 + (\nu_1 - \nu_2)]. \tag{3.2.14j}$$

The final result for the rotational strength is

$$R_{0n} = \frac{A}{8h}\left(\frac{e^2 h}{2mc}\right)(a_1 a_2 a_3)^2\left(\frac{1}{a_1^2} + \frac{1}{a_2^2}\right)(n_1+1)n_2 \left[\frac{2n_3+1}{\nu_3 - (\nu_1 - \nu_2)} + \frac{n_3+1}{\nu_3 + (\nu_1 - \nu_2)}\right]. \tag{3.2.15}$$

Since $\nu_3 > (\nu_1 - \nu_2)$, the sign of rotation is the same as that of A. The many electron oscillator affords numerous other examples, some in which the sign depends on the relative magnitudes of the n_i. It now remains to investigate the relation of the constant A to the physical situation.

If the dissymmetric potential arises from a point charge Q, the constant A may be evaluated explicitly. Let the coordinates of Q be X, Y, Z and those of the electron x, y, z. The perturbing potential is

$$V = \frac{-Qe^2}{\sqrt{(x-X)^2+(y-Y)^2+(z-Z)^2}}. \tag{3.2.16}$$

The xyz term is found from the Taylor expansion to be

$$\frac{1}{3!}\left(\frac{\partial^3 V}{\partial x \partial y \partial z}\right)_{000} xyz = -\frac{15}{6}\frac{XYZ}{R^7} xyzQe^2. \tag{3.2.17}$$

Equation 3.2.15 may therefore be written in the form

$$R_{0n} = -KQ\gamma_x \gamma_y \gamma_z, \tag{3.2.18}$$

where $\gamma_x = X/R$, etc., are the direction cosines of the charge.

This leads to an octant rule in which the eight regions formed by the three symmetry planes of the chromophore alternate in sign. This is an example of the general rule that the planes of symmetry of a chromophore divide it into regions of alternating sign. The choice of axis is made by requiring that the x_3- or z-axis be along the direction of polarization. The y-axis must be along the direction which loses charge and the x-axis along the direction which gains it. For example, a $2p \to 2p'$ transition is represented by (010) → (100). The situation is shown in Figure 3.3.

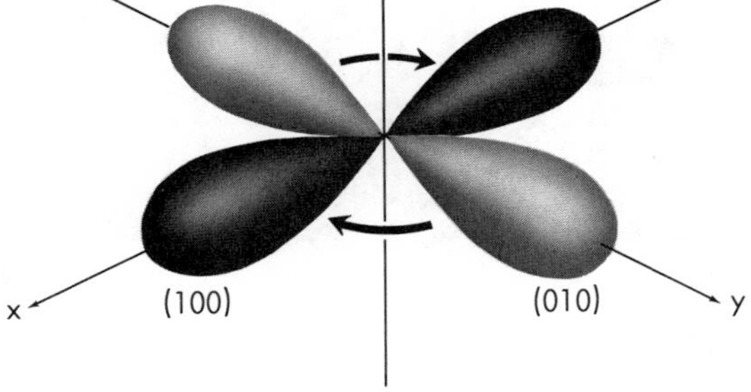

Figure 3.3. $2p \to 2p'$ transition.

There are several choices of axes, but they all lead to the same conclusion: If the observer stations himself at the position of the charge and rotates the half of the y-axis (original polarization direction) nearest him into the nearest half of the x-axis (final direction), the rotational strength is positive for a positive charge if this motion is counterclockwise. This is reminiscent of the classical model in Chapter 1.

If an infinitesimal perturbation is placed along the z-axis, the effective symmetry of the chromophore is still unchanged and this octant rule holds; but if the perturbation is made large enough, the symmetry will effectively become C_{2v}. The xy-plane is not even an approximate plane of symmetry; instead of an octant rule one obtains a quadrant rule. When the D_{2h} model is applied to the carbonyl chromophore, which has C_{2v} symmetry, qualitative agreement with experiment is obtained for substituents in the so-called front octants on the carbon side; but when compounds with substituents in the back octants were investigated, opposite signs to those predicted were found, indicating a quadrant rule.

3.3. The Coupled Oscillator

The second important mechanism to be investigated is the coupled oscillator, or electron correlation model. This will be presented here in its simplest form with the more general treatment being reserved for Chapter 4. We will consider two groups A and B, with attention initially focused on two electric transitions: $0 \rightarrow a$ in group A with transition moment $\boldsymbol{\mu}_{0a}$, and $0 \rightarrow b$ in group B with transition moment $\boldsymbol{\mu}_{0b}$. Each group will be assumed to contain one electron; the pertinent distances are shown in Figure 3.4. The

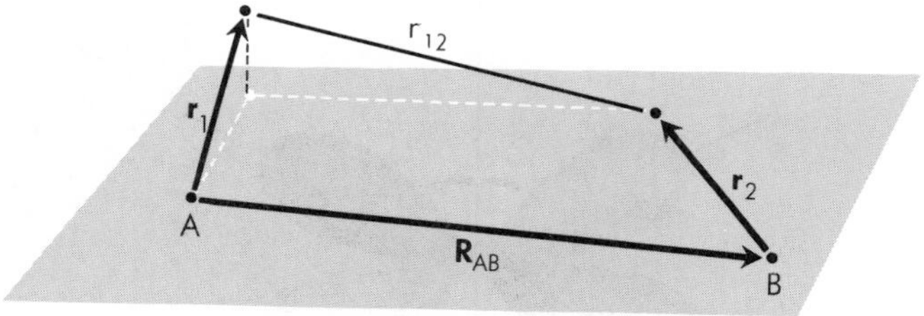

Figure 3.4. Distance vectors for the coupled oscillator.

two electrons will be considered to be under the influence of individual force fields $V_A(\mathbf{r}_1)$ and $V_B(\mathbf{r}_2)$, which confine them to their respective groups along with the repulsive interaction potential e^2/r_{12}; exchange phenomena are neglected and the groups are far enough apart to be considered in the Van der Waals region. The total potential energy will be written

$$V_T = V_0 + V = e[V_A(\mathbf{r}_1) + V_B(\mathbf{r}_2)] + e\left[V_A(\mathbf{r}_2) + V_B(\mathbf{r}_1) + \frac{e}{r_{12}}\right]. \quad (3.3.1)$$

The V_A and V_B terms depend only on individual electronic coordinates and not their products. The last term may be expanded

$$\frac{1}{r_{12}} = \frac{1}{R_{AB}}\left[1 + \left(\frac{\mathbf{r}_1^2 + \mathbf{r}_2^2 - 2\mathbf{r}_1 \cdot \mathbf{R}_{AB} + 2\mathbf{r}_2 \cdot \mathbf{R}_{AB} - 2\mathbf{r}_1 \cdot \mathbf{r}_2}{R_{AB}^2}\right)\right]$$

$$= \cdots + \frac{1}{R_{AB}^3}\left[\mathbf{r}_1 \cdot \mathbf{r}_2 - \frac{3(\mathbf{r}_1 \cdot \mathbf{R}_{AB})(\mathbf{r}_2 \cdot \mathbf{R}_{AB})}{R_{AB}^2}\right] + \cdots. \quad (3.3.2)$$

The relation $r_{12}^2 = (\mathbf{r}_2 + \mathbf{R}_{AB} - \mathbf{r}_1)^2$, derived with the aid of the figure, has been used, and only the lowest order quadratic terms in the products of the electronic coordinates have been retained.

As in the theory of Van der Waals forces, the zeroth order functions may be written

$$\begin{aligned} \psi_{00} &= \phi_0^{(A)}\phi_0^{(B)} \quad (a) \qquad & \psi_{a0} &= \phi_a^{(A)}\phi_0^{(B)} \quad (b) \\ \psi_{0b} &= \phi_0^{(A)}\phi_b^{(B)} \quad (c) \qquad & \psi_{ab} &= \phi_a^{(A)}\phi_b^{(B)}. \quad (d) \end{aligned} \quad (3.3.3)$$

In the perturbation theory treatment of the oscillator in the previous section the electric and magnetic moments were referred to a common origin, since all the electrons were localized to the same region. Here we have made the nonexchange approximation of localizing the electrons to the separate groups A and B. One can justify neither A nor B as the center of the system, and accordingly an arbitrary center will be chosen in which the centers of the two groups will have position vectors $\mathbf{R}_A$ and $\mathbf{R}_B$. These centers will be chosen so that the transitions $0 \to a$ and $0 \to b$ will have a purely electric dipole character and $\mathbf{m}_{b0}$, $\mathbf{m}_{a0}$ vanish. This may always be done for groups which are not themselves optically active. For inactive groups with low symmetry the choice of center will vary from one transition to another and an average position vector will be assumed.

Relative to the arbitrary origin the electric and magnetic moment operators are

$$\boldsymbol{\mu} = e(\mathbf{R}_A + \mathbf{R}_B) + \boldsymbol{\mu}_1 + \boldsymbol{\mu}_2 \quad (3.3.4a)$$

$$\mathbf{m} = \frac{e}{2mc}[(\mathbf{R}_A + \mathbf{r}_1) \times \mathbf{p}_1 + (\mathbf{R}_B + \mathbf{r}_2) \times \mathbf{p}_2]$$

$$= \frac{e}{2mc}\mathbf{R}_A \times \mathbf{p}_1 + \frac{e}{2mc}\mathbf{R}_B \times \mathbf{p}_2 + \mathbf{m}_1 + \mathbf{m}_2. \quad (3.3.4b)$$

The quantities $\boldsymbol{\mu}_1, \boldsymbol{\mu}_2, \mathbf{m}_1$, and $\mathbf{m}_2$ are local operators referred to the centers of the respective groups, and $\mathbf{p}_1, \mathbf{p}_2$ are momentum operators.

The rotational strength for the $0 \rightarrow a$ transition is given by

$$R_{0a} = \mathrm{Im}[\langle \psi'_{00} | \boldsymbol{\mu} | \psi'_{a0} \rangle \cdot \langle \psi'_{a0} | \mathbf{m} | \psi'_{00} \rangle]. \tag{3.3.5}$$

The zeroth order terms vanish, since $(\mathbf{p}_1)_{a0}$ and $(\boldsymbol{\mu}_1)_{0a}$ are collinear and $(\boldsymbol{\mu}_1)_{0a} \cdot (\mathbf{m}_1)_{a0} = 0$ for an inactive group. A preliminary perturbation expansion involving only the states a and b can be made. The contributions from the other states in group B can be determined by summing over b. The required expansions are

$$\psi'_{00} = \psi_{00} - \frac{V_{0a;\,0b}}{h(\nu_a + \nu_b)} \psi_{ab} \tag{3.3.6a}$$

$$\psi'_{a0} = \psi_{a0} - \frac{V_{0a;\,0b}}{h(\nu_b - \nu_a)} \psi_{0b}, \tag{3.3.6b}$$

where

$$V_{0a;\,0b} = \iint \phi_0^{(A)} \phi_a^{(A)} V \phi_0^{(B)} \phi_b^{(B)} \, d\tau_1 \, d\tau_2 .$$

The object of this investigation has been the derivation of the lowest order expression depending on products of individual group operators. From the initial discussion it follows that a potential proportional to terms like $x_1 x_2$ satisfies this requirement. The only nonvanishing terms are provided by the above expansion. With the appropriate substitutions and the familiar relation $\mathbf{p}_{0a} = (-2\pi i m/e)\nu_a \boldsymbol{\mu}_{0a}$, (3.3.5) becomes

$$\begin{aligned} R_{0a}^{(b)} &= \frac{2\pi}{ch} V_{0a;\,0b} \frac{\nu_a \nu_b}{\nu_a^2 - \nu_b^2} \boldsymbol{\mu}_{0a} \cdot \mathbf{R}_{AB} \times \boldsymbol{\mu}_{0b} \\ &= \frac{2\pi}{ch} \frac{\nu_a \nu_b}{\nu_a^2 - \nu_b^2} \boldsymbol{\mu}_{0a} \times \mathbf{R}_{AB} \cdot \boldsymbol{\mu}_{0b} \boldsymbol{\mu}_{0b} \cdot \mathbf{T} \cdot \boldsymbol{\mu}_{0a}, \end{aligned} \tag{3.3.7}$$

where

$$\mathbf{T} = \frac{1}{R_{AB}^3} \left(\mathbf{T} - \frac{3\mathbf{R}_{AB}\mathbf{R}_{AB}}{R_{AB}^2} \right).$$

The summation over b may be arranged in the suggestive form

$$\begin{aligned} R_{0a} = \sum_b R_{0a}^{(b)} &= \frac{\pi}{c} \nu_a \mathbf{R}_{AB} \times \boldsymbol{\mu}_{0a} \cdot \left(\frac{2}{h} \sum_b \frac{\nu_b \boldsymbol{\mu}_{0b} \boldsymbol{\mu}_{0b}}{\nu_b^2 - \nu_a^2} \right) \cdot \mathbf{T} \cdot \boldsymbol{\mu}_{0a} \\ &= \frac{\pi}{c} [\mathbf{R}_{AB} \times \mathbf{b}_{0a} \cdot \boldsymbol{\alpha}_B(\nu_a) \cdot \mathbf{I} \cdot \mathbf{b}_{0a}] \nu_a \mu_{0a}^2, \end{aligned} \tag{3.3.8}$$

where $\alpha_B(\nu_a)$ is the polarizability tensor of group B at the frequency ν_a and $\mathbf{b}_{0a}$ is a unit vector along the direction of the transition. This predicts that when conditions allow the optical activity of a transition to be governed solely by its coupling with other transitions the rotational strength will be proportional to the oscillator strength. The factor in brackets depends only on molecular geometry and the polarizability of the neighboring group.

Since current optical activity theory is devoted to absorbing regions, it will not be useful to sum the contributions to the rotatory parameter over all bands to obtain an expression good only outside these bands. Instead it will be fruitful to discuss the applicability of the above result to circular dichroism. A further simplification takes place if group B is assumed to have cylindrical symmetry. The polarizability tensor may be written

$$\alpha = (\alpha_3 - \alpha_1)\mathbf{bb} + \mathbf{I}\alpha_1, \tag{3.3.9}$$

where α_1 and α_3 are the parallel and perpendicular polarizabilities and $\mathbf{b}$ is the symmetry axis. The substitution of (3.3.9) into (3.3.8) gives

$$R_{0a} = \frac{\pi}{c}\,\Delta\alpha_B(\nu_a)(\mathbf{R}_{AB} \times \mathbf{b}_{0a}\cdot\mathbf{b})\mathbf{b}\cdot\mathbf{T}\cdot\mathbf{b}_{0a}\,\nu_a\boldsymbol{\mu}_{0a}^2, \tag{3.3.10}$$

where

$$\Delta\alpha_B(\nu_a) = \alpha_3(\nu_a) - \alpha_1(\nu_a).$$

This form embodies most of the characteristic features of the polarizability theory, which has been applied extensively to molecules. It will be instructive to discuss the model with the configuration shown in Figure 3.5, in which both $\mathbf{b}$ and $\mathbf{b}_{0a}$ are perpendicular to $\mathbf{R}_{AB}$. In terms of θ, the angle between $\mathbf{b}_{0a}$ and $\mathbf{b}$, $\mathbf{R}_{AB} \times \mathbf{b}_{0a}\cdot\mathbf{b} = R_{AB}\sin\theta$. This may be called the dissymmetry factor, since it is zero when the vectors are parallel and maximum when they are perpendicular. From the definition of $\mathbf{T}$ it follows that $\mathbf{b}\cdot\mathbf{T}\cdot\mathbf{b}_{0a} = (1/R_{AB}^3)\mathbf{b}\cdot\mathbf{b}_{0a} = (1/R_{AB}^3)\cos\theta$. This is the coupling factor, which is maximum for the parallel orientation and zero for the perpendicular.

Equation 3.3.10 becomes

$$R_{0a}^{\ddagger} = \frac{\pi}{2c}\,\Delta\alpha_B(\nu_a)\frac{\nu_a\boldsymbol{\mu}_{0a}^2}{R_{AB}^2}\sin 2\theta, \tag{3.3.11}$$

from which it follows that the maximum rotational strength will be obtained for $\theta = 45°$. It also follows that the right-handed screw pattern in Figure 3.4 leads to positive values in agreement with the classical model in Chapter 1. A more detailed criticism of this model will be found in Chapter 4. For actual molecules one is often well advised to use the above result as a semiempirical method of investigation.

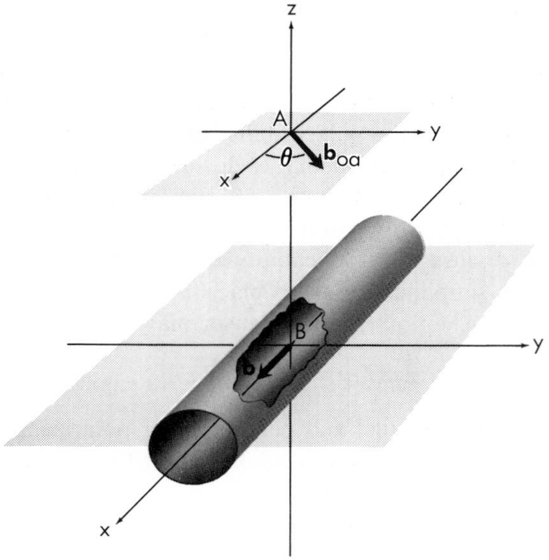

Figure 3.5. The perpendicular orientation.

3.4. Inherent Dissymmetry

A third important model is the inherently dissymmetric chromophore. In contradistinction to the previous two examples, where the dissymmetry was effected by the perturbation of one or two symmetrical systems, one will be dealing with a system in which all states are dissymmetric. Since the minimum number of points required for a dissymmetric configuration is four, the simplest model would be comprised of a single electron moving in the field of four protons.

A simplified LCAO method will be used with hydrogen 1s orbitals. If special configurations are avoided such as the nearly square planar or regular tetrahedral, the approximate linear combinations may be taken as

$$\psi_0 = \frac{1}{\sqrt{4}}(\phi_A + \phi_B + \phi_C + \phi_D) \tag{3.4.1a}$$

$$\psi_1 = \frac{1}{\sqrt{4}}(\phi_A + \phi_B - \phi_C - \phi_D) \tag{3.4.1b}$$

$$\psi_2 = \frac{1}{\sqrt{4}}(\phi_A - \phi_B - \phi_C + \phi_D) \tag{3.4.1c}$$

$$\psi_3 = \frac{1}{\sqrt{4}}(\phi_A - \phi_B + \phi_C - \phi_D). \tag{3.4.1d}$$

These functions are the solutions to the secular equation provided that $H_{AB} = H_{BC} = H_{CD} = \beta$, $H_{AA} = H_{BB} = H_{CC} = H_{DD} = \alpha$, and H_{AC}, etc., are zero. The normalization factors have all been taken to be equal. It may be verified that $H_{ij} = 0$ if $i \neq j$ and

$$\begin{aligned} H_{00} &= \alpha + \tfrac{3}{4}\beta \quad (a) \qquad & H_{11} &= \alpha + \tfrac{1}{4}\beta \quad (b) \\ H_{22} &= \alpha - \tfrac{1}{4}\beta \quad (c) \qquad & H_{33} &= \alpha - \tfrac{3}{4}\beta. \quad (d) \end{aligned} \tag{3.4.2}$$

The configuration is shown in Figure 3.6 with the center at B.

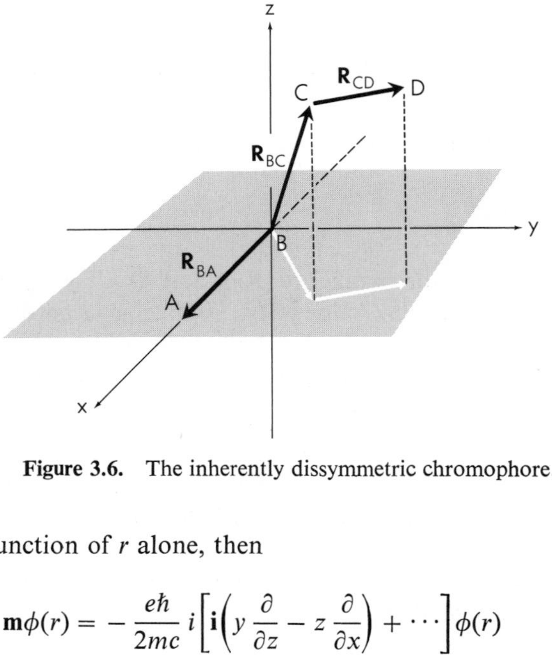

Figure 3.6. The inherently dissymmetric chromophore.

If ϕ is a function of r alone, then

$$\begin{aligned} \mathbf{m}\phi(r) &= -\frac{e\hbar}{2mc} i\left[\mathbf{i}\left(y\frac{\partial}{\partial z} - z\frac{\partial}{\partial x}\right) + \cdots\right]\phi(r) \\ &= -\frac{e\hbar}{2mc} i\left[\mathbf{i}\left(y\frac{\partial r}{\partial z} - z\frac{\partial r}{\partial x}\right) + \cdots\right]\frac{d\phi(r)}{\partial r} = 0. \end{aligned} \tag{3.4.3}$$

This means that the local magnetic moments $\langle\phi_A|\,\mathbf{m}_A\,|\phi_A\rangle$, etc., will vanish. In the calculation it will be convenient to express the $\mathbf{m}$, centered on B, in terms of the local operators at A, C, and D. With the aid of Figure 3.6 it follows that

$$\begin{aligned}\mathbf{m} &= \mathbf{m}_B \\ &= \mathbf{m}_A + \frac{e}{2mc}\mathbf{R}_{BA} \times \mathbf{p} \\ &= \mathbf{m}_C + \frac{e}{2mc}\mathbf{R}_{BC} \times \mathbf{p} \\ &= \mathbf{m}_D + \frac{e}{2mc}(\mathbf{R}_{BC} + \mathbf{R}_{CD}) \times \mathbf{p}.\end{aligned} \tag{3.4.4}$$

The local coordinate systems centered on A, C, and D will all have the same orientation as the central one on B in the computation of magnetic moments. A typical term is $\int \phi_D \mathbf{p} \phi_C \, d\tau = -i\hbar \int \phi_D \nabla \phi_C \, d\tau$. If $\phi = (1/\sqrt{\pi})a^{3/2}e^{-ar}$ one obtains

$$\begin{aligned}\int \phi_D \mathbf{p} \phi_C \, d\tau &= \frac{i\hbar}{\pi} a^4 \left[\mathbf{i}\left(\int \phi_D \frac{x_C}{r_C} \phi_C \, d\tau\right) + \mathbf{j}\left(\int \phi_D \frac{y_C}{r_C} \phi_C \, d\tau\right) + \mathbf{k}\left(\int \phi_D \frac{z_C}{r_C} \phi_C \, d\tau\right)\right] \\ &= \frac{i\hbar a^4}{\pi}(\mathbf{ii} \cdot \mathbf{b}_{CD} + \mathbf{jj} \cdot \mathbf{b}_{CD} + \mathbf{kk} \cdot \mathbf{b}_{CD})\Omega \\ &= \frac{i\hbar}{\pi} a^4 \Omega \mathbf{b}_{CD},\end{aligned} \tag{3.4.5}$$

where $\mathbf{b}_{CD}$ is a unit vector parallel to $\mathbf{R}_{CD}$ and $\Omega = \int \phi_D(z'_C/r_C)\phi_C \, d\tau$; the variable z'_C is measured from C along $\mathbf{R}_{CD}$ and Ω is accordingly positive. The final step occurs because only the components of x_C, y_C, and z_C along $\mathbf{R}_{CD}$ lead to a nonvanishing result. In a similar manner one obtains

$$\int \phi_C \mathbf{p} \phi_B \, d\tau = \frac{i\hbar}{\pi} a^4 \Omega \mathbf{b}_{BC} \tag{3.4.5a)'}$$

$$\int \phi_A \mathbf{p} \phi_B \, d\tau = \frac{i\hbar}{\pi} a^4 \Omega \mathbf{b}_{BA}. \tag{3.4.5b)'}$$

Nonadjacent matrix elements such as $\int \phi_A \mathbf{p} \phi_C \, d\tau$ will be set equal to zero. From (3.4.1) it follows that

$$\mathbf{m}_{20} = \tfrac{1}{4}(2\langle\phi_A|\, \mathbf{m}\, |\phi_B\rangle + 2\langle\phi_D|\, \mathbf{m}\, |\phi_C\rangle). \tag{3.4.6}$$

From (3.4.4), (3.4.5), and (3.4.5)′ we obtain

$$\langle\phi_A|\, \mathbf{m}\, |\phi_B\rangle = 0 \tag{3.4.7a}$$

$$\langle\phi_D|\, \mathbf{m}\, |\phi_C\rangle = \frac{ia^4}{\pi}\left(\frac{e\hbar}{2mc}\right)\Omega R \mathbf{b}_{BC} \times \mathbf{b}_{CD}, \tag{3.4.7b}$$

where R is the distance between adjacent nuclei. This leads to the result

$$\mathbf{m}_{20} = \frac{1}{2}\frac{a^4}{\pi}\frac{e\hbar}{2mc} i\Omega R \mathbf{b}_{BC} \times \mathbf{b}_{CD}.$$

The other magnetic moments are obtained in a similar manner; the summarized results are

$$\mathbf{m}_{10} = 0 \qquad (3.4.8a)$$

$$\mathbf{m}_{20} = iK\mathbf{b}_{BC} \times \mathbf{b}_{CD} \qquad (3.4.8b)$$

$$\mathbf{m}_{30} = -iK\mathbf{b}_{BC} \times \mathbf{b}_{CD}, \qquad (3.4.8c)$$

where $K = (a^4/2\pi)(e\hbar/2mc)\Omega R$.

The electric moments are obtained in a more straightforward manner; to lowest order

$$\boldsymbol{\mu}_{01} = eR(\mathbf{b}_{BA} + \mathbf{b}_{CD}) \qquad (3.4.9a)$$

$$\boldsymbol{\mu}_{02} = eR(\mathbf{b}_{BA} - 2\mathbf{b}_{BC} - \mathbf{b}_{CD}) \qquad (3.4.9b)$$

$$\boldsymbol{\mu}_{03} = eR(\mathbf{b}_{BA} - \mathbf{b}_{CD}). \qquad (3.4.9c)$$

The rotational strengths are found to be

$$R_{01} = 0 \qquad (3.4.10a)$$

$$R_{02} = eRK\mathbf{b}_{BA} \cdot \mathbf{b}_{BC} \times \mathbf{b}_{CD} \qquad (3.4.10b)$$

$$R_{03} = -eRK\mathbf{b}_{BA} \cdot \mathbf{b}_{BC} \times \mathbf{b}_{CD}. \qquad (3.4.10c)$$

In a more exact calculation R_{01} would not be exactly zero, but it would be much smaller than the other two. To this approximation the sum of the rotational strengths is zero; this often happens in calculations where the basis set is so restricted.

It is interesting to compare this result with the coupled oscillator in the previous section. In Figure 3.7 the two models are presented, both in the configuration of a right-handed screw pattern. The directions of relative motion of charge are shown for the $0 \rightarrow 2$ transition in the inherently dissymmetric chromophore. In the ground state the charge is more or less uniformly spread over all four nuclei; but in the excited state it is concentrated in the middle because ϕ_B and ϕ_C are the only adjacent wave functions with the same sign. From (3.4.10) it follows that the rotational strength for this transition is negative. In the coupled oscillator the two electrons move away from each other, leading to the opposite sign.

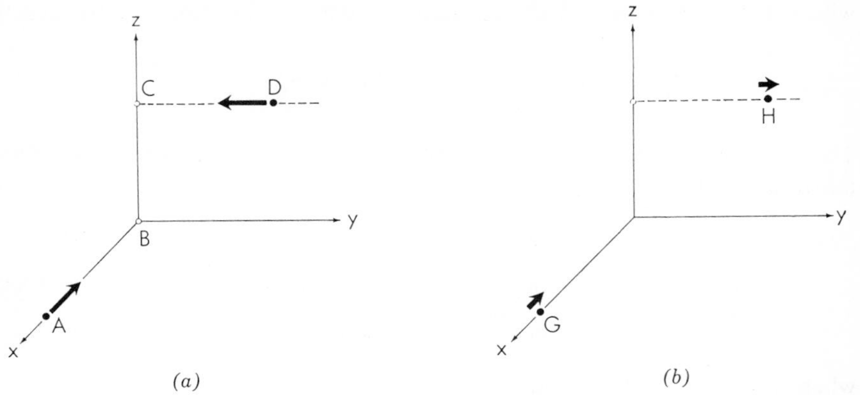

Figure 3.7. Comparison of inherently dissymmetric chromophore (*a*) and oscillator (*b*).

In this chapter we have presented in a relatively simplified form the principal mechanisms thought to be responsible for optical rotatory power. In the next chapter these themes will be explored in more detail along with general methods of investigating the properties of optically active molecules.

CHAPTER 4

The General Theory

4.1. The Nature of Approximations

Before embarking on a general theoretical investigation of optically active molecules, it is important to recognize the enormous obstacles which militate against the formulation of satisfactory quantitative methods from first principles. It must also be borne in mind that the most powerful techniques for obtaining wave functions have been focused upon the total energy criterion. Even the simplest examples of the variation method indicate the relative insensitivity of energy to the wave function. The use of a Gaussian trial function for the hydrogen atom leads to an error in the energy of no more than 15%. Such precision would be welcomed in optical activity theory. Unfortunately an error of 1% or 2% in the energy often brings the rotational strength off by an order of magnitude. Experience has shown that wave functions giving impressive agreement with experiment in the energy can give disappointing results in the determination of transition dipole moments. The plight of optical activity is even worse, where not one, but two, transition moments must be found. The difficulties in determining the origin of the 3-kcal barrier in ethane should engender a greater respect for the case of rotational strengths, which are often strongly affected by interaction energies of less than 1 kcal.

In this situation it is often prudent to speak in terms of extremes. This opportunity is furnished by the models in the previous chapter. The charge clouds of both the one electron and coupled oscillator were considered to be only slightly distorted by the presence of a distant group. A single electron was considered localized to a largely symmetric environment with perturbation theory employed to assess its degree of distortion.

The inherently dissymmetric chromophore goes to the opposite extreme of allowing a single electron the maximum amount of delocalization over the extent of several atoms. This invariably leads to considerably larger rotational strengths.

When properly formulated and thoroughly treated, both these theories tend toward the same result. When incompletely handled almost any desired result can be obtained in view of the peculiarities of convergence, as the following simple examples will demonstrate. The wave functions of multi-center one electron systems are often approximated as a sum of functions centered on the individual atoms; however, it is certainly true that the function may be obtained to any degree of approximation in terms of a complete set of functions centered on an arbitrary origin; the solutions to the hydrogen atom are an example.

In the hydrogen molecule ion the use of all linear combinations of atomic orbitals on the two protons in the variation method would finally lead to the same result as a single complete set of hydrogen functions referred to the midpoint of the internuclear axis. The main difference in the two methods is the rapidity of convergence, which is much faster for the two center calculation. To obtain a feeling for the possible errors in such calculations, consider the attempt to approximate the ground state of the hydrogen atom in terms of hydrogen functions centered on an origin at a distance R from the proton. Letting the desired ground state be ψ_{1s} and the remote set be ϕ_n, one obtains the expansion $\psi_{1s} = \sum_n c_n(R)\phi_n$, where $c_n(R) = \int \psi_{1s}\phi_n \, d\tau$. The coefficient of the ϕ_{1s} term is

$$\int \psi_{1s}\phi_{1s} \, d\tau = \frac{1}{\pi} \int e^{-r_A} e^{-r_B} \, d\tau,$$

where A and B are the two centers. This integral is the familiar overlap integral in the theory of H_2^+ whose value is $e^{-R}(1 + R + R^2/3)$ in atomic units. The first approximation to the desired expansion is then

$$\psi_{1s} = \frac{1}{\sqrt{\pi}} e^{-r_A} \sim \frac{1}{\sqrt{\pi}} e^{-r_B} e^{-R}\left(1 + R + \frac{R^2}{3}\right). \tag{4.1.1}$$

At the second origin, where $r_B = 0$, for $R = 3$ Å this approximation is more than an order of magnitude too high. The lesson to be learned here is that in an attempt to approximate many center functions it is quite easy to place undue emphasis on a particular region by taking an insufficient number of terms. In a many electron problem the situation is even more complicated.

If in the inherently dissymmetric chromophore of the preceding chapter one takes the four attractive centers to be protons, the first pair of electrons will be completely delocalized in the manner described; but when four electrons are present, the repulsions are mainly responsible for splitting the system into a pair of hydrogen molecules. If the distance is larger, the wave function will describe four separate hydrogen atoms. In the latter instance the rotational strength per electron would be much smaller than that of the original one electron system. The degree of delocalization profoundly affects the rotational strength and is in turn very strongly governed by electron repulsions. In general there is no simple way of assessing this crucial degree of delocalization; and incomplete many center calculations can often obscure the situation.

4.2. Approximate Summation Methods

An instructive procedure is to assume that the total molecular wave functions are a properly antisymmetrized set of SCF orbitals, where for each state one has obtained the best possible approximation to the true functions under the restrictions that the result be expressed as a product of single electron functions. This leads to what would be termed uncorrelated wave functions, since the probability of finding a given electron at an arbitrary point is independent of the positions of the other electrons. For a system of N electrons the functions will have the form

$$\Psi_n = \frac{S_n}{\sqrt{N!}} \left| \phi_{A_n}(1) \cdots \phi_{Z_n}(N) \right|, \tag{4.2.1}$$

where $S_n = 1$ only if the orbitals are all orthogonal.

The ϕ's will generally be orthogonal for the ground state, but there is no guarantee that they will be for excited states. The only rigid quantum requirement is that all the ψ_n shall be orthogonal; this does not necessarily mean that all the individual ϕ's shall be also, although by symmetry many of them will be. In the simplest approximations excited states are described by a function in which they differ from the ground in only one of the ϕ's. Even within the framework of the functions in (4.2.1) this neglects the changes which must occur in the other $N - 1$ functions. If these are now recalculated by the standard methods of self-consistent field theory, a modified set of orbitals is obtained.

Let the ground and excited states be given by

$$\Psi_0 = \frac{S_0}{\sqrt{N!}} \left| \phi_{A_0}(1) \cdots \phi_{Z_0}(N) \right| \tag{4.2.2a}$$

$$\Psi_1 = \frac{S_1}{\sqrt{N!}} \left| \phi_{A_1}(1) \cdots \phi'_{Z_0}(N) \right|. \tag{4.2.2b}$$

The labeling is meant to indicate that the major change in the excited state is in the functions ϕ_{A_0} and ϕ_{A_1} with lesser changes in the others indicated by primes. In an optically active molecule none of these functions will be orthogonal, although ϕ_{A_0} and ϕ_{A_1} will nearly be.

This formulation is capable of assessing all important contributions to optical activity with the exception of the electron correlation effects treated by the coupled oscillator model in Chapter 3. The lack of electron correlation was the main deficiency of this type of wave function. The methods of perturbation theory may conveniently be used on any set of functions with significantly different expectation values of the total Hamiltonian of the system including all electron repulsions.

At the present stage of advancement of quantum technology it is still worthwhile to dispense with certain mathematical amenities in order to gain a theoretically inspired empirical foothold in this subtle branch of spectroscopy. Determinantal states with nonorthogonal one electron functions are unwieldy. A general treatment of the subject is more readily forthcoming if the determinants in (4.2.2) are modified so as to contain only orthogonal functions. It will be assumed that these functions have been chosen by a variational procedure and represent the best approximations subject to the given restrictions.

In more general terms it will happen that a set of orthogonal one electron functions will be available. The set may be finite or infinite. As a simple but not very practical example it is possible in principle to solve a many electron problem by means of hydrogenlike functions and perturbation or variation methods. This procedure will make use of all possible N electron determinants and the calculation done to infinite order.

At the other extreme one may start with only two wave functions representing often only a semiquantitative approximation to the problem. These will be considered to be part of a complete, but unspecified, set of orthogonal functions, which need not be eigenfunctions of any Hamiltonian. (In general it is not always possible to find an H for which $H\psi_1 = E_1\psi_1$ and $H\psi_2 = E_2\psi_2$ for any values of E_1 and E_2.) Additional orthogonal orbitals with increasing numbers of nodes may be introduced and from these a set of determinantal functions constructed for use in a variation calculation. With only a few such orbitals the procedure becomes quite tedious, and an alternative is desirable. Below we shall first develop the first and second order expressions for optical activity with an outline of those of higher order. Then by use of an admittedly drastic summation approximation expressions will be obtained which depend only on the ground and excited states and the total Hamiltonian of the system.

For the sake of developing the formalism it will be most convenient to assume the existence of a set of functions ψ_q which satisfy the eigenvalue equation $H_0\psi_q = E_q\psi_q$, where $H_0 = \sum_{i=1}^{N} - (\hbar^2/2m)\nabla_i^2 + V^{(0)}$. In optical activity calculations matrix elements are sought between the eigenfunctions of the exact Hamiltonian of the dissymmetric molecule $H = \sum_{i=1}^{N}(-\hbar^2/2m) \times \nabla_i^2 + V'$. When $H = H_0 + V' - V^{(0)} = H_0 + V$ and ψ_0 and ψ_n are the wave functions for the zeroth order ground and excited states, standard perturbation methods give

$$\psi_n' = \psi_n + \sum_{q\neq n}\left[\frac{V_{qn}}{E_n - E_q} + \sum_{r\neq n}\frac{V_{qr}V_{rn}}{(E_n - E_q)(E_n - E_r)} + \cdots \right.$$
$$\left. + \sum_{\substack{r,s,t\ldots\\ \neq n}}\frac{V_{qr}V_{rs}\cdots V_{tn}}{(E_n - E_q)(E_n - E_r)\cdots(E_n - E_t)} + \cdots\right]\psi_q, \tag{4.2.3}$$

where the E_q, E_r, etc., are the zeroth order energies, and E_n is the exact energy of the excited state.

In order to conform to convention the rotational strength has been presented in the form $R_{0n} = \mathrm{Im}(\boldsymbol{\mu}_{0n} \cdot \mathbf{m}_{n0})$. It is worthwhile to examine the dependence of this expression on the choice of origin. Let $\mathbf{r}$ and $\mathbf{r}^{\ddagger}$ be the electronic coordinates in two arbitrary systems for which $\mathbf{r}^{\ddagger} = \mathbf{r} + \mathbf{R}$; then one may write $\boldsymbol{\mu}_{0n}^{\ddagger} = \boldsymbol{\mu}_{0n} + \mathbf{R}\langle\psi_0 \mid \psi_n\rangle$ and $\mathbf{m}_{n0}^{\ddagger} = \mathbf{m}_{n0} + (e/2mc)\mathbf{R} \times \mathbf{p}_{n0}$. If ψ_0 and ψ_n are both solutions to the same eigenvalue problem with energies E_0 and E_n, the general quantum relation, $\mathbf{p}/m = d\mathbf{r}/dt = i(H\mathbf{r} - \mathbf{r}H)/\hbar$, gives $\boldsymbol{\mu}_{0n} = e\mathbf{r}_{0n} = ie\hbar\mathbf{p}_{0n}/m(E_n - E_0)$. Assuming the orthogonality of ψ_0 and ψ_n this gives the result

$$\boldsymbol{\mu}_{0n}^{\ddagger} \cdot \mathbf{m}_{n0}^{\ddagger} = \boldsymbol{\mu}_{0n} \cdot \mathbf{m}_{n0},$$

since

$$\mathrm{Im}(i\mathbf{p}_{0n} \times \mathbf{p}_{n0}) = \mathrm{Im}[i(\mathbf{p}_{0n}^{(R)} + i\mathbf{p}_{0n}^{(I)}) \times (\mathbf{p}_{0n}^{(R)} - i\mathbf{p}_{0n}^{(I)})] = 2\,\mathrm{Im}[\mathbf{p}_{0n}^{(R)} \times \mathbf{p}_{0n}^{(I)}] = 0.$$

It is important to recognize that the only requirement behind the validity of this result is the relation of the two functions to the same Hamiltonian; whether or not this Hamiltonian is identical with that of the system being studied is immaterial. In many approximate treatments it is not always convenient to use eigenfunctions of the same Hamiltonian; in fact, the majority of molecular calculations to date have not done so. This in itself is no indictment of such methods, because one may equally well approach the true eigenfunctions by relating them to a single approximate Hamiltonian or two separate ones. In an iterative process these approximate Hamiltonians can approach the true one equally well.

Under the above conditions $\boldsymbol{\mu}_{0n}$ is no longer simply related to $\mathbf{p}_{0n}$, and the above arguments do not apply. The way out of the difficulty is to write the rotational strength in terms of $\mathbf{p}_{0n}$ instead of $\boldsymbol{\mu}_{0n}$. The magnetic moment is, of course, still dependent on the origin, but the product $\mathbf{p}_{0n} \cdot \mathbf{m}_{n0}$ is not:

$$\mathrm{Im}(i\mathbf{p}_{0n}^{\ddagger} \cdot \mathbf{m}_{n0}^{\ddagger}) = \mathrm{Im}(i\mathbf{p}_{0n} \cdot \mathbf{m}_{n0}) + \frac{e}{2mc}\,\mathrm{Im}(i\mathbf{p}_{0n} \cdot \mathbf{R} \times \mathbf{p}_{n0}) = \mathrm{Im}(i\mathbf{p}_{0n} \cdot \mathbf{m}_{n0}).$$

The desired form for the rotational strength is

$$R_{0n} = Re\left[\frac{e\hbar}{m(E_n - E_0)}\,\mathbf{p}_{0n} \cdot \mathbf{m}_{n0}\right],$$

where E_n and E_0 are taken to be the exact eigenvalues.

With the use of (4.2.3) for the excited and ground states the successive corrections to the trial product $\mathbf{p}_{0n}\cdot\mathbf{m}_{n0}$ may be obtained and arranged according to terms of increasing order:

$$\begin{aligned}\mathbf{p}'_{0n}\cdot\mathbf{m}'_{n0} = \mathbf{p}_{0n}\cdot\mathbf{m}_{n0} &+ (\mathbf{p}_{0n}\cdot\mathbf{m}^{(1)}_{n0} + \mathbf{p}^{(1)}_{0n}\cdot\mathbf{m}_{n0}) \\ &+ (\mathbf{p}_{0n}\cdot\mathbf{m}^{(2)}_{n0} + \mathbf{p}^{(1)}_{0n}\cdot\mathbf{m}^{(1)}_{n0} + \mathbf{p}^{(2)}_{0n}\cdot\mathbf{m}_{n0}) + \cdots \\ &+ \sum_{P=0}^{Q}\mathbf{p}^{(P)}_{0n}\cdot\mathbf{m}^{(Q-P)}_{n0} + \cdots . \end{aligned}\tag{4.2.4}$$

The explicit form in terms of the matrix elements V_{qn} is

$$\begin{aligned}\mathbf{p}'_{0n}\cdot\mathbf{m}'_{n0} = \mathbf{p}_{0n}\cdot\mathbf{m}_{n0} &+ \left[\mathbf{p}_{0n}\cdot\left(\sum_q \frac{V_{nq}\mathbf{m}_{q0}}{E_n - E_q} + \sum_q \frac{\mathbf{m}_{nq}V_{q0}}{E_0 - E_q}\right)\right. \\ &+ \left.\left(\sum_q \frac{\mathbf{p}_{0q}V_{qn}}{E_n - E_q} + \sum_q \frac{V_{0q}\mathbf{p}_{qn}}{E_0 - E_q}\right)\cdot\mathbf{m}_{n0}\right] \\ &+ \left\{\mathbf{p}_{0n}\cdot\left[\sum_{q,r}\frac{V_{nq}V_{qr}\mathbf{m}_{r0}}{(E_n - E_q)(E_n - E_r)} + \sum_{q,r}\frac{V_{nq}\mathbf{m}_{0q}V_{r0}}{(E_n - E_q)(E_0 - E_r)}\right.\right. \\ &+ \left.\sum_{q,r}\frac{\mathbf{m}_{nq}V_{qr}V_{r0}}{(E_0 - E_q)(E_0 - E_r)}\right] + \left(\sum_q \frac{\mathbf{p}_{0q}V_{qn}}{E_n - E_q} + \sum_q \frac{V_{0q}\mathbf{p}_{qn}}{E_0 - E_q}\right) \\ &\cdot\left(\sum_q \frac{V_{nq}\mathbf{m}_{q0}}{E_n - E_q} + \sum_q \frac{\mathbf{m}_{nq}V_{q0}}{E_0 - E_q}\right) + \left[\sum_{q,r}\frac{\mathbf{p}_{0q}V_{qr}V_{rn}}{(E_n - E_q)(E_n - E_r)}\right. \\ &+ \left.\left.\sum_{q,r}\frac{V_{0q}\mathbf{p}_{qr}V_{rn}}{(E_0 - E_q)(E_n - E_r)} + \sum_{q,r}\frac{V_{0q}V_{qr}\mathbf{p}_{rn}}{(E_0 - E_q)(E_0 - E_r)}\right]\cdot\mathbf{m}_{n0}\right\} \\ &+ \cdots + \sum_{P=0}^{Q}\left\{\left[\sum_{\substack{q\ldots \\ r,s \\ \ldots t}}\frac{\mathbf{p}_{0q}\cdots V_{rs}\cdots V_{tn}}{(E_n - E_q)\cdots(E_n - E_r)(E_n - E_s)\cdots(E_n - E_t)}\right.\right. \\ &+ \cdots \cdot \sum_{\substack{q\ldots \\ r,s,t,u \\ \ldots v}}\frac{V_{oq}\cdots V_{rs}\mathbf{p}_{st}V_{tu}\cdots V_{vn}}{(E_0 - E_q)\cdots(E_0 - E_r)(E_0 - E_s)\times(E_n - E_t)(E_n - E_u)\cdots(E_n - E_v)} \\ &+ \cdots\left.\sum_{\substack{q\ldots \\ r,s \\ \ldots t}}\frac{V_{0q}\cdots V_{rs}\cdots\mathbf{p}_{tn}}{(E_0 - E_q)\cdots(E_0 - E_r)(E_0 - E_s)\cdots(E_0 - E_t)}\right]_P \\ &\cdot\left[\sum_{\substack{q\ldots \\ r,s \\ \ldots t}}\frac{V_{nq}\cdots V_{rs}\cdots\mathbf{m}_{t0}}{(E_n - E_q)\cdots(E_n - E_r)(E_n - E_s)\cdots(E_n - E_t)}\right.\end{aligned}$$

$$+\cdots \sum_{\substack{q\ldots\\ r,s,t,u\\ \ldots v}} \frac{V_{nq}\cdots V_{rs}\mathbf{m}_{st}V_{tu}\cdots V_{v0}}{(E_n - E_q)\cdots(E_n - E_r)(E_n - E_s) \times (E_0 - E_t)(E_0 - E_u)\cdots(E_0 - E_v)}$$

$$\left.\left. + \cdots \sum_{\substack{q\ldots\\ r,s\\ \ldots t}} \frac{\mathbf{m}_{nq}\cdots V_{rs}\cdots V_{t0}}{(E_0 - E_q)\cdots(E_0 - E_r)(E_0 - E_s)\cdots(E_0 - E_t)}\right]_{Q-P}\right\}$$

$$+\cdots, \tag{4.2.5}$$

where $[\quad]_P$ indicates that all terms to order P in H are to be included. The summations are over all states which lead to nonvanishing denominators.

Close attention should be paid to the order of the terms in an individual summation as well as to the factors E_n and E_0 in the denominators. As seen from the general term, matrix elements of V which precede those of $\mathbf{p}$ are associated with $E_0 - E_q$, etc., while those which follow have $E_n - E_q$ in the denominator. The reverse is true for $\mathbf{m}$. Despite the seeming complexity of (4.2.5) the principles behind it are quite straightforward. The cumbersome terms involving diagonal elements of V are absent from (4.2.5), since E_n and E_0 are the exact energies of the ground and excited states, while all the E_q's are the expectation values of H for the approximate state functions.

Equation 4.2.5 is exact, subject to certain by-no-means trivial convergence conditions. This must not be construed to mean that this is the exact expression for the optical activity of a molecule, since $\mathbf{p}_{0n}\cdot\mathbf{m}_{n0}$ is only the lowest order term arising from a multipole expansion. In most problems of interest ψ_n is one of the lowest states; for the present it will be assumed that ψ_n is the lowest excited state for which there are nonvanishing matrix elements in (4.2.5). The energy denominators $E_n - E_q$ and $E_0 - E_q$ are all negative, and an approximate expression particularly suitable for empirical purposes may be obtained by replacing $E_n - E_q$ and $E_0 - E_q$ by the average quantities $E_n - \bar{E}$ and $E_0 - \bar{E}$ and using the matrix multiplication rule in the resulting summations. When it is found in the course of the calculation that lower states than ψ_n must be used the appropriate terms may be added and subtracted. The details of this procedure will become clearer in the examples to be discussed in the following chapter.

We are now in a position to sum over all states to obtain an expression which depends only on the two approximate state functions ψ_0 and ψ_n, the average energy denominators $E_0 - \bar{E}$ and $E_n - \bar{E}$, and the exact Hamiltonian H. The first summation in (4.2.5) will be

$$\sum_{q\neq n} \frac{V_{nq}\mathbf{m}_{q0}}{E_n - E_q} \simeq \frac{1}{E_n - \bar{E}} \sum_{q\neq n} V_{nq}\mathbf{m}_{q0} = \frac{1}{E_n - \bar{E}}\left(\sum_q V_{nq}\mathbf{m}_{q0} - V_{nn}\mathbf{m}_{n0}\right)$$

$$= \frac{1}{E_n - \bar{E}}[(V\mathbf{m})_{n0} - V_{nn}\mathbf{m}_{n0}]. \tag{4.2.6}$$

In the remaining summations one must always remember to subtract the appropriate terms where an index equals 0 or n.

A typical term is

$$\sum_{\substack{q\ldots\\ r,s\neq 0;\\ t,u\\ \ldots v\neq n}} \frac{\overbrace{V_{0q}\cdots V_{rs}}^{N}\mathbf{p}_{st}\overbrace{V_{tu}\cdots V_{vn}}^{P-N}}{(E_0-E_q)\cdots(E_0-E_r)(E_0-E_s)(E_n-E_t)(E_n-E_u)\cdots(E_n-E_v)}$$

$$\simeq \frac{1}{(E_0-\bar{E})^N(E_n-\bar{E})^{P-N}} \sum_{\substack{q\ldots\\ r,s\neq 0;\\ t,u\\ \ldots v\neq n}} \overbrace{V_{0q}\cdots V_{rs}}^{N}\mathbf{p}_{st}\overbrace{V_{tu}\cdots V_{vn}}^{P-N}, \quad (4.2.7)$$

where $\overbrace{\quad}^{N}$ indicates that N successive matrix elements of V precede $\boldsymbol{\mu}_{st}$; the term is evidently of order P.

Not only must all terms for which only one of the energy denominators vanishes be subtracted but also those for which 2, 3, ..., P of them vanish. The first term is the summation over all indices:

$$\sum_{\substack{q\ldots\\ r,s,t,u\\ \ldots v}} \overbrace{V_{0q}\cdots V_{rs}}^{N}\mathbf{p}_{st}\overbrace{V_{tu}\cdots V_{vn}}^{P-N} = (V^N\mathbf{p}V^{P-N})_{0n}. \quad (4.2.8)$$

Next one must exclude in succession terms for which each of the indices q, r, s equals 0 or t, u, v equals n. A typical term in this series is

$$\sum_{\substack{q\ldots\\ r,s\\ t,u,v,w\\ \ldots x}} \overbrace{V_{0q}\cdots V_{r0}}^{T}\overbrace{V_{0s}\cdots V_{tu}}^{N-T}\mathbf{p}_{uv}\overbrace{V_{vw}\cdots V_{xn}}^{P-N} = (V^T)_{00}(V^{N-T}\mathbf{p}V^{P-N})_{0n}. \quad (4.2.9)$$

The sum of such terms is seen to be

$$\sum_{T=1}^{N}(V^T)_{00}(V^{N-T}\,\mathbf{p}V^{P-N})_{0n} + \sum_{T=1}^{P-N}(V^N\mathbf{p}V^{P-N-T})_{0n}(V^T)_{nn}.$$

It is not worthwhile to display an iterated expression containing these corrections to the leading term $(V^N\mathbf{p}V^{P-N})_{0n}$, since there are a total of 2^P terms in the above example, a great many of which must be explicitly represented. It is only important to recognize that all such terms contain lower order corrections to the given electric or magnetic moments. Generally only the lowest order nonvanishing terms are of interest and such corrections would not be necessary. It does not follow that this will always be true, since it is quite conceivable that $\mathbf{p}_{0n}\cdot\mathbf{m}_{n0}\neq 0$ for the given choice of zeroth order functions. The best set of SCF one electron orbitals still fails to account for electron correlation effects; the complete correction terms would have to be used in order to prevent counting terms more than once.

The highest reasonable order which appears feasible is the fourth; this may be justified by observing that a good estimate to the direction of an originally forbidden transition is not always obtained by first order perturbation terms, particularly when the chromophore is polysubstituted. In order for both the magnetic and electric transition moments to obey a non-linear substitution rule, they must both be calculated to second order. It is not expected that such a drastic procedure will be necessary for strong electric or magnetic dipole transitions. If it is assumed that a fourth order calculation is only necessary when both $\boldsymbol{\mu}_{0n}$ and $\mathbf{m}_{n0}$ vanish, an abbreviated expression of the form

$$(\mathbf{p}_{0n} + \mathbf{p}_{0n}^{(1)} + \mathbf{p}_{0n}^{(2)} + \mathbf{p}_{0n}^{(3)}) \cdot (\mathbf{m}_{n0} + \mathbf{m}_{n0}^{(1)} + \mathbf{m}_{n0}^{(2)} + \mathbf{m}_{n0}^{(3)})$$

may be used with the retention of terms up to fourth order.

The most complex terms will be of the form

$$\sum_{\substack{q,\, r \neq 0 \\ s \neq n}} V_{0q} V_{qr} \mathbf{p}_{rs} V_{sn}.$$

The summation may be made over all indices without restriction and the excluded terms subtracted. Not only must the term $V_{00}^2 \mathbf{p}_{0n} V_{nn}$ be excluded, where all three indices have their forbidden values, but also those where only one or two indices take on these values. There are three ways of giving one index and three ways of giving two indices their forbidden values. The summation reduces to

$$\begin{aligned}\sum_{\substack{q,\, r \neq 0 \\ s \neq n}} V_{0q} V_{qr} \mathbf{p}_{rs} V_{sn} &= (V^2 \mathbf{p} V)_{0n} - V_{00}^2 V_{nn} \mathbf{p}_{0n} \\ &\quad - V_{00} \sum_{\substack{r \neq 0 \\ s \neq n}} V_{0r} \mathbf{p}_{rs} V_{sn} - \sum_{\substack{q \neq 0 \\ s \neq n}} V_{0q} V_{q0} \mathbf{p}_{0s} V_{sn} - V_{nn} \sum_{\substack{q \neq 0 \\ r \neq 0}} V_{0q} V_{qr} \mathbf{p}_{rn} \\ &\quad - V_{00}^2 \sum_{s \neq n} \mathbf{p}_{0s} V_{sn} - \mathbf{p}_{0n} V_{nn} \sum_{q \neq 0} V_{0q} V_{q0} - V_{00} V_{nn} \sum_{r \neq 0} V_{0r} \mathbf{p}_{rn}.\end{aligned} \quad (4.2.10)$$

The one and two index summations may be reduced by a similar process; for example,

$$\begin{aligned}\sum_{\substack{r \neq 0 \\ s \neq n}} V_{0r} \mathbf{p}_{rs} V_{sn} &= (V\mathbf{p}V)_{0n} - V_{00} V_{nn} \mathbf{p}_{0n} - V_{00} \sum_{s \neq n} \mathbf{p}_{0s} V_{sn} - V_{nn} \sum_{r \neq 0} V_{0r} \mathbf{p}_{rn} \\ &= (V\mathbf{p}V)_{0n} - V_{00} V_{nn} \mathbf{p}_{0n} - V_{00} [(\mathbf{p}V)_{0n} - \mathbf{p}_{0n} V_{nn}] \\ &\quad - V_{nn} [(V\mathbf{p})_{on} - V_{00} \mathbf{p}_{0n}] \\ &= (V\mathbf{p}V)_{0n} - V_{00} (\mathbf{p}V)_{0n} - V_{nn} (V\mathbf{p})_{0n} + V_{00} V_{0n} \mathbf{p}_{0n}.\end{aligned} \quad (4.2.11)$$

The completely reduced form of (4.2.10) is

$$\sum_{\substack{q,r\neq 0\\ s\neq n}} V_{0q}V_{qr}\mathbf{p}_{rs}V_{sn} = (V^2\mathbf{p}V)_{0n} - V_{nn}(V^2\mathbf{p})_{0n} - V_{00}(V\mathbf{p}V)_{0n}$$

$$+ [V_{00}^2 - (V^2)_{00}](\mathbf{p}V)_{0n} + V_{00}V_{nn}(V\mathbf{p})_{0n}$$

$$+ V_{nn}((V^2)_{00} - V_{00}^2)\mathbf{p}_{0n}. \qquad (4.2.12)$$

From the preceding discussion it follows that the rotational strength may be arranged in terms of ascending order:

$$\frac{m(E_n - E_0)}{e\hbar} R_{0n} = \mathrm{Re}[(\mathbf{p}_{0n} + \mathbf{p}_{0n}^{(1)} + \mathbf{p}_{0n}^{(2)} + \mathbf{p}_{0n}^{(3)} + \cdots)$$

$$\cdot (\mathbf{m}_{n0} + \mathbf{m}_{n0}^{(1)} + \mathbf{m}_{n0}^{(2)} + \mathbf{m}_{n0}^{(3)} + \cdots)]$$

$$= \frac{m(E_n - E_0)}{e\hbar}(R_{0n}^{(0)} + R_{0n}^{(1)} + R_{0n}^{(2)} + R_{0n}^{(3)} + R_{0n}^{(4)\ddagger} + \cdots),$$

where

$$\frac{m(E_n - E_0)}{e\hbar} R_{0n}^{(0)} = \mathrm{Re}(\mathbf{p}_{0n}\cdot\mathbf{m}_{n0}) \qquad (4.2.13a)$$

$$\frac{m(E_n - E_0)}{e\hbar} R_{0n}^{(1)} = \mathrm{Re}(\mathbf{p}_{0n}\cdot\mathbf{m}_{n0}^{(1)} + \mathbf{p}_{0n}^{(1)}\cdot\mathbf{m}_{n0}) \qquad (4.2.13b)$$

$$\frac{m(E_n - E_0)}{e\hbar} R_{0n}^{(2)} = \mathrm{Re}(\mathbf{p}_{0n}\cdot\mathbf{m}_{n0}^{(2)} + \mathbf{p}_{0n}^{(1)}\cdot\mathbf{m}_{n0}^{(1)} + \mathbf{p}_{0n}^{(2)}\cdot\mathbf{m}_{n0}) \qquad (4.2.13c)$$

$$\frac{m(E_n - E_0)}{e\hbar} R_{0n}^{(3)} = \mathrm{Re}(\mathbf{p}_{0n}\cdot\mathbf{m}_{n0}^{(3)} + \mathbf{p}_{0n}^{(1)}\cdot\mathbf{m}_{n0}^{(2)} + \mathbf{p}_{0n}^{(2)}\cdot\mathbf{m}_{n0}^{(1)} + \mathbf{p}_{0n}^{(3)}\cdot\mathbf{m}_{n0}) \qquad (4.2.13d)$$

$$\frac{m(E_n - E_0)}{e\hbar} R_{0n}^{(4)\ddagger} = \mathrm{Re}(\mathbf{p}_{0n}^{(1)}\cdot\mathbf{m}_{n0}^{(3)} + \mathbf{p}_{0n}^{(2)}\cdot\mathbf{m}_{n0}^{(2)} + \mathbf{p}_{0n}^{(3)}\cdot\mathbf{m}_{n0}^{(1)}). \qquad (4.2.13e)$$

The last term is given the symbol $R_{0n}^{(4)\ddagger}$ to emphasize the fact that it is not the complete fourth order term, the $\mathbf{p}_{0n}\cdot\mathbf{m}_{n0}^{(4)}$ and $\mathbf{p}_{0n}^{(4)}\cdot\mathbf{m}_{n0}$ terms being absent. In accordance with the discussion above this term should only be used when both $\boldsymbol{\mu}_{0n}$ and $\mathbf{m}_{n0}$ vanish.

The discussion centered on (4.2.5) and the example of (4.2.12) should be sufficient to verify that the first, second, and third order electric dipole moments are

$$\mathbf{p}_{0n}^{(1)} = \frac{1}{E_n - \bar{E}}[(\mathbf{p}V)_{0n} - V_{nn}\mathbf{p}_{0n}] + \frac{1}{E_0 - \bar{E}}[(V\mathbf{p})_{0n} - V_{00}\mathbf{p}_{0n}] \qquad (4.2.14a)$$

$$\mathbf{p}_{0n}^{(2)} = \frac{1}{(E_n - \bar{E})^2}\{(\mathbf{p}V^2)_{0n} - (\mathbf{p}V)_{0n}V_{nn} - [(V^2)_{nn} - V_{nn}^2]\mathbf{p}_{0n}\}$$

$$+ \frac{1}{(E_0 - \bar{E})(E_n - \bar{E})}[(V\mathbf{p}V)_{0n} - V_{00}(\mathbf{p}V)_{0n} - (V\mathbf{p})_{0n}V_{nn} + V_{nn}V_{00}\mathbf{p}_{0n}]$$

$$+ \frac{1}{(E_0 - \bar{E})^2}\{(V^2\mathbf{p})_{0n} - V_{00}(V\mathbf{p})_{0n} - [(V^2)_{00} - V_{00}^2]\mathbf{p}_{0n}\} \qquad (4.2.14b)$$

$$\mathbf{p}_{0n}^{(3)} = \frac{1}{(E_n - \bar{E})^3}\{(\mathbf{p}V^3)_{0n} - V_{nn}(\mathbf{p}V^2)_{0n} - [(V^2)_{nn} - V_{nn}^2](\mathbf{p}V)_{0n}$$

$$+ [2(V^2)_{nn}V_{nn} - (V^3)_{nn} - V_{0n}^3]\mathbf{p}_{0n}\} + \frac{1}{(E_n - \bar{E})^2(E_0 - \bar{E})}\{(V\mathbf{p}V^2)_{0n}$$

$$- V_{nn}(V\mathbf{p}V)_{0n} - V_{00}(\mathbf{p}V^2)_{0n} + V_{00}V_{nn}(\mathbf{p}V)_{0n} - [(V^2)_{nn} - V_{nn}^2](V\mathbf{p})_{0n}$$

$$+ [(V^2)_{nn} - V_{nn}^2]V_{00}\mathbf{p}_{0n}\} + \frac{1}{(E_n - \bar{E})(E_0 - \bar{E})^2}\{(V^2\mathbf{p}V)_{0n}$$

$$- V_{nn}(V^2\mathbf{p})_{0n} - V_{00}(V\mathbf{p}V)_{0n} + V_{00}V_{nn}(V\mathbf{p})_{0n} - [(V^2)_{00} - V_{00}^2](\mathbf{p}V)_{0n}$$

$$+ [(V^2)_{00} - V_{00}^2]V_{nn}\mathbf{p}_{0n}\} + \frac{1}{(E_0 - \bar{E})^3}\{(V^3\mathbf{p})_{0n} - V_{00}(V^2\mathbf{p})_{0n}$$

$$- [(V^2)_{00} - V_{00}^2](V\mathbf{p})_{0n} + [2V_{00}(V^2)_{00} - (V^3)_{00} - V_{00}^3]\mathbf{p}_{0n}\}. \qquad (4.2.14c)$$

The magnetic moment terms are obtained by substituting **m** for **p** and interchanging 0 and n.

4.3. Exchange Terms and the SCF Method

Equations 4.2.13 and 4.2.14 are the focal point of a general theory of optical activity for low energy transitions. Even when they are not numerically reliable they provide a systematic method for obtaining empirical relations which would not be readily inferred through other approaches; however, they are not yet in their most useful form.

As in the discussion of (4.2.1) and (4.2.2) it will be assumed that the zeroth order wave functions will be antisymmetrized products of orthogonal one electron orbitals which differ in only one index:

$$\Psi_0 = \frac{1}{\sqrt{N!}}\left|\phi_{A_1}(1)\bar{\phi}_{A_2}(2)\cdots\phi_{A_{i-1}}(i-1)\bar{\phi}_{A_i}(i)\cdots\phi_{A_{N-1}}(N-1)\bar{\phi}_{A_N}(N)\right| \qquad (4.3.1a)$$

$$\Psi\begin{pmatrix} A_1 \\ a_1 \end{pmatrix} = \frac{1}{\sqrt{N!}} \left| \phi_{a_1}(1)\bar{\phi}_{A_2}(2)\cdots\phi_{A_{i-1}}(i-1)\bar{\phi}_{A_i}(i)\cdots\phi_{A_{N-1}}(N-1)\bar{\phi}_{A_N}(N) \right|. \tag{4.3.1b}$$

In cases of degeneracy, as is often encountered for chromophores of high symmetry, the zeroth order excited state is a sum of terms:

$$\Psi_n \sim \sum_{i=1}^{N} c\begin{pmatrix} A_i \\ a_i \end{pmatrix} \Psi\begin{pmatrix} A_i \\ a_i \end{pmatrix}.$$

There will always be spin degeneracy for excited states. It is not necessary to assume that the molecule is divided into distinct groups; in fact, the ambiguity of this procedure has often proved to be a disadvantage. No assumptions will be made about the individual orbitals beyond their orthogonality. In most instances each orbital will contain two electrons with opposite spins and $A_1 = A_2$, etc.

The molecular operators V, $\mathbf{p}$, and $\mathbf{m}$ are the sums of one and two electron operators:

$$V = \sum_{i=1}^{N} (V_i - V_{0i}) + \sum_{i>j=1}^{N} \left(\frac{1}{r_{ij}} - V_{0ij} \right) \tag{4.3.2a}$$

$$\mathbf{p} = \sum_{i=1}^{N} \mathbf{p}_i \tag{4.3.2b}$$

$$\mathbf{m} = \sum_{i=1}^{N} \mathbf{m}_i . \tag{4.3.2c}$$

In the most general case $V_0 = \sum_i V_{0i} + \sum_{i,j} V_{0i_j}$, but the most practical cases are where the ϕ_i are eigenfunctions of one electron operators. One then writes

$$V = \sum_{i=1}^{N} V_i + \sum_{i>j=1}^{N} \frac{1}{r_{ij}}.$$

where V_i is the difference between the true potential of the fixed nuclei and the one electron potential. For the present the nuclei will be regarded as fixed in their equilibrium positions, and nuclear repulsion terms will be omitted in H. It is emphasized that the momentum and magnetic moments are always computed relative to the same fixed center.

There are $N!$ terms in each of the determinants of (4.3.1). As in the theory of chemical bonding, there will be nonexchange, single exchange, and multiple exchange integrals corresponding to the permutation of indices. The determinant may be written in terms of a permutation operator P, which interchanges indices,

$$\Psi_0 = \frac{1}{\sqrt{N!}} \sum_P (-1)^{\sigma_P} P[\phi_{A_1}(1)\bar{\phi}_{A_2}(2)\cdots\bar{\phi}_{A_N}(N)], \tag{4.3.3}$$

where σ_P is $+1$ for an even permutation and -1 for an odd one. The sum is over all $N!$ permutations. For a three electron system the even permutations are 123, 231, and 312, while the odd ones are 213, 132, and 321.

The product operators in (4.2.14) will be the sums of one, two, and many electron operators; for example, the operator $V^3\mathbf{p}$ may depend on the simultaneous values of as many as seven electronic coordinates through such terms as $(1/r_{12})(1/r_{34})(1/r_{56})\mathbf{p}_7$. Let Ω be a general quantum mechanical operator; it may be resolved as the sum of many electron operators as follows:

$$\Omega = \sum_i \Omega_i + \sum_{i \neq j} \Omega_{ij} + \sum_{\substack{i \neq j, \\ \text{etc.}}} \Omega_{ijk} + \cdots. \tag{4.3.4}$$

If $\Omega = V$ only the first two sums are used; for $\Omega = \mathbf{p}$ only the first sum applies; and for $\Omega = V\mathbf{p}$ the first three are necessary.

A matrix element of a one electron operator between Ψ_0 and the first determinant of $\Psi\binom{A_1}{a_1}$ in (4.3.1) will be written

$$\frac{1}{N!}\sum_{\mathbf{P}}\sum_{\mathbf{P}'}(-1)^{\sigma_P}(-1)^{\sigma_{P'}}$$

$$\times \left\langle P[\phi_{A_1}(1)\cdots\bar{\phi}_{A_N}(N)] \middle| \sum_{i=1}^{N}\Omega_i \middle| P'[\phi_{a_1}(1)\cdots\bar{\phi}_{A_N}(N)]\right\rangle.$$

There are $N \times (N!)^2$ terms in this expression, but only one unique nonvanishing quantity. Let P be the identity element and consider P' to range over its $N!$ operations. Since ϕ_{A_1} is orthogonal to all the functions in the second determinant, the only surviving terms must include Ω_1 for all permutations P'. The interchange of any pair of electronic coordinates in the second determinant leads to the integration of a pair of orthogonal functions; hence, the only term out of the $N \times N!$ possible for fixed P (in this case the identity element) is

$$\langle\phi_{A_1}(1)\cdots\bar{\phi}_{A_N}(N)|\,\Omega_1\,|\phi_{a_1}(1)\cdots\bar{\phi}_{A_N}(N)\rangle$$
$$= \langle\phi_{A_1}(1)|\,\Omega_1\,|\phi_{a_1}(1)\rangle = (\Omega_1)_{A_1a_1}. \tag{4.3.5}$$

When P undergoes its $N!$ permutations this same term is obtained $N!$ times with a positive sign, because in order to obtain a nonvanishing term P and P' must be the same permutation. Similar reasoning applies to any excitation, since the order of the factors in the determinant is irrelevant so long as both states have the same order. The general result is

$$\left\langle\Psi_0\middle|\sum_{i=1}\Omega_i\middle|\Psi\begin{pmatrix}A_k\\a_k\end{pmatrix}\right\rangle = (\Omega_k)_{A_ka_k}. \tag{4.3.6}$$

In the consideration of two electron operators it is possible to exchange one pair of electron coordinates leading to a nonexchange and a single exchange term. The standard term to be evaluated is

$$\frac{1}{N!}\sum_P\sum_{P'}(-1)^{\sigma_P}(-1)^{\sigma_{P'}}\left\langle P[\phi_{A_1}(1)\cdots\bar{\phi}_{A_N}(N)]\left|\sum_{i>j=1}^{N}\Omega_{ij}\right| P'[\phi_{a_1}(1)\cdots\bar{\phi}_{A_N}(N)]\right\rangle.$$

Since there are $[N(N-1)/2]\Omega_{ij}$ operators, there will be $[N(N-1)/2](N!)^2$ terms in this expression.

Again P will remain fixed and P' will undergo all permutations. Owing to the orthogonality of $\phi_{A_1}(1)$ to all of the ϕ functions, one of the indices in Ω_{ij} must always be 1; that is,

$$\sum_{i>j=1}^{N}\Omega_{ij}\rightarrow\sum_{j=2}^{N}\Omega_{1j}.$$

The nonexchange term is

$$\left\langle\phi_{A_1}(1)\cdots\bar{\phi}_{A_N}(N)\left|\sum_{j=2}^{N}\Omega_{1j}\right|\phi_{a_1}(1)\cdots\bar{\phi}_{A_N}(N)\right\rangle$$
$$=\left\langle\phi_{A_1}(1)\left|\sum_{j=2}^{N}[\langle\phi_{A_j}(2)|\Omega_{12}|\phi_{A_j}(2)\rangle]\right|\phi_{a_1}(1)\right\rangle=(\Omega_{12})_{A_1a_1}, \quad (4.3.7)$$

where the variable of integration j has been changed to 2. There are $N!$ such terms, all identical, corresponding to P and P' as the same permutation.

A single interchange of electron coordinates may be performed; the only nonvanishing terms are those for which the interchanged indices are i and 1 for the operator Ω_{ij}. This leads to the terms

$$-\sum_{j=3,5\ldots}^{N}\langle\phi_{A_1}(1)\cdots\phi_{A_j}(j)\cdots\bar{\phi}_{A_N}(N)|\Omega_{1j}|\phi_{A_j}(1)\cdots\phi_{a_1}(j)\cdots\bar{\phi}_{A_N}(N)\rangle$$
$$=-\sum_{j=3,5\ldots}^{N}\langle\phi_{A_1}(1)\phi_{A_j}(2)|\Omega_{12}|\phi_{A_j}(1)\phi_{a_1}(2)\rangle=-(\Omega_{21})_{A_1a_1}. \quad (4.3.8)$$

The summation is over only odd values of the index because of spin orthogonality. It will henceforth be assumed that only singlet states of even electron molecules are being considered, for which the ground state contains two electrons in each orbital with opposite spin. For N electrons there will be $N/2$ distinct orbitals, each with two electrons, in the ground state. The summation in (4.3.8) includes each orbital only once, whereas that in (4.3.7) counts each orbital twice. It will always be assumed unless explicit mention to the contrary is made that the ground state consists of such an array of doubly occupied orbitals, and the excited states are a sum of functions differing from the ground state in only a single orbital.

It will be necessary to deal with three-way interactions embodied in the terms $\sum_{i,j,k}\Omega_{ijk}$. This leads to the $[N(N-1)(N-2)/3!](N!)^2$ terms

$$\frac{1}{N!}\sum_{P}\sum_{P'}(-1)^{\sigma_P}(-1)^{\sigma_{P'}}$$
$$\times\left\langle P[\phi_{A_1}(1)\cdots\bar{\phi}_{A_N}(N)]\left|\sum_{\substack{i\neq j\\ i\neq k\\ j\neq k}}\Omega_{ijk}\right|P'[\phi_{a_1}(1)\cdots\bar{\phi}_{A_N}(N)]\right\rangle.$$

As before, P will first be the identity element and P' will be allowed all its $N!$ values. Again nonvanishing terms will be obtained only when one of the indices is 1. This allows us to write $\sum_{j>k=2}^{N}\Omega_{1jk}$ for the interaction operator. The nonexchange term is

$$\left\langle\phi_{A_1}(1)\cdots\bar{\phi}_{A_N}(N)\left|\sum_{j>k=2}^{N}\Omega_{1jk}\right|\phi_{a_1}(1)\cdots\bar{\phi}_{A_N}(N)\right\rangle$$
$$=\left\langle\phi_{A_1}(1)\left|\sum_{j>k=2}^{N}\langle\phi_{A_j}(2)\phi_{A_k}(3)|\,\Omega_{123}\,|\phi_{A_j}(2)\phi_{A_k}(3)\rangle\right|\phi_{a_1}(1)\right\rangle$$
$$=(\Omega_{123})_{A_1a_1}. \tag{4.3.9}$$

There will be two types of single exchange integral involving the ϕ_{a_1} orbital and a ϕ_{A_i} orbital or involving two other orbitals ϕ_{A_i} and ϕ_{A_j}. The first is given by

$$(\Omega_{213})_{A_1a_1}=\sum_{k\neq j=2}^{N}\sum_{j=3,5,\ldots}^{N}\langle\phi_{A_1}(1)\phi_{A_j}(2)\phi_{A_k}(3)|\,\Omega_{123}\,|\phi_{A_j}(1)\phi_{a_1}(2)\phi_{A_k}(3)\rangle. \tag{4.3.10}$$

The second is

$$(\Omega_{132})_{A_1a_1}=\sum_{j>k=2}^{N}\langle\phi_{A_1}(1)\phi_{A_j}(2)\phi_{A_k}(3)|\,\Omega_{123}\,|\phi_{a_1}(1)\phi_{A_k}(2)\phi_{A_j}(3)\rangle. \tag{4.3.11}$$

Both these terms will appear with a negative sign, because a single permutation of indices has been made.

4.4. Final Form of General Equations

The results of the preceding section may now be used to further reduce the matrix elements in (4.2.14). Consider the term

$$\mathbf{p}V=\sum_{i,j=1}^{N}\mathbf{p}_i V_j+\sum_{\substack{i,j,k=1\\ j\neq k}}^{N}\mathbf{p}_i\frac{1}{r_{jk}}. \tag{4.4.1}$$

In view of the discussion in the preceding section the nonexchange terms are given by the single integral

$$\int \cdots \int \phi_{A_1}(1) \cdots \phi_{A_N}(N) \mathbf{p} V \phi_a(1) \cdots \phi_{A_N}(N)\, d\tau_1 \cdots d\tau_N .$$

Since $\int \phi_{A_1}(1)\phi_{a_1}(1)\, d\tau_1 = 0$, it will be convenient to display the operators depending on the first coordinate explicitly:

$$\mathbf{p}V = \mathbf{p}_1 \sum_{i=2}^{N} V_i + \mathbf{p}_1 V_1 + \sum_{i,\,j=2}^{N} \mathbf{p}_i V_j + \sum_{i=2}^{N} \mathbf{p}_i V_1 + \mathbf{p}_1 \sum_{i,\,j=2}^{N} \frac{1}{r_{ij}}$$
$$+ \sum_{i=2}^{N} \mathbf{p}_1 \frac{1}{r_{1i}} + \sum_{i,\,j,\,k=2}^{N} \mathbf{p}_i \frac{1}{r_{jk}} + \sum_{\substack{i,\,j=2\\ i\neq j}}^{N} \mathbf{p}_i \frac{1}{r_{ij}} + \sum_{i=2}^{N} \mathbf{p}_i \frac{1}{r_{1i}}. \qquad (4.4.2)$$

Matrix elements of the terms $\sum_{i=j,2}^{N} \mathbf{p}_i V_j$ and $\sum_{i,j,k=2} \mathbf{p}_i(1/r_{jk})$ vanish, because they do not depend on the coordinates of electron 1. The terms $\sum_{i=2}^{N} \mathbf{p}_i V_1$ and $\sum_{i,j=2,i\neq j}^{N} \mathbf{p}_i(1/r_{1j})$ also lead to vanishing matrix elements, because diagonal elements of the momentum operator are zero. This leads to the result

$$(\mathbf{p}V)_{0n} = (\mathbf{p}_1 V_1)_{A_1 a_1} + \left(\sum_{i=2}^{N} \mathbf{p}_1 \left\langle \frac{1}{r_{1i}} \right\rangle_{ii}\right)_{A_1 a_1} + \left(\sum_{i=2}^{N} \mathbf{p}_i \frac{1}{r_{1i}}\right)_{A_1 a_1,\, ii}$$
$$+ \mathbf{p}_{A_1 a_1}\left[\sum_{i=2}^{N} (V_i)_{ii} + \sum_{i,\,j=2}^{N} \left(\frac{1}{r_{ij}}\right)_{ii,\,jj}\right], \qquad (4.4.3)$$

where

$$(\mathbf{p}_1 V_1)_{A_1 a_1} = \int \phi_{A_1}(1) \mathbf{p}_1 V_1 \phi_{a_1}(1)\, d\tau,$$

$$\left\langle \frac{1}{r_{1i}} \right\rangle_{ii} = \int \phi_{A_i}(i) \frac{1}{r_{1i}} \phi_{A_i}(i)\, d\tau_i,$$

$$\left\langle \frac{1}{r_{ij}} \right\rangle_{ii,\,jj} = \iint \phi_{A_i}(i)\phi_{A_j}(j) \frac{1}{r_{ij}} \phi_{A_i}(i)\phi_{A_j}(j)\, d\tau_i\, d\tau_j .$$

It will be observed that $\langle(1/r_{1i})\rangle_{ii}$ depends only on the coordinates of electron 1.

In a similar fashion the more straightforward term $\mathbf{p}_{0n} V_{nn}$ is found to be

$$\mathbf{p}_{0n} V_{nn} = \mathbf{p}_{A_1 a_1}\left[(V_1)_{aa} + \left(\sum_{i=2}^{N} \left\langle \frac{1}{r_{1i}} \right\rangle_{ii}\right)_{aa} + \sum_{i=2}^{N} (V_i)_{ii} + \sum_{i,\,j=2}^{N} \left[\frac{1}{r_{ij}}\right]_{ii,\,jj}\right]. \qquad (4.4.4)$$

from which it follows that

$$(\mathbf{p}V)_{0n} - \mathbf{p}_{0n} V_{nn} = [\mathbf{p}_1(V_1^{\ddagger} - V_1^{(0)})]_{A_1a_1} + \left(\sum_{i=2}^{N} \mathbf{p}_i \frac{1}{r_{1i}}\right)_{A_1a_1,\, ii} - \mathbf{p}_{A_1a_1}(V_1^{\ddagger} - V_1^{(0)})_{A_1a_1}, \quad (4.4.5)$$

where $V_1^{\ddagger} = V_1' + \sum_{i=2}^{N} \langle 1/r_{1i}\rangle_{ii}$. The quantity $V_1^{\ddagger}$ is the self-consistent field potential in which the chromophoric electron moves; it is the sum of the potential of the fixed nuclei V_1' and the average field of the other electrons $\sum_{i=2}^{N} \langle 1/r_{1i}\rangle_{ii}$. The potential $V_1^{(0)}$ describes the approximate (in general arbitrary) field which determines the eigenfunctions ϕ_{A_1} and ϕ_{a_1}:

$$\left(-\frac{1}{2m}\hbar^2\nabla_1^2 + V_1^{(0)}\right)\begin{pmatrix}\phi_{A_1}\\ \phi_{a_1}\end{pmatrix} = \begin{pmatrix}E_{A_1}\phi_{A_1}\\ E_{a_1}\phi_{a_1}\end{pmatrix}.$$

It should be recognized that, while V_i' has the same functional form for all electrons, $V_i^{(0)}$ will differ from one zeroth order orbital to another. In the event that ϕ_{A_1} and ϕ_{a_1} are true SCF functions $V_1^{\ddagger} = V_1^{(0)}$, and the only surviving term is the electron correlation term

$$\left(\sum_{i=2}^{N} \mathbf{p}_i \frac{1}{r_{1i}}\right)_{A_1a_1,\, ii}.$$

In a similar manner the other first order terms for the electric and magnetic moments are obtained:

$$\mathbf{p}_{A_1a_1}^{(1)} = \frac{1}{E_n - \bar{E}}\left\{[\mathbf{p}_1(V_1^{\ddagger} - V_1^{(0)})]_{A_1a_1} + \left(\sum_{i=2}^{N} \mathbf{p}_i \frac{1}{r_{1i}}\right)_{A_1a_1,\, ii} - \mathbf{p}_{A_1a_1}(V_1^{\ddagger} - V_1^{(0)})_{a_1a_1}\right\} + \frac{1}{E_0 - \bar{E}}\left\{[(V_1^{\ddagger} - V_1^{(0)})\mathbf{p}_1]_{A_1a_1} + \left(\sum_{i=2}^{N} \frac{1}{r_{1i}} \mathbf{p}_i\right)_{A_1a_1,\, ii} - \mathbf{p}_{A_1a_1}(V_1^{\ddagger} - V_1^{(0)})_{A_1A_1}\right\} \quad (4.4.6a)$$

$$\mathbf{m}_{a_1A_1}^{(1)} = \frac{1}{E_n - \bar{E}}\left\{[(V_1^{\ddagger} - V_1^{(0)})\mathbf{m}_1]_{a_1A_1} + \left(\sum_{i=2}^{N} \frac{1}{r_{1i}} \mathbf{m}_i\right)_{a_1A_1,\, ii} - \mathbf{m}_{a_1A_1}(V_1^{\ddagger} - V_1^{(0)})_{a_1a_1}\right\} = \frac{1}{E_0 - \bar{E}}\left\{[\mathbf{m}_1(V_1^{\ddagger} - V_1^{(0)})]_{a_1A_1} + \left(\sum_{i=2}^{N} \mathbf{m}_i \frac{1}{r_{1i}}\right)_{a_1A_1,\, ii} - \mathbf{m}_{a_1A_1}(V_1^{\ddagger} - V_1^{(0)})_{A_1A_1}\right\}. \quad (4.4.6b)$$

In correlating the rotational strengths of a series of molecules one should make every effort to fit the data to as simple a rule as possible. On the other hand, it should be recognized that complex chromophores like aromatic systems do not lend themselves readily to simple linear pairwise interaction theories. Within the framework of the above method the next higher degree of complexity is attained either through the inclusion of first order exchange or second order nonexchange terms. It is likely that both will be useful in expanding the theory to its outer limits.

The operator $\mathbf{p}V^2$ may be expanded as follows:

$$\mathbf{p}V^2 = \sum_{i,j,k=1}^{N} \mathbf{p}_i V_j V_k + \sum_{i,j,k,l=1}^{N} \mathbf{p}_i V_j \frac{1}{r_{kl}} + \sum_{i,j,k,l,m=1}^{N} \mathbf{p}_i \frac{1}{r_{jk}} \frac{1}{r_{lm}}, \tag{4.4.7}$$

where the indices range over all meaningful values. As before, it will be necessary to distinguish between the index 1 and the other $N-1$ indices. The appropriate resolution of (4.4.7) is

$$\begin{aligned}
\mathbf{p}V^2 = {} & \sum_{i,j,k=2}^{N} \mathbf{p}_i V_j V_k + 2V_1 \sum_{i,j=2}^{N} \mathbf{p}_i V_j + V_1^2 \sum_{i=2}^{N} \mathbf{p}_i + \mathbf{p}_i \sum_{i,j=2}^{N} V_i V_j \\
& + 2\mathbf{p}_1 V_1 \sum_{i=2}^{N} V_i + \mathbf{p}_1 V_1^2 + 2 \sum_{i,j,k,l=2}^{N} \mathbf{p}_i V_j \frac{1}{r_{kl}} + 2V_1 \sum_{i,j,k=2}^{N} \mathbf{p}_i \frac{1}{r_{jk}} \\
& + 2 \sum_{i,j,k=2}^{N} \mathbf{p}_i V_j \frac{1}{r_{1k}} + 2V_1 \sum_{i,j=2}^{N} \frac{\mathbf{p}_i}{r_{1j}} + 2\mathbf{p}_1 \sum_{i,j,k=2}^{N} V_i \frac{1}{r_{jk}} \\
& + 2\mathbf{p}_1 V_1 \sum_{i,j=2}^{N} \frac{1}{r_{ij}} + 2 \sum_{i,j=2}^{N} \mathbf{p}_1 \frac{1}{r_{1i}} V_j + 2\mathbf{p}_1 V_1 \sum_{i=2}^{N} \frac{1}{r_{1i}} \\
& + \sum_{i,j,k,l,m=2}^{N} \mathbf{p}_i \frac{1}{r_{ij}} \frac{1}{r_{kl}} + \sum_{i,j,k,l=2}^{N} \mathbf{p}_i \frac{1}{r_{1j}} \frac{1}{r_{kl}} + \sum_{i,j,k=2}^{N} \mathbf{p}_i \frac{1}{r_{1j}} \frac{1}{r_{1k}} \\
& + \mathbf{p}_1 \sum_{i,j,k,l=2}^{N} \frac{1}{r_{ij}} \frac{1}{r_{kl}} + \mathbf{p}_1 \sum_{t,j,k=2}^{N} \frac{1}{r_{1i}} \frac{1}{r_{jk}} + \mathbf{p}_1 \sum_{i,j=2}^{N} \frac{1}{r_{1i}} \frac{1}{r_{1j}}.
\end{aligned} \tag{4.4.8}$$

The complete treatment of this expression is quite cumbersome, and unnecessary, if one assumes that second order terms will be included only when they describe some unique and important aspect of the intramolecular interactions. The above terms will be divided into two categories: those which describe corrections to the first order matrix elements with essentially the same geometrical dependence and the unique second order terms which describe perturbations of the chromophore depending on the simultaneous values of two intergroup distances.

The first category may be omitted from the second order expression and considered to be a small modification of the first order. The second category will consist of all terms in (4.4.8) which cannot be factored into products of independent variables. For example,

$$\left(\mathbf{p}_1 V_1 \sum_{i=2}^{N} V_i\right)_{0n} = (\mathbf{p}_1 V_1)_{A_1 a_1} \left[\sum_{i=2}^{N} (V_i)_{ii}\right]$$

is factorable and represents a correction to the first order, one electron term $[\mathbf{p}_1(V_1^{\ddagger} - V_1^{(0)})]_{A_1a_1}$; but $\mathbf{p}_1 V_1^2$ is a unique second order term. In reducing the terms of (4.4.8) it should be borne in mind that matrix elements of all products independent of electron 1 vanish because of the orthogonality of ϕ_{A_1} and ϕ_{a_1}. The required expression is

$$(\mathbf{p}V^2)_{0n} \cong (\mathbf{p}_1 V_1^2)_{A_1a_1} + 2\sum_{i=2}^{N}\left[\left(\mathbf{p}_i V_i \frac{1}{r_{1i}}\right)_{A_1a_1,\,ii} + \left(\mathbf{p}_i V_1 \frac{1}{r_{1j}}\right)_{A_1a_1,\,ii}\right.$$

$$\left. + \left(\mathbf{p}_1 V_i \frac{1}{r_{1i}}\right)_{A_1a_1,\,ii} + \left(\mathbf{p}_1 V_1 \frac{1}{r_{1i}}\right)_{A_1a_1,\,ii}\right]$$

$$+ 2\sum_{i\neq j}^{N}\left[\left(\mathbf{p}_i \frac{1}{r_{1i}}\frac{1}{r_{ij}}\right)_{A_1a_1,\,ii,\,jj} + \left(\mathbf{p}_i \frac{1}{r_{1i}}\frac{1}{r_{1j}}\right)_{A_1a_1,\,ii,\,jj}\right.$$

$$+ \left(\mathbf{p}_1 \frac{1}{r_{1i}}\frac{1}{r_{ij}}\right)_{A_1a_1,\,ii,\,jj} + \left(\mathbf{p}_1 \frac{1}{r_{1i}}\frac{1}{r_{1j}}\right)_{A_1a_1,\,ii,\,jj}$$

$$\left. + \left(\mathbf{p}_i \frac{1}{r_{1j}}\frac{1}{r_{1j}}\right)_{A_1a_1,\,ii,\,jj}\right]. \tag{4.4.9}$$

The first three terms in the two summations may be combined; a typical term is

$$\sum_{i=2}^{N}\left(\mathbf{p}_i V_i \frac{1}{r_{1i}}\right)_{A_1a_1,\,ii} + \sum_{i\neq j}^{N}\left(\mathbf{p}_i \frac{1}{r_{ij}}\frac{1}{r_{1i}}\right)_{A_1a_1,\,ii,\,jj}$$

$$= \sum_{i=2}^{N}\left[\mathbf{p}_i\left(V_i + \sum_{j=1}^{N}\left\langle\frac{1}{r_{ij}}\right\rangle_{jj} - \left\langle\frac{1}{r_{1i}}\right\rangle_{a_1a_1}\right)\frac{1}{r_{1i}}\right]_{A_1a_1,\,ii}$$

$$= \sum_{i=2}^{N}\left[\mathbf{p}_i(V_i^{\ddagger} - V_i^{(0)})\frac{1}{r_{1i}}\right]_{A_1a_1,\,ii} - \sum_{i=2}^{N}\left(\mathbf{p}_i \frac{1}{r_{1i}}\left\langle\frac{1}{r_{1i}}\right\rangle_{a_1a_1}\right)_{A_1a_1,\,ii}$$

$$\cong \sum_{i=2}^{N}\left[\mathbf{p}_i(V_i^{\ddagger} - V_i^{(0)})\frac{1}{r_{1i}}\right]_{A_1a_1,\,ii}. \tag{4.4.10}$$

The term $\sum_{i=2}^{N}[\mathbf{p}_i(1/r_{1i})\langle 1/r_{1i}\rangle_{a_1a_1}]_{A_1a_1,ii}$ has been absorbed into the first order expression, because the summand depends on only one vicinal group at a time. It tends to be cancelled by similar terms encountered in the more detailed theory.

By a similar process one obtains the important second order, one electron term

$$(\mathbf{p}_1 V_1^2)_{A_1a_1} + 2\left[\sum_{i=2}^{N}\left(\mathbf{p}_1 V_1 \frac{1}{r_{1i}}\right)_{A_1a_1,\,ii} + \sum_{i\neq j}^{N}\left(\mathbf{p}_1 \frac{1}{r_{1i}}\frac{1}{r_{1j}}\right)_{A_1a_1,\,ii,\,jj}\right]$$

$$\cong [\mathbf{p}_1(V_1^{\ddagger} - V_1^{(0)})^2]_{A_1a_1}. \tag{4.4.11}$$

Equation 4.4.9 may therefore be written

$$(\mathbf{p}V^2)_{0n} \cong [\mathbf{p}_1(V_1^\ddagger - V_1^{(0)})^2]_{A_1a_1} + 2\sum_{i=2}^{N}\left\{\left[\mathbf{p}_i \frac{1}{r_{1i}}(V_1^\ddagger - V_1^{(0)})\right]_{A_1a_1,\,ii} + \left[\mathbf{p}_i \frac{1}{r_{1i}}(V_1^\ddagger - V_1^{(0)})\right]_{A_1a_1,\,ii} + \left[\mathbf{p}_1 \frac{1}{r_{1i}}(V_i^\ddagger - V_i^{(0)})\right]_{A_1a_1,\,ii}\right\} + 2\sum_{i\neq j}\left(\mathbf{p}_i \frac{1}{r_{ij}}\frac{1}{r_{1j}}\right)_{A_1a_1,\,ii,\,jj} \tag{4.4.12}$$

One last simplification can be made by observing that the chromophore is relatively insensitive to minor modifications in the shape of the vicinal groups; it is their location which is of primary importance. The term $V_i^\ddagger - V_i^{(0)}$ represents the difference between the SCF force field in the presence of the chromophore and the approximate one used to obtain the zeroth order vicinal functions. For empirical purposes one may generally assume that the vicinal orbitals satisfy the SCF requirement $V_i^{(0)} = V_i^\ddagger$. This may not be said of $V_1^{(0)}$, for that would defeat the purpose of the theory by initially assuming the degree of dissymmetry we are seeking to calculate. Equation 4.4.12 becomes

$$(\mathbf{p}V^2)_{0n} \cong [\mathbf{p}_1(V_1^\ddagger - V_1^{(0)})^2]_{A_1a_1} + 2\left\{\sum_{i=2}^{N}\left[\mathbf{p}_i \frac{1}{r_{1i}}(V_1^\ddagger - V_1^{(0)})\right]_{A_1a_1,\,ii} + \sum_{i\neq j}^{N}\left(\mathbf{p}_i \frac{1}{r_{ij}}\frac{1}{r_{1j}}\right)_{A_1a_1,\,ii,\,jj}\right\}. \tag{4.4.13}$$

The terms $(V\mathbf{p}V)_{0n}$ and $(V^2\mathbf{p})_{0n}$ are evaluated in an analogous manner with the result

$$\begin{aligned}\mathbf{p}_{0n}^{(2)} = {} & \frac{1}{(E_n - \bar{E})^2}\left\{\left[\mathbf{p}_1(V_1^\ddagger - V_1^{(0)})^2\right]_{A_1a_1} + 2\sum_{i=2}^{N}\left[\mathbf{p}_i \frac{1}{r_{1i}}(V_1^\ddagger - V_1^{(0)})\right]_{A_1a_1,\,ii} \right.\\ & \left. + 2\sum_{i\neq j}^{N}\left(\mathbf{p}_i \frac{1}{r_{ij}}\frac{1}{r_{1j}}\right)_{A_1a_1,\,ii,\,jj}\right\} + \frac{1}{(E_n - \bar{E})(E_0 - \bar{E})}\left\{[(V_1^\ddagger - V_1^{(0)})\right.\\ & \times \mathbf{p}_1(V_1^\ddagger - V_1^{(0)})]_{A_1a_1} + \sum_{i=2}^{N}\left[\frac{1}{r_{1i}}\mathbf{p}_i(V_1^\ddagger - V_1^{(0)}) + (V_1^\ddagger - V_1^{(0)})\right.\\ & \left.\left. \times \mathbf{p}_i \frac{1}{r_{1i}}\right]_{A_1a_1,\,ii} + \sum_{i\neq j}^{N}\left(\frac{1}{r_{ij}}\mathbf{p}_i\frac{1}{r_{1j}} + \frac{1}{r_{1j}}\mathbf{p}_i\frac{1}{r_{ij}}\right)_{A_1a_1,\,ii,\,jj}\right\}\\ & + \frac{1}{(E_0 - E)^2}\left\{[(V_1^\ddagger - V_1^{(0)})^2\mathbf{p}_1]_{A_1a_1} + 2\sum_{i=2}^{N}\left[(V_1^\ddagger - V_1^{(0)})\frac{1}{r_{1i}}\mathbf{p}_i\right]_{A_1a_1,\,ii}\right.\\ & \left. + 2\sum_{i\neq j}^{N}\left(\frac{1}{r_{ij}}\frac{1}{r_{1j}}\mathbf{p}_i\right)_{A_1a_1,\,ii,\,jj}\right\}.\end{aligned} \tag{4.4.14}$$

The first order exchange terms are tractable and well worth including. The complete integral to be considered is

$$\left\langle \Psi_0 | \mathbf{p}V | \Psi\begin{pmatrix} A_1 \\ a_1 \end{pmatrix} \right\rangle = \frac{1}{N!} \int_1 \cdots \int_N \Bigg[|\phi_{A_1}(1)\bar{\phi}_{A_1}(2) \cdots$$

$$\phi_{A_i}(2i-1)\bar{\phi}_{A_i}(2i) \cdots \phi_{A_{N/2}}(N-1)\bar{\phi}_{A_{N/2}}(N)| \left(\sum_{i=1}^{N} \mathbf{p}_i \right) \left(\sum_{i=1}^{N} V_i + \sum_{i>j=1}^{N} \frac{1}{r_{ij}} \right)$$

$$\times |\phi_{a_1}(1)\bar{\phi}_{A_1}(2) \cdots \phi_{A_i}(2i-1)\bar{\phi}_{A_i}(2i) \cdots \phi_{A_{N/2}}(N-1)\bar{\phi}_{A_{N/2}}(N)| \Bigg] d\tau_1 \cdots d\tau_N. \tag{4.4.15}$$

The single exchange terms are obtained by interchanging one pair of coordinates. If electron 1 is involved, the terms will be

$$-\sum_{i=2}^{N/2} \iint \phi_{A_1}(1)\phi_{A_i}(2) \left[(\mathbf{p}_1 + \mathbf{p}_2) \left(V_1 + V_2 + \sum_{j \neq 2}^{N} \frac{1}{r_{1j}} + \sum_{j \neq 1}^{N} \frac{1}{r_{2j}} + \frac{1}{r_{12}} \right) \right]$$

$$\times \phi_{A_i}(1)\phi_{a_1}(2)\, d\tau_1\, d\tau_2,$$

where it is understood that this is to be integrated with respect to the other $N-2$ coordinates.

Since both $\int \phi_{A_1}(1)\phi_{A_i}(1)\, d\tau_1$ and $\int \phi_{A_i}(2)\phi_{a_1}(2)\, d\tau_2$ are assumed to be zero, the matrix elements of operators not depending on both coordinates will vanish. This leads to the result

$$\iint \phi_{A_1}(1)\phi_{A_i}(2)(\mathbf{p}V)\phi_{Ai}(1)\phi_{a_1}(2)\, d\tau_1\, d\tau_2$$

$$= \mathbf{p}_{A_1A_i}\left(V_1 + \sum_{j \neq 1}^{N} \left\langle \frac{1}{r_{1j}} \right\rangle_{jj} \right)_{A_ia_1} + \mathbf{p}_{A_ia_1}\left(V_1 + \sum_{j \neq i}^{N} \left\langle \frac{1}{r_{1j}} \right\rangle_{jj} \right)_{A_1a_i}$$

$$+ \left(\mathbf{p}_1 \frac{1}{r_{12}} + \mathbf{p}_2 \frac{1}{r_{12}} \right)_{A_1A_i,\, A_ia_1}$$

$$= \mathbf{p}_{A_1A_i}[V^{\ddagger}(1i)]_{A_ia_1} + \mathbf{p}_{A_ia_1}[V^{\ddagger}(1i)]_{A_1A_i}$$

$$+ \left(\mathbf{p}_1 \frac{1}{r_{12}} + \mathbf{p}_2 \frac{1}{r_{12}} \right)_{A_1A_i,\, A_ia_1}, \tag{4.4.16}$$

where $V^{\ddagger}(1i)$ is understood to be the difference between the zeroth order potential and the SCF potential excluding the orbitals ϕ_{A_1}, ϕ_{a_1}, and ϕ_{A_i}.

A second type of single exchange term is obtained when the coordinates of ϕ_{A_i} and ϕ_{A_j} are permuted. This leads to the integral

$$-\sum_{i,j=2}^{N/2} \iiint \phi_{A_1}(1)\phi_{A_i}(2)\phi_{A_j}(3)(\mathbf{p}V)\phi_{a_1}(1)\phi_{A_j}(2)\phi_{A_i}(3)\, d\tau_1\, d\tau_2\, d\tau_3.$$

The only surviving terms are

$$-\sum_{i,j=2}^{N/2}\left(\mathbf{p}_1\frac{1}{r_{23}}+\mathbf{p}_2\frac{1}{r_{13}}+\mathbf{p}_3\frac{1}{r_{12}}\right)_{A_1a_1,\,A_iA_j,\,A_jA_i}$$

The term $\mathbf{p}_{A_1a_1}(1/r_{12})_{A_iA_j,A_jA_i}$ is merely a correction to the zeroth order transition moment and may be omitted. The other terms cancel in pairs, because

$$\int\phi_{A_i}(2)\mathbf{p}_2\phi_{A_j}(2)\,d\tau_2=-\int\phi_{A_j}(3)\mathbf{p}_3\phi_{A_i}(3)\,d\tau_3.$$

The only other nonvanishing exchange terms arise from the double permutation of three coordinates, leading to the terms

$$\sum_{i,j=2}^{N/2}\left[\iiint\phi_{A_1}(1)\phi_{A_i}(2)\phi_{A_j}(3)\left(\mathbf{p}_1\frac{1}{r_{23}}+\mathbf{p}_2\frac{1}{r_{13}}+\mathbf{p}_3\frac{1}{r_{12}}\right)\right.$$
$$\times\,\phi_{A_i}(1)\phi_{A_j}(2)\phi_{a_1}(3)\,d\tau_1\,d\tau_2\,d\tau_3+\iiint\phi_{A_1}(1)\phi_{A_i}(2)\phi_{A_j}(3)$$
$$\left.\times\left(\mathbf{p}_1\frac{1}{r_{23}}+\mathbf{p}_2\frac{1}{r_{13}}+\mathbf{p}_3\frac{1}{r_{12}}\right)\phi_{A_j}(1)\phi_{a_1}(2)\phi_{A_i}(3)\,d\tau_1\,d\tau_2\,d\tau_3\right].$$

The complete first order exchange terms are

$$\mathbf{p}^{(1)}(E)=\left(\frac{1}{E_n-\bar{E}}+\frac{1}{E_0-\bar{E}}\right)\left\{-\left[\sum_{i=2}^{N/2}\mathbf{p}_{A_1A_i}[V^{\ddagger}(1i)]_{A_ia_1}\right.\right.$$
$$\left.+\,\mathbf{p}_{A_ia_1}[V^{\ddagger}(1i)]_{A_1A_i}+\left\langle A_1A_i\left|\,\mathbf{p}_1\frac{1}{r_{1i}}+\mathbf{p}_i\frac{1}{r_{1i}}\right|A_ia_1\right\rangle\right]$$
$$+\sum_{i,j=2}^{N/2}\left\langle A_1A_iA_j\left|\,\mathbf{p}_1\frac{1}{r_{ij}}+\mathbf{p}_i\frac{1}{r_{1j}}+\mathbf{p}_j\frac{1}{r_{1i}}\right|A_iA_ja_1\right\rangle$$
$$\left.+\sum_{i,j=2}^{N/2}\left\langle A_1A_iA_j\left|\,\mathbf{p}_1\frac{1}{r_{ij}}+\mathbf{p}_i\frac{1}{r_{1j}}+\mathbf{p}_j\frac{1}{r_{1i}}\right|A_ja_1A_i\right\rangle\right\}\qquad(4.4.17a)$$

$$\mathbf{m}^{(1)}(E)=\left(\frac{1}{E_n-\bar{E}}+\frac{1}{E_0-\bar{E}}\right)\left\{-\left[\mathbf{m}_{A_iA_1}[V^{\ddagger}(1i)]_{a_1A_i}\right.\right.$$
$$\left.+\,\mathbf{m}_{a_1A_i}[V^{\ddagger}(1i)]_{A_1A_i}+\left\langle a_1A_i\left|\,\frac{1}{r_{1i}}\mathbf{m}_1+\frac{1}{r_{1i}}\mathbf{m}_i\right|A_iA_1\right\rangle\right]$$
$$+\sum_{i,j=2}^{N/2}\left\langle A_i\;A_ja_1\left|\,\frac{1}{r_{ij}}\mathbf{m}_1+\frac{1}{r_{1j}}\mathbf{m}_i+\frac{1}{r_{1i}}\mathbf{m}_j\right|A_1A_iA_j\right\rangle$$
$$\left.+\sum_{i,j=2}^{N/2}\left\langle A_ja_1A_i\left|\,\frac{1}{r_{ij}}\mathbf{m}_1+\frac{1}{r_{1j}}\mathbf{m}_i+\frac{1}{r_{1i}}\mathbf{m}_j\right|A_1A_iA_j\right\rangle\right\}.\qquad(4.4.17b)$$

The $E_n - \bar{E}$ and $E_0 - \bar{E}$ terms are identical because

$$\mathbf{p}_1 \frac{1}{r_{1i}} + \mathbf{p}_i \frac{1}{r_{1i}} = 0 \qquad \text{and} \qquad \mathbf{m}_1 \frac{1}{r_{1i}} + \mathbf{m}_i \frac{1}{r_{1i}} = 0.$$

The general perturbation terms to first order in exchange and second order in nonexchange are embodied in (4.4.6), (4.4.14), and (4.4.17). It is probably not profitable to attempt a general derivation of higher order terms, but there is one relatively simple addition which may have far-reaching consequences. The most efficient way for effects to be propagated through unconjugated bonds is via a correlation chain where one electron acts on a second, which in turn acts on a third, etc. This immediately suggests the consideration of the term

$$\frac{1}{(E_n - \bar{E})^Q} \sum \left(\mathbf{p}_i \overbrace{\frac{1}{r_{ij}} \frac{1}{r_{jk}} \cdots \frac{1}{r_{st}} \frac{1}{t_{t1}}}^{Q}\right)_{A_1a_1,\, ii,\, jj,\, kk,\, \ldots\, ss,\, tt},$$

where $\overbrace{\quad}^{Q}$ indicates that Q factors are present. The effect of each intervening bond is described by a factor $1/(E_n - \bar{E})r_{ij}$ in the integrand, which introduces an approximately constant attenuation factor for each bond between the chromophore and the dissymmetrically oriented perturbing group. Such a term is much more likely to be of importance as a contribution to the magnetic moment, where it would behave in a similar manner to the classical coupled oscillator effect.

4.5. Critique of the Approximations

It is not possible to give general completely reduced expressions for all the terms derived in the previous section. We can, however, outline general methods, the details of which will depend on the molecular system. There is one prevalent shortcoming which must be guarded against. It is possible to lose important terms depending on energy differences; this immediately follows from the nature of the approximation, in which the denominators $(E_n - E_i)$ in a summation are replaced by an average $(E_n - \bar{E})$. This can often be remedied by converting from $\mathbf{p}$ to $\boldsymbol{\mu}$, provided no origin dependence is introduced.

For example, consider the evaluation of

$$\sum_{i=2}^{N} \left(\frac{1}{r_{1i}} \mathbf{m}_i\right)_{a_1A_1,\, ii} = \sum_{i=2}^{N} \int \phi_{A_1}(1)\phi_{a_1}(1) \left\langle \phi_{A_i} \left| \frac{1}{r_{1i}} \mathbf{m}_i \right| \phi_{A_i} \right\rangle d\tau_1. \quad (4.5.1)$$

Since $\langle \phi_{A_i} | (1/r_{1i})\mathbf{m}_i | \phi_{A_i} \rangle = \langle \phi_{A_i} | \mathbf{m}_i(1/r_{1i}) | \phi_{A_i} \rangle^*$ for diagonal matrix elements of operator products, the use of a simple identity allows one to write

$$\left\langle \phi_{A_i} \left| \frac{1}{r_{1i}} \mathbf{m}_i \right| \phi_{A_i} \right\rangle = \frac{1}{2}\left(\left\langle \phi_{A_i} \left| \frac{1}{r_{1i}} \mathbf{m}_i \right| \phi_{A_i} \right\rangle + \left\langle \phi_{A_i} \left| \mathbf{m}_i \frac{1}{r_{1i}} \right| \phi_{A_i} \right\rangle \right.$$
$$\left. + \left\langle \phi_{A_i} \left| \frac{1}{r_{1i}} \mathbf{m}_i - \mathbf{m}_i \frac{1}{r_{1i}} \right| \phi_{A_i} \right\rangle \right)$$
$$= -\frac{1}{2} \left\langle \phi_{A_i} \left| -i \left[\frac{e\hbar}{2mc} \right] \frac{\mathbf{r}_i \times \mathbf{r}_1}{r_{1i}^3} \right| \phi_{A_i} \right\rangle. \tag{4.5.2}$$

The last step occurs because the matrix elements of real wave functions are pure imaginary, and the sum of such a quantity and its complex conjugate is zero. The remaining term is the commutator of $1/r_{1i}$ and $\mathbf{m}_i$. Equation 4.5.1 then becomes

$$\sum_{i=2}^{N} \left(\frac{1}{r_{1i}} \mathbf{m}_i \right)_{a_1 A_1, ii} \simeq \frac{i\hbar}{4mc} \frac{\mathbf{R}_i}{R_{1i}^3} \times \boldsymbol{\mu}_{a_1 A_1}. \tag{4.5.3}$$

The scalar product of this leading term with $\mathbf{p}_{A_1 a_1}$ vanishes, unlike the coupled oscillator term to which it is an approximation. The alternative procedure is to first write the original perturbation summation as

$$\int \phi_{A_1}(1)\phi_{a_1}(1) \left[\sum_q \left(\frac{1}{r_{1i}} \right)_{0q} (\mathbf{m}_i)_{q0} \frac{1}{h(\nu_{0n} - \nu_{oq})} \right] d\tau_1$$
$$\simeq \frac{\pi i \mathbf{R}_i}{hc} \times \left\{ \int \phi_{A_1}(1)\phi_{a_1}(1) \left[\sum_q \left(\frac{1}{r_{1i}} \right)_{0q} \boldsymbol{\mu}_{q0} \frac{\nu_{0q}}{\nu_{0n} - \nu_{oq}} \right] d\tau_1 \right\}.$$

A result comparable to the polarizability formula in Chapter 3 may be derived in terms of the quadrupole moment tensor. One may replace $\nu_{0q}/(\nu_{0n} - \nu_{0q})$ by an average value $\bar{\nu}_n/(\nu_{0n} - \bar{\nu}_n)$ and carry out the summation

$$\sum_{q \neq 0} \left(\frac{1}{r_{1i}} \right)_{0q} (\boldsymbol{\mu}_i)_{q0} = \left(\frac{\boldsymbol{\mu}_i}{r_{1i}} \right)_{00} - (\boldsymbol{\mu})_{00}(r_{1i}^{-1})_{\upsilon 0}.$$

The development now proceeds along the lines of Chapter 3, where the expansion $1/r_{1i} - \mathbf{r}_1 \cdot \mathbf{T} \cdot \mathbf{r}_i$ $[\mathbf{T} = (1/R_{1i}^3)(\mathbf{I} - 3\mathbf{R}_{1i}\mathbf{R}_{1i})]$ is used. This gives

$$\int \phi_{A_1}(1)\phi_{a_1}(1) \left[\sum_q \left(\frac{1}{r_{1i}} \right)_{0q} (\mathbf{m}_i)_{q0} \frac{1}{h(\nu_{0n} - \nu_{0q})} \right]$$
$$\cong \frac{\pi i \mathbf{R}_i}{hc} \times \left(\frac{\bar{\nu}_n}{\nu_{0n} - \bar{\nu}_n} \mathbf{Q} \cdot \mathbf{T} \cdot \boldsymbol{\mu}_{A_1 a_1} \right), \tag{4.5.4}$$

where $\mathbf{Q} = (\mathbf{r}_i\,\mathbf{r}_i)_{ii}$ is the quadrupole moment tensor contribution from the ith orbital. This result is entirely equivalent to the polarizability formula and has the same geometrical dependence.

The term above is accompanied by the first order correction to the momentum

$$\int \phi_{A_1}(1)\phi_{a_1}(1)\left[\sum_q (\mathbf{p}_i)_{0q}\left(\frac{1}{r_{1i}}\right)_{q0}\frac{1}{h(\nu_{0n}-\nu_{0q})}\right] d\tau_1$$

$$\cong -\,2\pi i m \frac{\bar{\nu}_n}{\nu_{0n}-\bar{\nu}_n}\,\mathbf{Q}\cdot\mathbf{T}\cdot\boldsymbol{\mu}_{A_1a_1}. \qquad (4.5.5)$$

The sum of the two appropriate scalar products is

$$\mathbf{p}_{A_1a_1}\cdot\mathbf{m}^{(1)}_{a_1A_1} + \mathbf{p}^{(1)}_{A_1a_1}\cdot\mathbf{m}_{a_1A_1}$$

$$= \frac{\pi i}{hc}\frac{\bar{\nu}_n}{\nu_{0n}-\bar{\nu}_n}\,\mathbf{p}_{A_1a_1}\times(\mathbf{R}_i-\mathbf{R}_1)\cdot\mathbf{Q}\cdot\mathbf{T}\cdot\boldsymbol{\mu}_{A_1a_1}, \qquad (4.5.6)$$

which is independent of origin despite the conversion from momentum to electric moment operators.

The nature of this type of approximation can be seen by considering the polarizability tensor itself:

$$\boldsymbol{\alpha} = \frac{2}{h}\sum_n \frac{\nu_{0n}\,\boldsymbol{\mu}_{0n}\,\boldsymbol{\mu}_{n0}}{\nu_{0n}^2-\nu^2}. \qquad (4.5.7)$$

If one first assumes that $\nu_{0n}/(\nu_{0n}-\nu^2) \simeq \bar{\nu}/(\bar{\nu}^2-\nu^2)$, then

$$\boldsymbol{\alpha}' = \frac{2}{h}\frac{\bar{\nu}}{\bar{\nu}^2-\nu^2}\left[(\boldsymbol{\mu}\boldsymbol{\mu})_{00} - \boldsymbol{\mu}_{00}\,\boldsymbol{\mu}_{00}\right]. \qquad (4.5.8)$$

On the other hand if it is assumed that $1/(\nu_{0n}^2-\nu^2) \cong 1/(\bar{\nu}^2-\nu^2)$, one obtains

$$\boldsymbol{\alpha}'' = \frac{2}{h}\frac{1}{\bar{\nu}^2-\nu^2}\sum_{n\neq 0}\nu_{0n}\,\boldsymbol{\mu}_{0n}\,\boldsymbol{\mu}_{n0}$$

$$= \frac{2}{h}\frac{1}{\bar{\nu}^2-\nu^2}\frac{e}{2\pi i m}\sum_{n\neq 0}\boldsymbol{\mu}_{0n}\,\mathbf{p}_{n0} = N\frac{e^2}{4\pi^2 m}\frac{1}{\bar{\nu}^2-\nu^2}\,\mathbf{I}, \qquad (4.5.9)$$

where N is the number of electrons.

The second approximation, which embodies the argument of the Kuhn-Thomas sum rule, gives an isotropic result proportional to the number of electrons; whereas the first approximation preserves the anisotropic property of the group by relating the polarizability to the quadrupole moment tensor. A relation to the number of electrons is also to be found, since

$$[(\boldsymbol{\mu}_1+\boldsymbol{\mu}_2+\cdots)(\boldsymbol{\mu}_1+\boldsymbol{\mu}_2+\cdots)]_{00}$$

increases with N just as does

$$[(\boldsymbol{\mu}_1 + \boldsymbol{\mu}_2 + \cdots)(\mathbf{p}_1 + \mathbf{p}_2 + \cdots)]_{00}.$$

A second type of difficulty is encountered when $[\mathbf{p}(V^{\ddagger} - V^{(0)})]_{A_1a_1}$ or $[\mathbf{p}(V^{\ddagger} - V^{(0)})^2]_{A_1a_1}$ vanishes. Invariably this is a peculiar manifestation of the model and zeroth order wave function. For example, in the theory of transition metal complexes zeroth order functions with octahedral ($\mathcal{O}_h$) symmetry have generally been used. For certain types of perturbation both first and second order terms vanish. One could equally well use distorted $3d$ orbitals in the zeroth order functions to avoid this difficulty.

The evaluation of the term $\sum_{q\neq n} 1/(E_n - E_2)(\mathbf{p}_i)_{0q}[(1/r_{1i})_{qn}]$ proceeds in a similar manner. It may be summed in two alternative ways:

$$\sum_{q\neq n} \frac{1}{E_n - E_q} (\mathbf{p}_i)_{0q} \left(\frac{1}{r_{1i}}\right)_{qn} \simeq \frac{1}{E_n - \bar{E}} \left(\mathbf{p}_i \frac{1}{r_{1i}}\right)_{0n} = \frac{1}{2} \frac{-i\hbar}{E_n - \bar{E}} \left(\frac{\mathbf{r}_1 - \mathbf{r}_i}{r_{1i}^3}\right)_{0n} \tag{4.5.10a}$$

$$\sum_{q\neq n} \frac{1}{E_n - E_q} (\mathbf{p}_i)_{0q} \left(\frac{1}{r_{1i}}\right)_{qn} = -2\pi i m \sum_{q\neq n} \frac{\nu_{0q}}{E_n - E_q} (\mathbf{r}_i)_{0q} \left(\frac{1}{r_{1i}}\right)_{qn}$$

$$\cong -\frac{2\pi i m}{E_n - \bar{E}} \bar{\nu}_n \left[\left(\mathbf{r}_i \frac{1}{r_{1i}}\right)_{0n} - (\mathbf{r}_i)_{00} \left(\frac{1}{r_{1i}}\right)_{0n}\right]. \tag{4.5.10b}$$

The term $(\mathbf{r}_i)_{00}(1/r_{1i})_{0n}$ appears in the second part because $\nu_{00} = 0$, and one is not entitled to include it in the summation. This has the effect of ensuring that (4.5.10*b*) is independent of origin.

The factors $\mathbf{r}_i/r_{1i}$ and $\mathbf{r}_{1i}/r_{1i}^3$ may be approximated by the multipole expansion; the origins for measuring $\mathbf{r}_1$ and $\mathbf{r}_i$ will be taken as the center of charges for the ground state. If $\mathbf{R}_{1i}$ is the vector distance from 1 to i, one has

$$\mathbf{r}_{1i} = \mathbf{R}_{1i} + \mathbf{r}_i - \mathbf{r}_1 \tag{4.5.11a}$$

$$r_{1i} = R_{1i}\sqrt{1 + (1/R_{1i}^2)(r_1^2 + r_i^2 + 2\mathbf{R}_{1i}\cdot\mathbf{r}_i - 2\mathbf{R}_{1i}\cdot\mathbf{r}_1 - 2\mathbf{r}_i\cdot\mathbf{r}_1)}. \tag{4.5.11b}$$

Owing to the choice of origin the second term in (4.5.10*b*) is zero. In the expansion of $1/r_{1i}$ one must seek those terms with the factor $\mathbf{r}_i$, since $(\mathbf{r}_i)_{ii} = 0$. Furthermore the orthogonality of ϕ_{A_1} and ϕ_{a_1} requires the presence of factors in $\mathbf{r}_1$ or $\mathbf{r}_1\mathbf{r}_1$. The appropriate terms will contain both r_1 and r_i factors. The result is

$$\frac{\mathbf{r}_i}{r_{1i}} = \frac{\mathbf{r}_i}{R_{1i}}\left\{1 + \mathbf{r}_1 \cdot \frac{\mathbf{r}_i}{R_{1i}^2} + \frac{3}{R_{1i}^4}[(\mathbf{R}_{1i}\cdot\mathbf{r}_1)(\mathbf{r}_1\cdot\mathbf{r}_i) - (\mathbf{R}_{1i}\cdot\mathbf{r}_i)(\mathbf{R}_{1i}\cdot\mathbf{r}_1)] - \frac{15}{2R_{1i}^6}[(\mathbf{R}_{1i}\cdot\mathbf{r}_1)(\mathbf{R}_{1i}\cdot\mathbf{r}_1)(\mathbf{R}_{1i}\cdot\mathbf{r}_i)] + \cdots\right\}. \tag{4.5.12}$$

A typical term is

$$[(\mathbf{R}_{1i}\cdot\mathbf{r}_1)(\mathbf{r}_1\cdot\mathbf{R}_{1i})(\mathbf{R}_{1i}\cdot\mathbf{r}_i)\mathbf{r}_i]_{0n} = \mathbf{R}_{1i}\cdot(\mathbf{Q}_1)_{A_1a_1}\cdot\mathbf{R}_{1i}\mathbf{R}_{1i}\cdot(\mathbf{Q}_i)_{ii},$$

where $\mathbf{Q}_1 = \mathbf{r}_1\mathbf{r}_1$ and $\mathbf{Q}_i = \mathbf{r}_i\mathbf{r}_i$ are the quadrupole moment operators. The desired expression is

$$\left(\frac{\mathbf{r}_i}{r_{1i}}\right)_{0n} = \frac{1}{R_{1i}^3}(\mathbf{r}_1)_{A_1a_1}\cdot\left(\mathbf{I} - \frac{3\mathbf{R}_{1i}\mathbf{R}_{1i}}{R_{1i}^2}\right)\cdot(\mathbf{Q}_i)_{ii} + \frac{3}{R_{1i}^5}$$
$$\times\,[\mathbf{R}_{1i}\cdot(\mathbf{Q}_1)_{A_1a_1}\cdot(\mathbf{Q}_i)_{ii} - (\tfrac{5}{2}\mathbf{R}_{1i}\cdot(\mathbf{Q}_1)_{A_1a_1}\cdot\mathbf{R}_{1i}\mathbf{R}_{1i}\cdot(\mathbf{Q}_i)_{ii})R_{1j}^{-2}] \quad (4.5.13)$$

In a similar manner one obtains

$$\frac{\mathbf{r}_{1i}}{r_{1i}^3} = (\mathbf{R}_{1i} + \mathbf{r}_i - \mathbf{r}_1)\frac{1}{R_{1i}^3}\left\{1 - \frac{3}{2R_{1i}^2}[-2(\mathbf{R}_{1i}\cdot\mathbf{r}_1)] + \frac{15}{8R_{1i}^4}[4(\mathbf{R}_{1i}\cdot\mathbf{r}_1)(\mathbf{R}_{1i}\cdot\mathbf{r}_1)] + \cdots\right\}, \quad (4.5.14)$$

from which it follows that

$$\left(\frac{\mathbf{r}_{1i}}{r_{1i}^3}\right)_{0n} = 3\mathbf{R}_{1i}\left[\frac{\mathbf{R}_{1i}\cdot(\mathbf{r}_1)_{A_1a_1}}{R_{1i}^5}\right] - \frac{3}{R_{1i}^5}$$
$$\times\,[\mathbf{R}_{1i}\cdot(\mathbf{Q}_1)_{A_1a_1} - \tfrac{5}{2}(\mathbf{R}_{1i}\mathbf{R}_{1i}\cdot(\mathbf{Q}_1)_{A_1a_1}\cdot\mathbf{R}_{1i})R_{1j}^{-2}] \quad (4.5.15)$$

The expressions 4.5.13 and 4.5.15 are nearly equivalent as can be seen by reversing the approximation process in (4.5.10). One obtains

$$-2\pi i m\bar{v}_n(\mathbf{r}_i\mathbf{r}_i)_{ii} \simeq \sum_q (\mathbf{p}_i)_{iq}(\mathbf{r}_i)_{qi} = (\mathbf{pr})_{ii}$$
$$= \tfrac{1}{2}(\mathbf{pr} + \mathbf{rp})_{ii} + \tfrac{1}{2}(\mathbf{pr} - \mathbf{rp})_{ii} = -\frac{i\hbar}{2}\mathbf{I}, \quad (4.5.16)$$

where q labels a complete set of one-electron functions. When this approximation is used, both alternatives in (4.5.10) give identical results, as they must. [The term $(\mathbf{r}_1)_{A_1a_1}\cdot\mathbf{I}\cdot(\mathbf{Q}_i)_{ii}$ in (4.5.13) becomes $(\mathbf{r}_1)_{A_1a_1}\cdot\mathbf{I}\cdot\mathbf{I} = (\mathbf{r}_1)_{A_1a_1}$; and it has been omitted in view of its presumed orthogonality to $\mathbf{m}_{a_1A_1}$.] It then follows that the original procedure will be modified only for an $\mathbf{m}_i/\mathbf{r}_{1i}$ term.

The electron correlation term will be discussed in terms of the simpler form of (4.5.10*a*):

$$\frac{1}{E_n - \bar{E}}\left(\mathbf{p}_i\frac{1}{r_{1i}}\right)_{0n} = \frac{1}{2}\frac{i\hbar}{E_n - \bar{E}}$$
$$\times\left\{\frac{3\mathbf{R}_{1i}}{R_{1i}^5}[\mathbf{R}_{1i}\cdot(\mathbf{r}_1)_{A_1a_1}] - \frac{3}{R_{1i}^5}[\mathbf{R}_{1i}\cdot(\mathbf{Q}_1)_{A_1a_1} - \tfrac{5}{2}(\mathbf{R}_{1i}\mathbf{R}_{1i}\cdot(\mathbf{Q}_1)_{A_1a_1}\cdot\mathbf{R}_{1i})]R_{1i}^{-2}\right\}$$
$$(4.5.17)$$

If we confine ourselves to inactive zeroth order systems, there are two distinct cases when $\mathbf{m}_{a_1A_1} \neq 0$: either $\boldsymbol{\mu}_{A_1a_1} = 0$ or $\boldsymbol{\mu}_{A_1a_1} \neq 0$ with $\boldsymbol{\mu}_{A_1a_1} \cdot \mathbf{m}_{a_1A_1} = 0$. In the symmetry groups $C_{nv}(n = 3, 4, \ldots)$, C_{1h}, and D_{2d} certain transitions will have perpendicular electric and magnetic moments; this will be true of all transitions with C_{1h} symmetry. For such systems the leading term in (4.5.17) leads to a rotational strength contribution proportional to $(\boldsymbol{\mu}_{A_1a_1} \cdot \mathbf{R}_{1i})(\mathbf{R}_{1i} \cdot \mathbf{m}_{a_1A_1})/R_{1i}^5$.

If $\boldsymbol{\mu}_{A_1a_1} = 0$, the second term will be nonvanishing whenever $\mathbf{Q}$ has components in the same representation as the appropriate component of $\mathbf{m}$. For example, this will occur for C_{2v} and D_{2h} but not for an $A_{1g} \rightarrow A_{2g}$ transition in $D_{nh}(n > 2)$. It is expected that this term could only be important when $(\boldsymbol{\mu}_1)_{A_1a_1} \neq 0$.

In this chapter the complete exposition of the first and second order contributions to optical activity has been undertaken. This has led to both exchange and nonexchange terms in which the distinction between one electron or SCF contributions and electron correlation effects has proved useful. It is anticipated that each chromophore has its unique characteristics, which will require the emphasis of certain terms at the expense of the others.

CHAPTER 5

Applications to Specific Chromophores

5.1. The Carbonyl Chromophore

It will now be our task to illustrate the use of the formulas developed in Chapter 4 with specific examples. First the carbonyl chromophore will be discussed. The essential features of the general problem are embodied in the cyclopentanone skeleton (Figure 5.1). The zeroth order system will consist

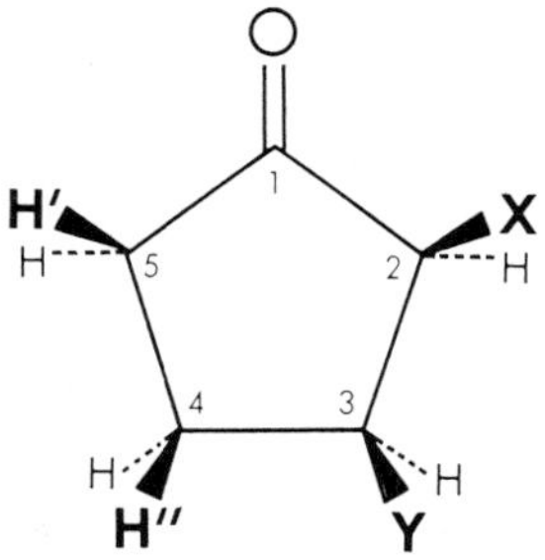

Figure 5.1. The optically active cyclopentanone derivative.

of the nuclei and core electrons, the 14 σ-bonds, the nonbonding electrons, and the two orbitals of the π-system, the ground π and the excited π^*. They are listed in Table 5.1.

This model will also serve for the discussion of single substitution where X or Y is replaced by H'. In the interest of reasonable simplification the practice of considering only exchange effects between the chromophore and α-substituents will be adopted. Since it is simpler, the effect of β-substitution will first be considered. If it is assumed that the n, π, π^*, and σ orbitals of the chromophoric system have the C_{2v} symmetry of formaldehyde, the parallel component of $\mathbf{p}_{A_{1a_1}}$ will be zero. In (4.4.6*a*) the first term to be considered is

$$\frac{1}{E_n - \bar{E}} [\mathbf{p}_1(V_1^{\ddagger} - V_1^{(0)})]_{n\pi^*}.$$

When an empirical relation is desired, a great deal more latitude is available in the choice of zeroth order function. In each instance strong consideration

TABLE 5.1

The Cyclopentanone Orbitals

Orbital Type	Location	Symbol
σ	Carbon atoms 1 and 2	σ_{12}
$\vdots$	$\vdots$	$\vdots$
σ	Carbon atoms 1 and 5	σ_{15}
σ	X and carbon atom 2	σ_{2X}
σ	Y and carbon atom 3	σ_{3Y}
σ	H and carbon atom 2	σ_{2H}
σ	H and carbon atom 3	σ_{3H}
σ	H' and carbon atom 4	$\sigma_{4H'}$
$\vdots$	$\vdots$	$\vdots$
σ	H' and carbon atom 5	$\sigma_{5H'}$
σ	Carbon and oxygen	σ
π	Carbon and oxygen	π
π^*	Carbon and oxygen	π^*
n	Oxygen	n

should be given to dissymmetric functions. No general rule can be given; it will often be wise to think in terms of active and inactive zeroth order states. In this first example C_{2v} symmetry will be considered the starting point. The logical choice here is the unsubstituted cyclopentanone. The n, π, π^*, and σ functions will be solutions to this SCF problem. It then follows that

$$V_1^{\ddagger} - V_1^{(0)} = \int \frac{\sigma_{3y}^2(2)}{r_{12}}\, d\tau_2 - \int \frac{\sigma_{3H'}^2(2)}{r_{12}}\, d\tau_2 + \sum_i \int \frac{\psi_{Yi}^2(2)}{r_{12}}\, d\tau_2 - \sum_i \frac{Z_{Yi}}{r_{Yi}}, \tag{5.1.1}$$

where the ψ_{Yi} are the other orbitals in group Y and Z_{Yi} are the various nuclear charges.

For the moment various refinements in the estimation of V will be overlooked in favor of the simpler approach of replacing the group with a monopole, dipole, and quadrupole moment. These will be scalar, vector, and tensor quantities respectively with symbols ε, $\boldsymbol{\sigma}$, and $\boldsymbol{\Omega}$. Let us assume that the SCF potential of any group may be approximated by the form

$$V_i = -\left(\frac{\varepsilon_i}{r_{1i}} + \frac{\sigma_i \cdot \mathbf{r}_{1i}}{r_{1i}^3} + \frac{\mathbf{r}_{1i} \cdot \boldsymbol{\Omega}_i \cdot \mathbf{r}_{1i}}{r_{1i}^5} + \cdots\right). \tag{5.1.2}$$

The reciprocal powers of $r_{1i}(\mathbf{r}_{1i} = \mathbf{R}_{1i} - \mathbf{r}_1)$ may be obtained by the usual power series method in which r_1^2 terms are omitted, because only the lowest order nonvanishing terms are meaningful. For the purposes of this expansion one may write

$$\frac{1}{r_{1i}} = \frac{1}{R_{1i}}\left(1 + \frac{r_1^2 - 2\mathbf{r}_1 \cdot \mathbf{R}_{1i}}{R_{1i}^2}\right)^{-1/2} \simeq \frac{1}{R_{1i}}\left(1 - \frac{2\mathbf{r}_1 \cdot \mathbf{R}_{1i}}{R_{1i}^2}\right)^{-1/2} \tag{5.1.3}$$

The power series expansions of $(1 - x)^{-1/2}$, $(1 - x)^{-3/2}$, and $(1 - x)^{-5/2}$, where $x = 2\mathbf{r}_1 \cdot \mathbf{R}_{1i}/R_{1i}^2$, allow us to write

$$\frac{1}{r_{1i}} = \frac{1}{R} + \frac{\mathbf{r}_1 \cdot \mathbf{R}}{R^3} + \frac{3}{2R^5}\mathbf{R} \cdot \mathbf{Q}_1 \cdot \mathbf{R} + \cdots \tag{5.1.4a}$$

$$\frac{\boldsymbol{\sigma} \cdot \mathbf{r}_{1i}}{r_{1i}^3} = \left[\frac{3(\boldsymbol{\sigma} \cdot \mathbf{R})(\mathbf{R} \cdot \mathbf{r}_1)}{R^2} - \boldsymbol{\sigma} \cdot \mathbf{r}_1\right]\frac{1}{R^3} + \left[\frac{15}{2}\frac{(\boldsymbol{\sigma} \cdot \mathbf{R})(\mathbf{R} \cdot \mathbf{Q}_1 \cdot \mathbf{R})}{R^2} - 3(\boldsymbol{\sigma} \cdot \mathbf{Q}_1 \cdot \mathbf{R})\right]\frac{1}{R^5} + \cdots \tag{5.1.4b}$$

$$\frac{\mathbf{r}_{1i} \cdot \boldsymbol{\Omega}_i \cdot \mathbf{r}_{1i}}{r_{1i}^5} = \left[\frac{5(\mathbf{R} \cdot \boldsymbol{\Omega} \cdot \mathbf{R})(\mathbf{r}_1 \cdot \mathbf{R})}{R^3} - \frac{2(\mathbf{r}_1 \cdot \boldsymbol{\Omega} \cdot \mathbf{R})}{R}\right]\frac{1}{R^4} + \left[\frac{35}{2}\frac{(\mathbf{R} \cdot \boldsymbol{\Omega} \cdot \mathbf{R})(\mathbf{R} \cdot \mathbf{Q}_1 \cdot \mathbf{R})}{R^4} - \frac{10(\mathbf{R} \cdot \boldsymbol{\Omega} \cdot \mathbf{Q}_1 \cdot \mathbf{R})}{R^2} + \mathbf{r}_1 \cdot \boldsymbol{\Omega} \cdot \mathbf{r}_1\right]\frac{1}{R^5}, \tag{5.1.4c}$$

where $Q_1 = \mathbf{r}_1\mathbf{r}_1$ is $1/e$ times the quadrupole moment for electron 1 and the subscript **R** has been dropped.

In cyclopentanone the $n \to \pi^*$ transition is $A_1 \to A_2$ in the C_{2v} symmetry group. The product $\phi_{A_1}\phi_{a_1}$ transforms like xy. The matrix element $e(\mathbf{p}_1 V_1)_{A_1a_1}$ may be written in terms of the electric moment in the usual manner:

$$e(\mathbf{p}_1 V_1)_{A_1a_1} = -2\pi i m \sum_q \nu_{A_1q}\boldsymbol{\mu}_{A_1q}V_{qa_1}$$

$$\simeq -2\pi i m\bar{\nu}_{A_1}[(\boldsymbol{\mu}_1 V_1)_{A_1a_1} - \boldsymbol{\mu}_{A_1A_1}V_{A_1a_1}]. \tag{5.1.5}$$

The subtraction of the $\boldsymbol{\mu}_{A_1A_1}V_{A_1a_1}$ term compensates for the vanishing of $\mathbf{p}_{A_1A_1}$ and $\nu_{A_1A_1}$. It is emphasized that $\boldsymbol{\mu}_{A_1A_1}$ is the dipole moment of the ϕ_{A_1} orbital and not the entire group or molecule. In view of the C_{2v} symmetry the center of the ϕ_{A_1} orbital ($\boldsymbol{\mu}_{A_1A_1} = 0$) does not in general coincide with the center of the product $\phi_{A_1}\phi_{a_1}$; this would only be true for D_{2h} symmetry. If z is measured along the carbonyl bond axis,

$$\langle\phi_{A_1}| x_1y_1z_1 |\phi_{a_1}\rangle \neq 0.$$

The lowest order nonvanishing terms in the expansions of (5.1.4) will involve the quadripole moment, which takes the form $(\mathbf{ij}+\mathbf{ji})x_1y_1$. In view of the empirical nature of this investigation one is justified only in retaining the symmetrical $\mathbf{R}\cdot\mathbf{Q}_1\cdot\mathbf{R}$ terms for simplicity; others may be added if this initial attempt absolutely fails to correlate the experimental data. This leads to the result

$$(\mathbf{p}_1V_1)_{A_1a_1} = +2\pi im\bar{v}_{A_1}\mathbf{k}\langle\phi_{A_1}|\,x_1y_1z_1\,|\phi_{a_1}\rangle \times 2\gamma_X\gamma_Y\left[\frac{3\varepsilon}{2R^3}+\frac{15}{2R^5}(\boldsymbol{\sigma}\cdot\mathbf{R})+\frac{35}{2R^7}\mathbf{R}\cdot\boldsymbol{\Omega}\cdot\mathbf{R}\right]. \quad (5.1.6)$$

This embodies the familiar quadrant rule so often used in the study of the carbonyl group along with additional terms having an orientation dependence.

For the α-substituent it will be necessary to investigate the exchange terms in (4.4.17*a*). Exchange may take place among the orbitals n, π, π^*, σ, σ_{12}, σ_{2X}, and σ_{2H}. The symmetry of the system reduces the problem to a consideration of the difference between the exchange properties of the σ_{2X} and $\sigma_{2H'}$ orbitals.

The situation is simplified by considering overlap only between orbitals on adjacent atoms. For the $n\rightarrow\pi^*$ transition this will eliminate the single exchange terms, because they will all depend upon the overlap between the σ_{2X} or $\sigma_{2H'}$ and the nonbonding orbital, which may be considered to be centered primarily on oxygen. Any such integrals must include either the σ_{2X} or $\sigma_{2H'}$ orbital in addition to the n and π^* orbitals; otherwise the resulting charge distribution will have a plane of symmetry. This leaves for the intermediate state the π, σ, or σ_{12} orbitals. The double exchange terms for the π-orbital from (4.4.17*a*) are

$$\left\langle n(1)\pi(2)\sigma_{2X}(3)\left|\,\mathbf{p}_1\frac{1}{r_{23}}+\mathbf{p}_2\frac{1}{r_{13}}+\mathbf{p}_3\frac{1}{r_{12}}\right|\pi(1)\sigma_{2X}(2)\pi^*(3)\right\rangle$$
$$= \mathbf{p}_{n\pi}\left\langle\pi(1)\sigma_{2X}(2)\left|\frac{1}{r_{12}}\right|\sigma_{2X}(1)\pi^*(2)\right\rangle+\mathbf{p}_{\pi\sigma_{2X}}\left\langle n(1)\sigma_{2X}(2)\left|\frac{1}{r_{12}}\right|\pi(1)\pi^*(2)\right\rangle$$
$$+\mathbf{p}_{\sigma_{2X}\pi^*}\left\langle n(1)\pi(2)\left|\frac{1}{r_{12}}\right|\pi(1)\sigma_{2X}(2)\right\rangle \quad (5.1.7a)$$

$$\left\langle n(1)\pi(2)\sigma_{2X}(3)\left|\,\mathbf{p}_1\frac{1}{r_{23}}+\mathbf{p}_2\frac{1}{r_{13}}+\mathbf{p}_3\frac{1}{r_{12}}\right|\sigma_{2X}(1)\pi^*(2)\pi(3)\right\rangle$$
$$= \mathbf{p}_{n\sigma_{2X}}\left\langle\pi(1)\sigma_{2X}(2)\left|\frac{1}{r_{12}}\right|\pi^*(1)\pi(2)\right\rangle+\mathbf{p}_{\pi\pi^*}\left\langle n(1)\sigma_{2X}(2)\left|\frac{1}{r_{12}}\right|\sigma_{2X}(1)\pi(2)\right\rangle$$
$$+\mathbf{p}_{\sigma_{2X}\pi}\left\langle n(1)\pi(2)\left|\frac{1}{r_{12}}\right|\sigma_{2X}(1)\pi^*(2)\right\rangle. \quad (5.1.7b)$$

The second set of terms may be neglected in comparison to the first because of the small overlap between the n and σ_{2X} orbitals. The moment $\mathbf{p}_{n\pi}$ vanishes by symmetry, leaving only two terms, which tend to cancel by virtue of the fact that $\mathbf{p}_{\pi\sigma_{2X}} \simeq \mathbf{p}_{\sigma_{2X}\pi^*}$ and

$$\left\langle n(1)\sigma_{2X}(2)\left|\frac{1}{r_{12}}\right|\pi(1)\pi^*(2)\right\rangle \simeq \left\langle n(1)\pi(2)\left|\frac{1}{r_{12}}\right|\pi(1)\sigma_{2X}(2)\right\rangle.$$

A similar set of terms is encountered for the σ and σ_{12} orbitals. Again the σ terms may be neglected, because the σ-orbital is unfavorably oriented for overlap with the σ_{2X}. In any event a more detailed analysis shows that these neglected terms have essentially the same geometrical dependence as the σ_{12} principal term.

As above, only three terms need be considered:

$$\begin{aligned}
&\left\langle n(1)\sigma_{12}(2)\sigma_{2X}(3)\left|\mathbf{p}_1\frac{1}{r_{23}} + \mathbf{p}_2\frac{1}{r_{13}} + \mathbf{p}_3\frac{1}{r_{12}}\right|\sigma_{12}(1)\sigma_{2X}(2)\pi^*(3)\right\rangle \\
&\quad = \mathbf{p}_{n\sigma_{12}}\left\langle \sigma_{12}(1)\sigma_{2X}(2)\left|\frac{1}{r_{12}}\right|\sigma_{2X}(1)\pi^*(2)\right\rangle \\
&\qquad + \mathbf{p}_{\sigma_{12}\sigma_{2X}}\left\langle n(1)\sigma_{2X}(2)\left|\frac{1}{r_{12}}\right|\sigma_{12}(1)\pi^*(2)\right\rangle \\
&\qquad + \mathbf{p}_{\sigma_{2X}\pi^*}\left\langle n(1)\sigma_{12}(2)\left|\frac{1}{r_{12}}\right|\sigma_{12}(1)\sigma_{2X}(2)\right\rangle.
\end{aligned} \tag{5.1.8}$$

Even with simple mathematical forms the multiple center integrals in these expressions have a somewhat complex geometrical dependence; however, if only the orientation of the σ_{2X} or $\sigma_{2H'}$ bond is considered to vary, as is reasonable, a particularly simple result is obtained. For example, $\mathbf{p}_{n\sigma_{12}}$ will be a constant, independent of the nature of σ_{2X}; $\mathbf{p}_{\sigma_{2X}\pi^*}$ will be most sensitive to the $2p_z$ component of σ_{2X} and will have the form $A\gamma_z$; $\mathbf{p}_{\sigma_{12}\sigma_{2X}}$ will be insensitive to relatively small variations in the orientation of σ_{2X}. The integrals $\langle\sigma_{12}(1)\sigma_{2X}(2)|\,1/r_{12}\,|\sigma_{2X}(1)\pi^*(2)\rangle$ and $\langle n(1)\sigma_{2X}(2)|\,1/r_{12}\,|\sigma_{12}(1)\pi^*(2)\rangle$ will be dependent on the $2p_z$ component of σ_{2X}, since both $n(1)$ and σ_{12} lie in the xy-plane; the integral $\langle n(1)\sigma_{12}(2)|\,1/r_{12}\,|\sigma_{12}(1)\sigma_{2X}(2)\rangle$ will be insensitive to the orientation of σ_{2X}.

As a result, one may write for the exchange terms the simple expression

$$p_{n\pi^*}(\text{exchange}) = iA\gamma_z, \tag{5.1.9}$$

where γ_z is the direction cosine of the σ_{2X} bond. If the α-substituent is of a complex structure, such as a propyl group, a geometrical factor of the form (5.1.6) will be necessary. It then follows that an empirical expression embodying (5.1.6) and the exchange effects of (5.1.9) will have the form

$$R_{n\pi*} = A\gamma_z(\alpha) + B\gamma_z(\alpha') + \sum_i \left(\frac{a_i}{R_i^3} + b_i \frac{\mathbf{k}_i \cdot \mathbf{R}_i}{R_i^5}\right)\gamma_X^{(i)}\gamma_Y^{(i)}, \qquad (5.1.10)$$

where α and α' refer to substituents on either side of the carbonyl and the summation is over all other perturbing orbitals with $\mathbf{k}_i$ generally along a bond symmetry axis. The sign of the constants A and B will depend on which side of the carbonyl group the substituent is located.

5.2. Benzene Derivatives

The benzene chromophore provides an opportunity to study a degenerate system. Even at the empirical level the situation can be made quite complicated by attempting to include all the terms of the previous chapter. It will be instructive to consider an abbreviated treatment, which includes only the important features of the problem. The simplified model is shown in Figure 5.2. Substitution has been arbitrarily divided into planar and perpendicular at the six vertices.

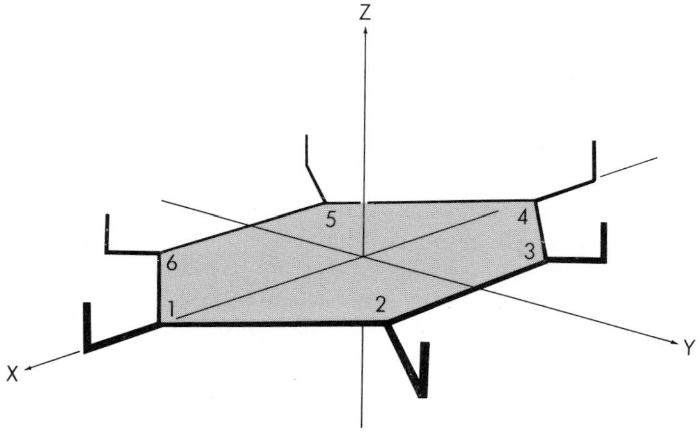

Figure 5.2. The benzene chromophore.

The greatest perturbation to the ring will come from the atoms in the plane. This will determine the electric moments in the B_{1u}, B_{2u}, and E_{1u} states. The vertical lines in the figure indicate uncompensated out-of-plane substituents, which will be responsible for planar components of magnetic moment.

By using the LCAO Hückel approximation it would be possible to derive a set of rules relating all three transitions to one or two parameters for each group. This procedure has two disadvantages: the treatment is more cumbersome in that the π-electrons are treated individually; and the relation of the three rotational strengths to the same parameters is of doubtful validity in view of the difficulty in explaining the relative ordering of energies by such a simple method. Accordingly, each transition will be given its own parameters.

Experience with benzene derivatives indicates that a linear rule is inadequate to correlate the transition moment directions. In this empirical theory it will be convenient to replace $\mathbf{p}$ with $\boldsymbol{\mu}$, since no absolute numerical results are to be calculated. In the notation of Chapter 4 $V^{\ddagger}$ will denote the SCF field of the ring substituents. The linear contribution of a transition $0 \rightarrow n$ will be given by the quantity $(\boldsymbol{\mu} V^{\ddagger})_{0n}$. All other linear terms such as through bond electron correlation will be initially presumed to have the same geometrical dependence.

The most effective nonlinear contributions will be made by terms which do not depend on the distance between ring substituents. This requirement will exclude $[\boldsymbol{\mu}(V^{\ddagger})^2]_{0n}$ and all correlation and exchange terms which depend on the product of two distances to a common point such as $(1/r_{12})(1/r_{13})$. The product $(1/r_{12})(1/r_{34})$ is the lowest order term which may be considered. Four separate orbitals are needed in general. The simplest procedure is to let electrons 2 and 4 be in the two substituent orbitals and electrons 1 and 3 in π-orbitals. The term

$$\left(\boldsymbol{\mu}_1 \frac{1}{r_{12}} \frac{1}{r_{34}}\right)_{A_1a_1,\, A_2A_2,\, A_3A_3,\, A_4A_4} = \left(\boldsymbol{\mu}_1 \frac{1}{r_{12}}\right)_{A_1a_1,\, A_2A_2} \left(\frac{1}{r_{34}}\right)_{A_3A_3,\, A_4A_4}$$

will not appear in the formalism of Chapter 4 because of the cancellation inherent in the difference $(\boldsymbol{\mu} V^2)_{0n} - (\boldsymbol{\mu} V)_{0n} V_{nn}$.

If χ_1 and χ_2 denote substituent orbitals, ϕ_1 and ϕ_1' are the ground and excited π-orbitals, and ϕ_2 is a second π-orbital, then the exchange integral

$$\left\langle \phi_1(1)\phi_2(2)\chi_1(3)\chi_2(4) \left| \boldsymbol{\mu}_1 \frac{1}{r_{13}} \frac{1}{r_{24}} \right| \chi_1(1)\chi_2(2)\phi_2(3)\phi_1'(4) \right\rangle$$

$$= \left\langle \phi_1(1)\chi_1(3) \left| \boldsymbol{\mu}_1 \frac{1}{r_{13}} \right| \chi_1(1)\phi_2(3) \right\rangle \left\langle \phi_2(2)\chi_2(4) \left| \frac{1}{r_{24}} \right| \chi_2(2)\phi_1'(4) \right\rangle \quad (5.2.1)$$

satisfies the overlap requirement; in addition it is a unique term that does not appear in $(\boldsymbol{\mu} V)_{0n} V_{nn}$. In the following empirical discussion such complex integrals will not be evaluated in detail; they will merely be introduced to demonstrate the existence of sizable second order terms depending on the product of parameters for two different substituents.

The phase relationship for the B_{1u} and B_{2u} states is shown in Figure 5.3. Instead of using the customary six π-orbitals we shall approximate the behavior of the system by single orbitals of the appropriate symmetry. Since it is slightly simpler, the B_{1u} transition will be discussed first. The integral $\int \Psi_{A_{1g}} \boldsymbol{\mu} V \Psi_{B_{2u}}\, d\tau$

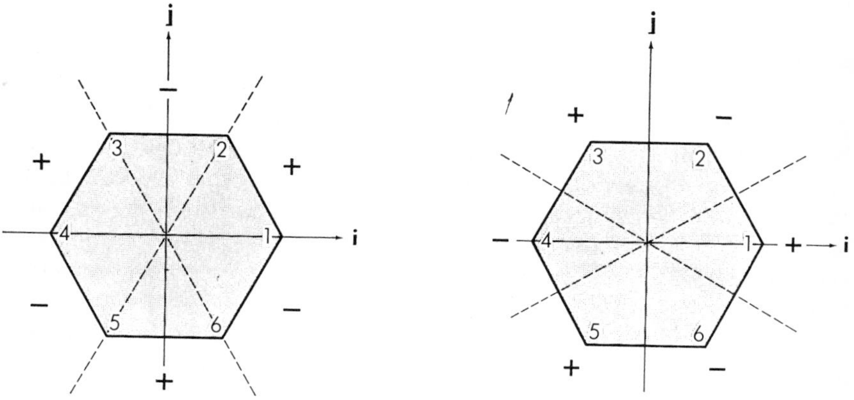

Figure 5.3. The (*a*) B_{2u} and (*b*) B_{1u} states.

is zero for benzene because the six oppositely signed sections (Figure 5.3) lead to cancellation. If the ring is substituted and the integration is carried out one section at a time, each substituent will make a contribution $\pm A_i \mathbf{b}_i$, where $\mathbf{b}_i$ is a unit vector through the substituted vertex; positions 1, 3, 5 will have a positive sign and positions 2, 4, 6 will have a negative sign. The result is

$$\boldsymbol{\mu}^{(1)}_{B_{1u}} = \mathbf{i}[A_1 + A_4 - \tfrac{1}{2}(A_2 + A_3 + A_5 + A_6)] + \sqrt{\tfrac{3}{2}}\,\mathbf{j}(-A_2 + A_3 - A_5 + A_6). \quad (5.2.2)$$

This predicts a simple linear relationship among the dipole moments of transitions in substituted benzene derivatives. To take into account the discrepancy between the observed and predicted values a nonlinear expression like (5.2.1) is needed. Although this expression is based on the simultaneous occupancy of two separate π-orbitals, the form of the second order term can be inferred by observing that (5.2.1) will lead to the same geometrical dependence as a term like $\langle 0|\,\boldsymbol{\mu} V|Q\rangle\langle Q|\,V|n\rangle$, where Q is an orbital with A_{1g} symmetry. By reasoning similar to the derivation of (5.2.2) one obtains

$$\langle \Psi_{A_{1g}}|\,\boldsymbol{\mu} V\,|Q\rangle = [B_1 - B_4 + \tfrac{1}{2}(B_2 - B_3 - B_5 + B_6)]\mathbf{i} + \sqrt{\tfrac{3}{2}}(B_2 + B_3 - B_5 - B_6)\mathbf{j} \quad (5.2.3a)$$

$$\langle Q|\,V\,|\Psi_{B_{1u}}\rangle = C_1 - C_2 + C_3 - C_4 + C_5 - C_6\,. \quad (5.2.3b)$$

The second order transition moment may now be written

$$\begin{aligned}\boldsymbol{\mu}_{B_{1u}} = \mathbf{i}\{&[A_1 + A_4 - \tfrac{1}{2}(A_2 + A_3 + A_5 + A_6)]\\ &+ (C_1 - C_2 + C_3 - C_4 + C_5 - C_6)\\ &\times [B_1 - B_4 + \tfrac{1}{2}(B_2 - B_3 - B_5 + B_6)]\}\\ &+ \mathbf{j}\sqrt{\tfrac{3}{2}}[(-A_2 + A_3 - A_5 + A_6) + (C_1 - C_2 + C_3 - C_4 + C_5 - C_6)\\ &\times (B_2 + B_3 - B_5 - B_6)]. \end{aligned} \qquad (5.2.4)$$

The magnetic moment may be obtained by observing that the charge is concentrated in the region of vertices and bonds on the periphery of the hexagon. The operator $\mathbf{r} \times \mathbf{p}$ may be considered to be effective only in this region. For the B_{1u} state the charge is concentrated at the vertices, and $\mathbf{r} \times \mathbf{p}$ may be replaced by $\mathbf{R} \times \mathbf{p}$, when $\mathbf{R}$ is the vector distance to the appropriate vertex. In order that there be a planar component of $\mathbf{m}_{B_{1u}}$ there must be perpendicular components of $\mathbf{p}_{B_{1u}}$ in one or more of the sectors. This will be true only for an uncompensated substituent above or below the plane.

In Figure 5.4 the relative directions of $\mathbf{R} \times \mathbf{p}$ in each sector for similarly

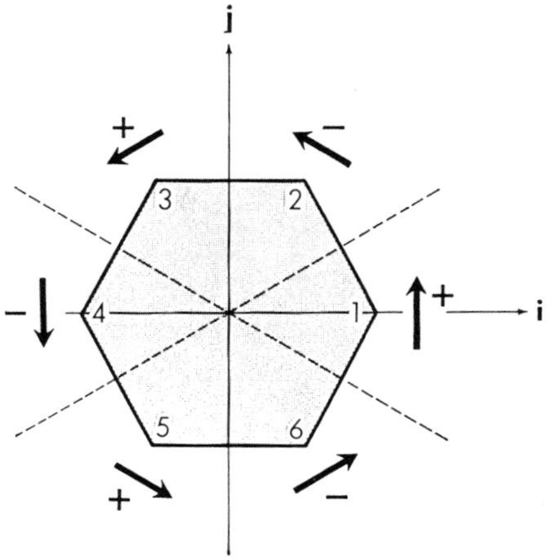

Figure 5.4. The magnetic behavior of the B_{1u} state.

behaving substituents are shown. Each dissymmetric substituent will make a contribution to **m** along the direction shown with the accompanying sign. Accordingly, one may write for the first order component of $\mathbf{m}_{B_{1u}}$

$$\mathbf{m}^{(1)}_{B_{1u}} = i\left\{\frac{\sqrt{3}}{2}(D_2 - D_3 + D_5 - D_6)\mathbf{i} + [D_1 + D_4 - \tfrac{1}{2}(D_2 + D_3 + D_5 + D_6)]\mathbf{j}\right\}. \qquad (5.2.5)$$

Substituents on the opposite side of the plane will make contributions of the opposite sign.

The second order magnetic moment may be found in a similar manner to the method employed on the electric moment. The terms to consider are of the form $\langle B_{1u}| V|Q\rangle\langle Q| V\mathbf{m}|A_{1g}\rangle$. The result is

$$\mathbf{m}^{(2)}_{B_{1u}} = i(F_1 - F_2 + F_3 - F_4 + F_5 - F_6)$$

$$\times \left\{\frac{\sqrt{3}}{2}(-E_2 - E_3 + E_5 + E_6)\mathbf{i} + [E_1 - E_4 + \tfrac{1}{2}(E_2 - E_3 - E_5 + E_6)]\mathbf{j}\right\}. \tag{5.2.6}$$

The combination of the two terms gives

$$\frac{1}{i}\mathbf{m}_{B_{1u}} = \frac{\sqrt{3}}{2}\mathbf{i}[(D_2 - D_3 + D_5 - D_6) + (F_1 - F_2 + F_3 - F_4 + F_5 - F_6)$$

$$\times(-E_2 - E_3 + E_5 + E_6)] + \mathbf{j}\{[D_1 + D_4 - \tfrac{1}{2}(D_2 + D_3 + D_5 + D_6)]$$

$$+(F_1 - F_2 + F_3 - F_4 + F_5 - F_6)$$

$$\times[E_1 - E_4 + \tfrac{1}{2}(E_2 - E_3 - E_5 + E_6)]\}. \tag{5.2.7}$$

The treatment of the B_{2u} proceeds similarly with a slight modification. Since the nodes are at the vertices, the contributions to $(\boldsymbol{\mu}V)_{0n}$ and $(V\mathbf{m})_{n0}$ from a given sector will be determined by the sum of two vertex parameters. This leads to the expression

$$\boldsymbol{\mu}^{(1)}_{B_{2u}} = \frac{\sqrt{3}}{2}[(A_1 + A_2) - (A_3 + A_4) + (A_4 + A_5) - (A_6 + A_1)]\mathbf{i}$$

$$+\{-(A_2 + A_3) - (A_5 + A_6) + \tfrac{1}{2}[(A_1 + A_2) + (A_3 + A_4) + (A_4 + A_5)$$

$$+(A_6 + A_1)]\}\mathbf{j}$$

$$= \frac{\sqrt{3}}{2}(A_2 - A_3 + A_5 - A_6)\mathbf{i}$$

$$+[A_1 + A_4 - \tfrac{1}{2}(A_2 + A_3 + A_5 + A_6)]\mathbf{j}. \tag{5.2.8}$$

The direction of the vector contribution has been taken to be perpendicular to the bond in each sector.

The positions of the nodes in the B_{2u} state precludes the second order treatment used on the B_{1u} state; however, unlike the B_{1u} state, the B_{2u} state is particularly susceptible to the interaction of adjacent ring substituents. Accordingly, terms of the form $(\boldsymbol{\mu}V^2)_{0n}$ will be employed. Such an integral may be approximated by the product of two factors; for example, the second order contribution from the first sector will be given by $B_1B_2[(\sqrt{3}/2)\mathbf{i} + \frac{1}{2}\mathbf{j}]$. The combined result of first and second order terms is

$$\boldsymbol{\mu}_{B_{2u}} = \frac{\sqrt{3}}{2}\mathbf{i}[(A_2 - A_3 + A_5 - A_6) + (B_1B_2 - B_3B_4 + B_4B_5 - B_6B_1)]$$
$$+ \mathbf{j}\{[A_1 + A_4 - \tfrac{1}{2}(A_2 + A_3 + A_5 + A_6)]$$
$$+ [-B_2B_3 - B_5B_6 + \tfrac{1}{2}(B_1B_2 + B_3B_4 + B_4B_5 + B_6B_1)]\}. \quad (5.2.9)$$

A similar set of second order terms may also prove necessary for the B_{1u} state. This example is meant to be instructive but by no means exhaustive. Further refinements may well include a detailed analysis of the six individual π-orbitals.

The first and second order magnetic contributions $(V\mathbf{m})_{n0}$ and $(V^2\mathbf{m})_{n0}$ are found by the above methods to be

$$\frac{1}{i}\mathbf{m}_{B_{2u}} = \{[-C_1 - C_4 + \tfrac{1}{2}(C_2 + C_3 + C_5 + C_6)]$$
$$+ [D_2D_3 + D_5D_6 - \tfrac{1}{2}(D_1D_2 + D_3D_4 + D_4D_5 + D_6D_1)]\}\mathbf{i}$$
$$+ \left[\frac{\sqrt{3}}{2}(C_2 - C_3 + C_5 - C_6) + (D_1D_2 - D_3D_4\right.$$
$$\left. + D_4D_5 - D_6D_1)\right]\mathbf{j}. \quad (5.2.10)$$

Owing to its degeneracy, the treatment of the E_{1u} band proceeds along different lines. The two functions ψ_X and ψ_Y may be considered to have the same transformation properties as the coordinates X and Y. Strictly speaking, the only group theoretical requirement is that the two transformation matrices be related by a similarity transformation. For empirical purposes we shall take this to be the identity. The correct linear combinations from standard doubly degenerate perturbation theory may be written

$$\Psi_A = \psi_X \cos\Omega + \psi_Y \sin\Omega \quad (5.2.11a)$$

$$\Psi_B = -\psi_X \sin\Omega + \psi_Y \cos\Omega, \quad (5.2.11b)$$

where

$$\cos\Omega = \left[\frac{1}{2}\left(1 + \frac{1}{\sqrt{1 + 4\Delta^2}}\right)\right]^{1/2}$$

$$\Delta = \frac{\langle X|V|Y\rangle}{\langle X|V|X\rangle - \langle Y|V|Y\rangle}. \quad (5.2.11b)$$

Using the same numbering as in Figure 5.3, consider a substituent at vertex 1. Since ψ_Y has a node in the XZ-plane, the quantity $\langle X|\, V_1\,|Y\rangle$ is zero. The quantity $\langle Y|\, V_1\,|Y\rangle$ does not vanish, but owing to the nodal plane it should be considerably smaller than $\langle X|\, V_1\,|X\rangle$; since its inclusion adds no essentially unique features to the theory, it will be omitted. Now $V = \sum_{i=1}^{6} V_i$; an integral such as $\int \psi_X V_2 \psi_Y \, d\tau$ can be evaluated by a rotation of coordinates through $-60°$. This produces the transformations

$$V_2 \to V_1 \tag{5.2.12a}$$

$$\psi_X \to \psi_X \cos 60° - \psi_Y \sin 60° \tag{5.2.12b}$$

$$\psi_Y \to \psi_X \sin 60° + \psi_Y \cos 60°. \tag{5.2.12c}$$

Since $\langle X|\, V_1\,|Y\rangle = 0$ and $\langle Y|\, V_1\,|Y\rangle$ is small, one obtains

$$\langle X|\, V_2\,|Y\rangle = \langle X|\, V_1\,|X\rangle \cos 60° \sin 60° = \frac{\sqrt{3}}{4} A_2, \tag{5.2.13}$$

where the designation A_2 indicates that the perturbing substituent is at the second vertex.

By analogy to (5.2.12) the general relations are obtained:

$$\langle X|\, V_i\,|Y\rangle = \cos(i-1)60° \sin(i-1)60° A_i \tag{5.2.14a}$$

$$\langle X|\, V_i\,|X\rangle = \cos^2(i-1)60° A_i \tag{5.2.14b}$$

$$\langle Y|\, V_i\,|Y\rangle = \sin^2(i-1)60° A_i, \tag{5.2.14c}$$

from which it follows that

$$\langle X|\, V\,|Y\rangle = \frac{\sqrt{3}}{4}(A_2 - A_3 + A_5 - A_6) \tag{5.2.15a}$$

$$\langle X|\, V\,|X\rangle - \langle Y|\, V\,|Y\rangle = [A_1 + A_4 - \tfrac{1}{2}(A_2 + A_3 + A_5 + A_6)]. \tag{5.2.15b}$$

If $\boldsymbol{\mu}_{GX} = \mu\mathbf{i}$, $\boldsymbol{\mu}_{GY} = \mu\mathbf{j}$, one obtains

$$\langle \Psi_{A_{1g}}|\, \boldsymbol{\mu}\,|\Psi_A\rangle = \mu(\cos\Omega\mathbf{i} + \sin\Omega\mathbf{j}) \tag{5.2.16a}$$

$$\langle \Psi_{A_{1g}}|\, \boldsymbol{\mu}\,|\Psi_B\rangle = \mu(-\sin\Omega\mathbf{i} + \cos\Omega\mathbf{j}). \tag{5.2.16b}$$

Initially no second order term is needed because the direction of the transition moment already has a nonlinear dependence on the A_i's; however, this is merely the simplest beginning and is by no means the last word on the subject.

Figure 5.4 may be used as a guide for determining the contributions of each substituent to the magnetic moment (the signs should be omitted). Here the perturbation V_i at each vertex serves to destroy the planar symmetry of the system by giving a nonvanishing component of p_z. By the same reasoning as above it is concluded that

$$\langle X| V_1\mathbf{m} |G\rangle = iB_1\mathbf{j} \tag{5.2.17a}$$

$$\langle Y| V_1\mathbf{m} |G\rangle = 0. \tag{5.2.17b}$$

By rotating the coordinate system one can obtain the general result that

$$\langle X| V_i\mathbf{m} |G\rangle = i\{\cos(i-1)60°[-\mathbf{i}\sin(i-1)60° + \mathbf{j}\cos(i-1)60°]\} \tag{5.2.18a}$$

$$\langle Y| V_i\mathbf{m} |G\rangle = i\{\sin(i-1)60°[-\mathbf{i}\sin(i-1)60° + \mathbf{j}\cos(i-1)60°]\}. \tag{5.2.18b}$$

From this it follows that

$$\langle X |V\mathbf{m}|G\rangle = i\left\{\frac{\sqrt{3}}{4}(-B_2 + B_3 - B_5 + B_6)\mathbf{i} + [B_1 + B_4 + \tfrac{1}{4}(B_2 + B_3 + B_5 + B_6)]\mathbf{j}\right\} \tag{5.2.19a}$$

$$\langle Y |V\mathbf{m}|G\rangle = i\left[-\tfrac{3}{4}(B_2 + B_3 + B_5 + B_6)\mathbf{i} + \frac{\sqrt{3}}{4}(B_2 - B_3 + B_5 - B_6)\mathbf{j}\right]. \tag{5.2.19b}$$

For simplicity the rotational strengths will be represented only to lowest order. The resulting expressions are nonlinear and may be adequate to correlate many systems. Further refinements may be introduced in a systematic manner by the methods outlined above. The behavior of the B_{1u} transition is obtained by the dot product of the vectors in (5.2.2) and (5.2.5):

$$\begin{aligned} R_{B_{1u}} &= i\frac{\sqrt{3}}{2}\{[A_1 + A_4 - \tfrac{1}{2}(A_2 + A_3 + A_5 + A_6)](D_2 - D_3 + D_5 - D_6) \\ &\quad - (A_2 - A_3 + A_5 - A_6)[D_1 + D_4 - \tfrac{1}{2}(D_2 + D_3 + D_5 + D_6)]\} \\ &= i\frac{\sqrt{3}}{2}[(A_1 + A_4)(D_2 + D_5) + (A_2 + A_5)(D_3 + D_6) + (A_3 + A_6) \\ &\quad \times (D_1 + D_4) - (A_1 + A_4)(D_3 + D_6) - (A_2 + A_5)(D_1 + D_4) \\ &\quad - (A_3 + A_6)(D_2 + D_5)]. \end{aligned} \tag{5.2.20}$$

This expression has the property of vanishing whenever the molecule has a vertical plane of symmetry either through opposite vertices or bonds. For example, if the XZ-plane is an element of symmetry, then $A_2 = A_6$, $A_3 = A_5$, $D_2 = D_6$, $D_3 = D_5$, and (5.2.20) vanishes. It will be recalled that the A_i's arise from the magnetic moments. Substituents on the opposite side of the plane will be described by a D_i with the opposite sign. Any attempt to correlate (5.2.20) with data from oscillator strengths will probably be unfruitful, because the nonlinear contributions to $\boldsymbol{\mu}$ have not been included; however, the expression may be quite useful in a purely empirical correlation of rotational strengths. The treatment of the B_{2u} band leads to an expression of exactly the same form, where in general different parameters must be used. It by no means follows that the B_{1u} and B_{2u} transitions have the same sign. More detailed information on this matter can be obtained by delving into the diverse structures of the individual π-orbitals.

Finally, the scalar product of (5.2.16) with the corresponding magnetic quantities found from (5.2.19) gives for the E_{1u} band

$$R_A = -R_B = \frac{i\mu}{2}\left\{[B_1 + B_4 - \tfrac{1}{2}(B_2 + B_3 + B_5 + B_6)]\sin 2\Omega - \frac{\sqrt{3}}{2}(B_2 - B_3 + B_5 - B_6)\cos 2\Omega\right\}, \quad (5.2.21)$$

where

$$\sin 2\Omega = \frac{2\Delta}{\sqrt{1 + 4\Delta^2}},$$

$$\cos 2\Omega = \frac{1}{\sqrt{1 + 4\Delta^2}},$$

$$\Delta = \frac{\sqrt{3}}{4}\frac{A_2 - A_3 + A_5 - A_6}{[A_1 + A_4 - \tfrac{1}{2}(A_2 + A_3 + A_5 + A_6)]}.$$

Again this can be put into a more symmetrical form:

$$\begin{aligned} R_A = -R_B = \frac{i\mu\sqrt{3}}{4} &\times \{[A_1 + A_4 - \tfrac{1}{2}(A_2 + A_3 + A_5 + A_6)]^2 + \tfrac{3}{4}(A_2 - A_3 + A_5 - A_6)^2\}^{1/2} \\ &\times [(A_1 + A_4)(B_2 + B_5) + (A_2 + A_5)(B_3 + B_6) + (A_3 + A_6)(B_1 + B_4) \\ &- (A_1 + A_4)(B_3 + B_6) - (A_2 + A_5)(B_1 + B_4) - (A_3 + A_6)(B_2 + B_5)]. \end{aligned} \quad (5.2.22)$$

This is identical in form to (5.2.20); however, when all the A_i's are equal this expression becomes indeterminate. The degeneracy has not been lifted, and neither $\boldsymbol{\mu}$ nor $\mathbf{m}$ has any specific direction. Some important points can be illustrated here: When the splitting of the degeneracy is quite pronounced, as we have tacitly assumed here by the division of the substitutents into electric and magnetic moment perturbations, the rotational strengths of the components tend to cancel. When an optically active molecule has threefold or higher rotational symmetry, the above method is not applicable. When the degeneracy remains, both components have the same sign and in fact are indistinguishable in the absence of external force fields.

The existence of high symmetry optically active molecules brings out an interesting point. Not every transition is symmetry allowed; this means that any observed dichroism in such a band will be solely a vibronic effect. It is well known that vibronic interactions cannot give rise to optical activity in molecules whose equilibrium configurations are not dissymmetric; but the question as to whether they can elicit optical activity from symmetry forbidden bands in dissymmetric molecules has not been conclusively decided.

Experimental reinforcement of this subject is not easily forthcoming, because either the existing compounds do not have forbidden bands in the accessible region of the spectrum or those which do are too difficult to synthesize. As a possible incentive to those who might be interested in getting a first-hand look at the situation, the synthesis of a compound such as the aromatic derivative in Figure 5.5 may not fall too far into the category of the outrageous. The B_{1u}, B_{2u}, and E_{1u} bands are all in the accessible region. The molecule itself has D_6 symmetry in which the B_{1u} and B_{2u} bands become the still forbidden B_1 and B_2 bands of the D_6 group.

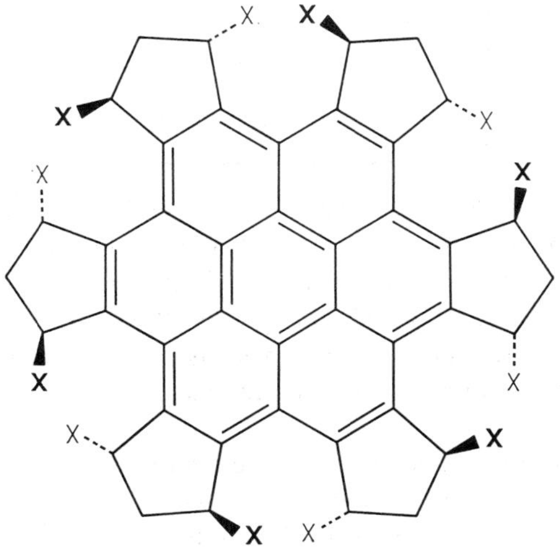

Figure 5.5. Optically active compound with D_6 symmetry.

5.3. Transition Metal Complexes

A rather fertile field in the general behavior of highly symmetrical chromophores is provided by transition metal complexes. In this section attention will be given to compounds with latent octahedral ($\mathcal{O}_h$) symmetry; in particular only complexes with six *d*-electrons will be considered. Starting from the full spherical symmetry of the *d*-orbitals one will be led through a progression of compounds of lower symmetry until any desired series of optically active molecules is reached.

The prototype of the basic chromophore is the $Co(NH_3)_6^{+3}$ ion. It belongs to the symmetry group $\mathcal{O}_h$, whose character table is given for reference in Table 5.2. The six ligands will be located at the positions (100), (−100),

TABLE 5.2

The $\mathcal{O}_h$ Symmetry Group

	$\mathcal{O}_h$	E	$8C_3$	$3C_2$	$6C_2'$	$6C_4$	i	$8S_3$	3σ	$6\sigma'$	$6S_4$
	A_{1g}	1	1	1	1	1	1	1	1	1	1
	A_{2g}	1	1	1	−1	−1	1	1	1	−1	−1
	E_g	2	−1	2	0	0	2	−1	2	0	0
m	T_{1g}	3	0	−1	−1	1	3	0	−1	−1	1
	T_{2g}	3	0	−1	1	−1	3	0	−1	1	−1
	A_{1u}	1	1	1	1	1	−1	−1	−1	−1	−1
	A_{2u}	1	1	1	−1	−1	−1	−1	−1	1	1
	E_u	2	−1	2	0	0	−2	1	−2	0	0
μ	T_{1u}	3	0	−1	−1	1	−3	0	1	1	−1
	T_{2u}	3	0	−1	1	−1	−3	0	1	−1	1

(010), (0−10), (001), (00−1). The four threefold axes (C_3) of symmetry pass through the points (111), (−1−11), (−111), (1−11); the **i**, **j**, and **k** axes are both twofold (C_2) and fourfold (C_4) axes; six additional twofold axes (C_2') pass through the points (001), (01−1), (101), (−101), (110), (1−10). The center of inversion leads to the rotation reflection axes S_3 and S_4, corresponding to the operations C_3 and C_4 and to the reflection planes σ and σ'.

The nine planes of symmetry divide the figure into $2^7 = 128$ sections, each with a sign opposite to that of its neighbors. From this standpoint a high degree of cancellation is inherent in the model.

In the optically active derivatives the strongest bands will generally arise from perturbations of parent T_{1g} or T_{1u} transitions. The lowest of the metal transitions is the magnetically allowed T_{1g}. In the absence of a definitive theoretical method for optically active complexes it is worthwhile to pursue a simple descriptive program. For this purpose crystal field theory will be adequate. The $3d_{yz}$ and $3d_{y^2-z^2}$ orbitals are shown in Figure 5.6.

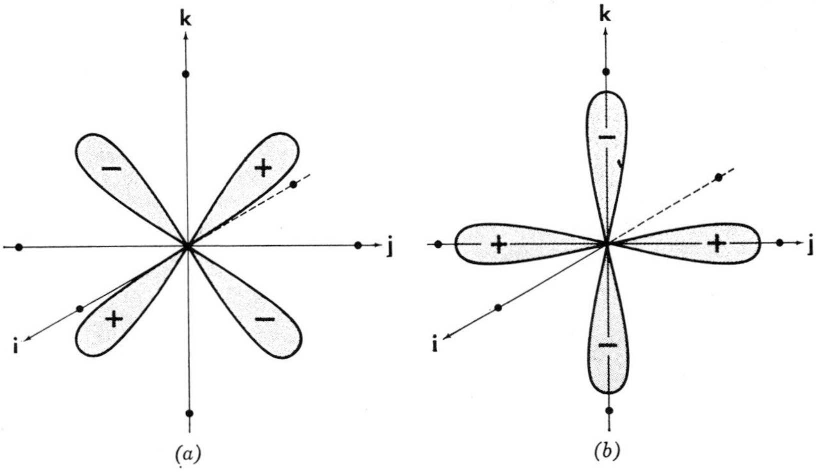

Figure 5.6. The $3d$ orbitals (*a*) $3d_{yz}$; (*b*) $3d_{y^2-z^2}$.

According to the usual argument the negative field of the six ligands leads to a lower energy for the $3d_{xy}$ orbital, because it places charge away from the ligand locations. The situation in the xy and xz planes is identical and a total of six orbitals requires consideration: $3d_{xy}$, $3d_{yz}$, $3d_{xz}$, $3d_{x^2-y^2}$, $3d_{y^2-z^2}$, $3d_{z^2-x^2}$. Only five of these are linearly independent, but in the multiple electron problem all six will be required.

For the ground state all six electrons are placed in the lower energy xy, yz, and xz orbitals. It happens that the desired T_{1g} state is obtained by promoting one of the electrons to one of the $x^2 - y^2$, $y^2 - z^2$, or $z^2 - x^2$ orbitals. The ground and triply degenerate excited T_{1g} state functions are

$$\psi_G = \frac{1}{\sqrt{6!}} |\phi_{xy}(1)\bar{\phi}_{xy}(2)\phi_{yz}(3)\bar{\phi}_{yz}(4)\phi_{xz}(5)\bar{\phi}_{xz}(6)| \tag{5.3.1a}$$

$$\psi_X = \frac{1}{\sqrt{6!}} |\phi_{xy}(1)\bar{\phi}_{xy}(2)\phi_{y^2-z^2}(3)\bar{\phi}_{yz}(4)\phi_{xz}(5)\bar{\phi}_{xz}(6)| \tag{5.3.1b}$$

$$\psi_Y = \frac{1}{\sqrt{6!}} |\phi_{xy}(1)\bar{\phi}_{xy}(2)\phi_{yz}(3)\bar{\phi}_{yz}(4)\phi_{z^2-x^2}(5)\bar{\phi}_{xz}(6)| \tag{5.3.1c}$$

$$\psi_Z = \frac{1}{\sqrt{6!}} |\phi_{x^2-y^2}(1)\bar{\phi}_{xy}(2)\phi_{yz}(3)\bar{\phi}_{yz}(4)\phi_{xz}(5)\bar{\phi}_{xz}(6)|, \tag{5.3.1d}$$

where spin degeneracy effects have been neglected. The direction of the magnetic moments has been anticipated in the labeling.

The indicated symmetry properties of these functions may be verified by observing that all the operations of the $\mathcal{O}_h$ group effect permutations of the coordinates x, y, z with no more than sign changes. For example, a counterclockwise rotation about the (111) C_3-axis transforms x into y, y into z, and z into x. From the elementary properties of determinants it follows that $\psi_G \to \psi_G$, $\psi_X \to \psi_Y$, $\psi_Y \to \psi_Z$, $\psi_Z \to \psi_X$, which leads to a zero trace for the transformation matrix of the T_{1g} functions in agreement with Table 5.2.

The simplicity of the hydrogenlike orbitals provides a strong temptation to treat the entire problem by means of point charge perturbations and the multipole expansion. A number of unforeseen complications bar the way to an attractive and instructive presentation. Despite the fact that only a few perturbing charges are required to describe the essential features of the system, the number of effective parameters becomes quite large, because the existence of the 128 oppositely signed sections requires the use of unduly high order multipole expansion terms. The $3d$ hydrogenlike orbitals have another serious drawback in that they are unsuitable zeroth order functions for dissymmetric perturbations. The effect of the octahedral field is not properly reflected, since the $3d$ functions have spherical symmetry instead of octahedral. This fact has led to the conclusion in some early theories of optically active complexes that the rotational strengths of the individual components sum to zero and the splitting of the degeneracy is responsible for the observed rotations.

As we have seen, degeneracy is not split in all optically active molecules (except for the small Jahn-Teller effect). This mechanism cannot be responsible for the activity of any degenerate band in a complex with $\mathcal{O}$ symmetry, since the degeneracy persists in the change from $\mathcal{O}_h$ to $\mathcal{O}$ symmetry. Unfortunately it is not very likely that a complex of exactly $\mathcal{O}$ symmetry will be isolated in the near future. One would be forced to wrestle with such intricate compounds as the Osmium complex in Figure 5.7, which may not necessarily be stable.

Pure $\mathcal{O}$ symmetry is not merely an idle consideration; it is an instructive aspect of the whole problem. Consider the idealized system in Figure 5.8. On opposite ends of each fourfold axis are four offset points at the corners of a square. The figure is brought into coincidence with itself by all the proper rotational operations of an octahedron; whereas the improper rotations produce the mirror image. This $\mathcal{O}$ symmetry is displayed so long as the crosses are all rotated through the same angle and the points do not lie in any of the symmetry planes, that is, $\theta \neq 45°$, $90°$, $135°$, etc.

By reference to Table 5.2 it may be verified that the T_{1g} states have the symmetry properties shown in Figure 5.9. The signs indicate the contribution from each segment to integrals such as $(zV)_X = \langle\psi_G|\, zV\,|\psi_X\rangle$. The plane is

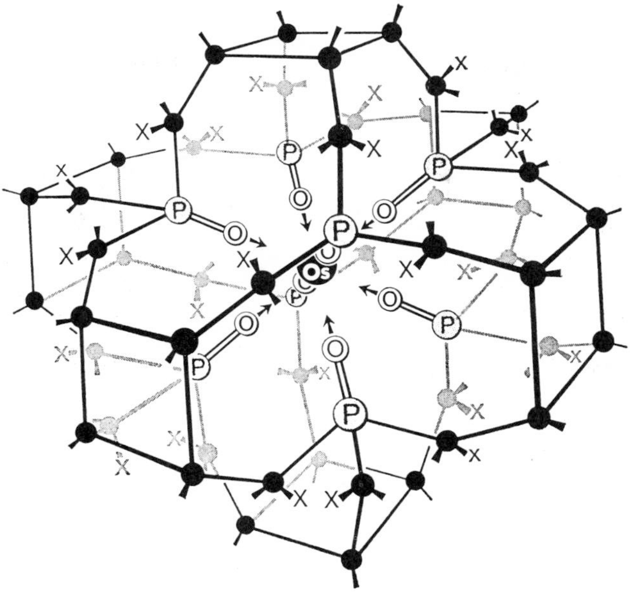

Figure 5.7. Transition metal complex with $\mathcal{O}$ symmetry.

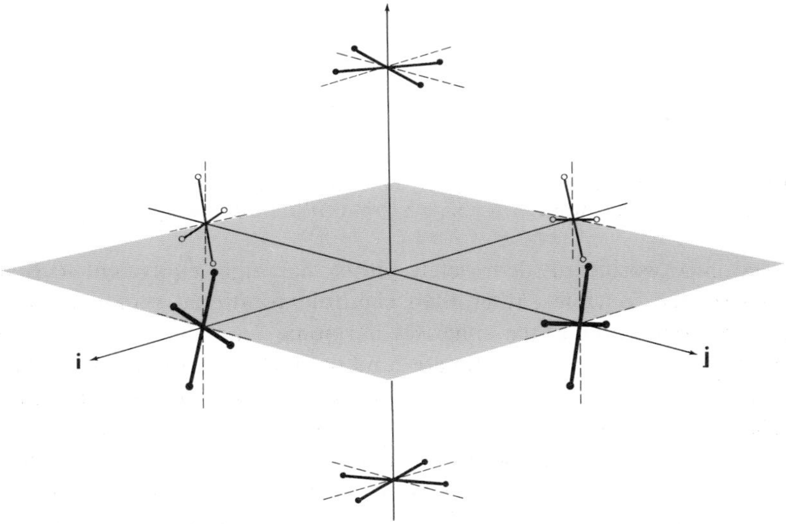

Figure 5.8. Schematic representation of $\mathcal{O}$ symmetry.

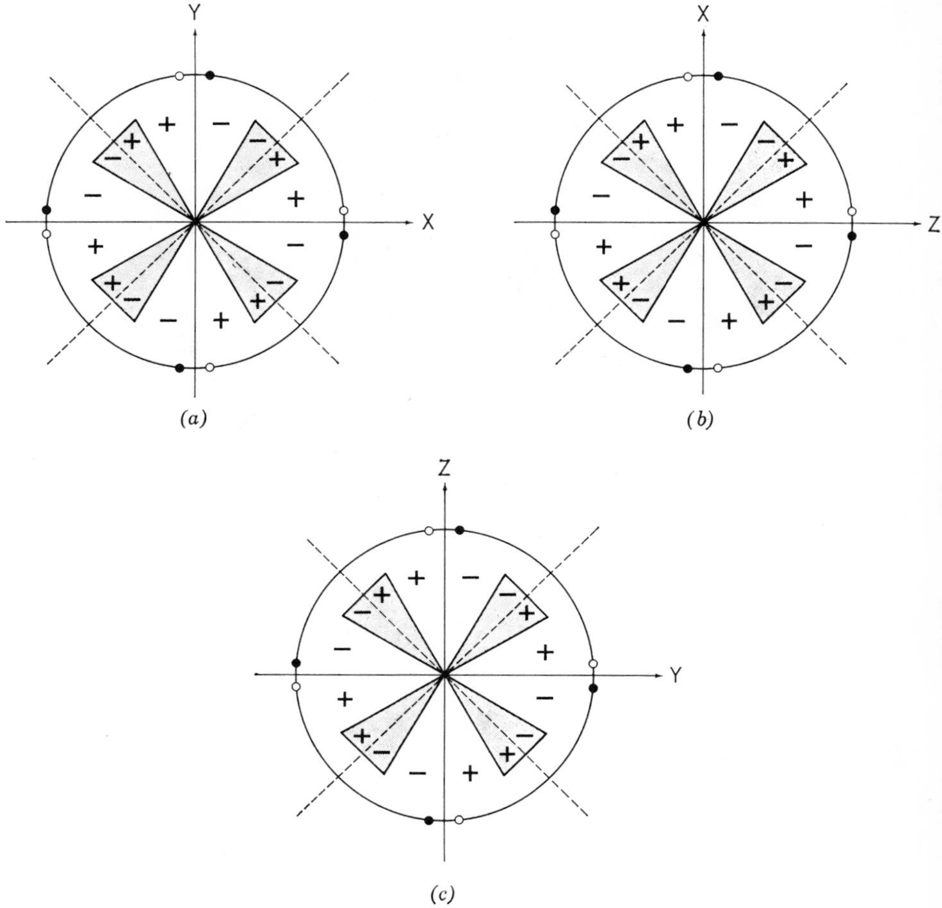

Figure 5.9. The analysis of $(\mu V)_{X,Y,Z}$ for an $\mathcal{O}$ symmetry complex. Black dots represent points above the plane, white dots points below. *(a)* ψ_Z; *(b)* ψ_Y; *(c)* ψ_X.

divided into two inequivalent octets rather than eight equivalent sections to emphasize the fourfold rather than eightfold rotational symmetry. As has been mentioned above, the spherical harmonic functions $x^2 - y^2$, xy, etc., imply too high a degree of symmetry and often lead to needless cancellation. In the figure the locations of the eight points associated with the perpendicular axis are indicated. In each case the four points above the plane lie in negative regions, while those below the plane lie in the positive regions.

This means that the contributions to V from charges in these positions will lead to nonvanishing values of $(xV)_X$, $(yV)_Y$, and $(zV)_Z$ which are equal and of the same sign. A similar analysis on the other 16 points leads to the same result with different values of the parameters. It is shown below that $(m_x)_X$, $(m_y)_Y$, and $(m_z)_Z$ are all of the same sign, from which it follows that

$$(\boldsymbol{\mu} V)_{GX} \cdot (m)_{XG} = (\boldsymbol{\mu} V)_{GY} \cdot (\mathbf{m})_{YG} = (\boldsymbol{\mu} V)_{GZ} \cdot (\mathbf{m})_{ZG} \neq 0.$$

Since the degeneracy remains, one is at liberty to use any linear combination of ψ_X, ψ_Y, and ψ_Z. In particular, the use of the individual functions immediately leads to the conclusion that in the absence of vibronic effects a truly degenerate transition will lead to a single circular dichroism band.

With this as background we will now outline the general theory of active transition metal complexes. Any perturbing potential V can be expanded in terms of a complete set of functions which span the representations of any given symmetry group. In general a different set of linear combinations is required for each group. In addition to what will be called the diagonal terms $(\mu_x V)_{GX}$, $(\mu_y V)_{GY}$, $(\mu_z V)_{GZ}$, there are the off diagonal terms $(\mu_x V)_{GY}$, $(\mu_y V)_{GX}$, $(\mu_y V)_{GZ}$, $(\mu_z V)_{GY}$, $(\mu_z V)_{GX}$, $(\mu_x V)_{GZ}$ which arise when the degeneracy is split.

From the theory of group character multiplication it is found that the nine possible products of μ_x, μ_y, μ_z with ψ_x, ψ_y, ψ_z span the $T_{1u} \times T_{1g} = T_{1u} + T_{2u} + E_u + A_{1u}$ representations. This means that a necessary condition for the nonvanishing of the above nine matrix elements is that the $\mathcal{O}_h$ expansion of V contain terms with T_{1u}, T_{2u}, E_u, or A_{1u} symmetry. The lowest order polynomial functions which lead to nonvanishing results are

$$V_{T_{1u}} = \left.\begin{matrix} x(y^2 + z^2) \\ y(z^2 + x^2) \\ z(x^2 + y^2) \end{matrix}\right\} f(r) \tag{5.3.2a}$$

$$V_{T_{2u}} = \left.\begin{matrix} x(y^2 - z^2) \\ y(z^2 - x^2) \\ z(x^2 - y^2) \end{matrix}\right\} g(r) \tag{5.3.2b}$$

$$V_{E_u} = \left.\begin{matrix} xyz(2z^2 - x^2 - y^2) \\ xyz(x^2 - y^2) \end{matrix}\right\} h(r) \tag{5.3.2c}$$

$$V_{A_{1u}} = xyz(x^2 - y^2)(y^2 - z^2)(z^2 - x^2)k(r). \tag{5.3.2d}$$

The products $x\psi_X$, $y\psi_Y$, $z\psi_Z$ change sign upon reflection in the xy, yz, zx, and two appropriate dihedral planes; the off diagonal products like $x\psi_Y$ change sign upon reflection in one of the planes xy, yz, zx.

This suggests that the diagonal matrix elements are determined by V_{E_s} and $V_{A_{1u}}$, and the off diagonal ones by $V_{T_{1u}}$ and $V_{T_{2u}}$. The x, y, z terms are unique among the T_{1_u} functions in that they restore antisymmetry in the dihedral planes for the products $x\psi_y$, etc., while destroying it in the principal planes.

The reason for the unwieldiness of a multipole expansion treatment may now be seen. An $\mathcal{O}$ field will transform like the totally symmetric representation (A_1) of the $\mathcal{O}$ symmetry group. This will include both $V_{A_{1g}}$ and $V_{A_{1u}}$ terms in the parent $\mathcal{O}_h$ group and no others. The totally symmetric $V_{A_{1g}}$ terms make no contribution to the optical activity, which leaves only the $V_{A_{1u}}$ terms. The lowest order multipole expansion term would be

$$xyz(x^2 - y^2)(y^2 - z^2)(z^2 - x^2)/R^{10}.$$

By similar reasoning it is found that this is also the lowest order term for the diagonal components of the commonly encountered D_3 complexes like $Co(en)_3^{+3}$.

The hydrogenlike functions of (5.3.1) are satisfactory for computing the magnetic moment directions. Since all the orbitals are orthogonal, only the 6! terms in which the functions differ for only one electron will be nonvanishing with the result

$$(\mathbf{m})_{XG} = -i\beta \int \phi_{y^2-z^2}\mathbf{r} \times \nabla\phi_{yz}\, d\tau = -i\beta\mathbf{i} \tag{5.3.3a}$$

$$(\mathbf{m})_{YG} = -i\beta \int \phi_{z^2-x^2}\mathbf{r} \times \nabla\phi_{xz}\, d\tau = -i\beta\mathbf{j} \tag{5.3.3b}$$

$$(\mathbf{m})_{ZG} = -i\beta \int \phi_{x^2-y^2}\mathbf{r} \times \nabla\phi_{xy}\, d\tau = -i\beta\mathbf{k}, \tag{5.3.3c}$$

where $\beta = e\hbar/2mc$. Whatever the actual form of the wave functions, it will be assumed that their phases lead to the above result, where β is a parameter not necessarily equal to the Bohr magneton.

In a degenerate system a perturbation will prescribe a certain set of basis functions which will lead to magnetic moments along definite directions. Often the axes are determined by symmetry such as in the D_3 complexes. Generally they must be found by calculating the matrix elements of the perturbation V_{XY}, etc. Let the prescribed linear combinations be given by

$$\Theta_i = g_{i1}\psi_X + g_{i2}\psi_Y + g_{i3}\psi_Z, \qquad i = 1, 2, 3, \tag{5.3.4}$$

from which it follows that

$$\langle\Theta_i|\,\mathbf{m}\,|\psi_G\rangle = -i\beta(g_{i1}\,\mathbf{i} + g_{i2}\,\mathbf{j} + g_{i3}\,\mathbf{k}). \tag{5.3.5}$$

Let V represent a perturbation to any order (i.e., $\overline{V}$, $\overline{V}^2$, etc.). Then the appropriate perturbed moments are

$$\begin{aligned}\langle\psi_G|\,\boldsymbol{\mu}V\,|\Theta_i\rangle = {} & [g_{i1}(xV)_X + g_{i2}(xV)_Y + g_{i3}(xV)_Z]\mathbf{i} \\ & + [g_{i1}(yV)_X + g_{i2}(yV)_Y + g_{i3}(yV)_Z]\mathbf{j} \\ & + [g_{i1}(zV)_X + g_{i2}(zV)_Y + g_{i3}(zV)_Z]\mathbf{k}.\end{aligned} \tag{5.3.6}$$

The scalar product of the electric and magnetic moments is given by

$$\begin{aligned}\operatorname{Im}(\langle\psi_G|\,\boldsymbol{\mu}V\,|\Theta_i\rangle\cdot\langle\Theta_i|\,\mathbf{m}\,|\psi_G\rangle)\\ = -\beta\{[g_{i1}^2(xV)_X + g_{i2}^2(yV)_Y + g_{i3}^2(zV)_Z]\\ + g_{i1}g_{i2}[(xV)_Y + (yV)_X] + g_{i1}g_{i3}[(xV)_Z + (zV)_X]\\ + g_{i2}\,g_{i3}[(yV)_Z + (zV)_Y]\}.\end{aligned} \tag{5.3.7}$$

It will be recalled that the nine coefficients g_{i1}, g_{i2}, g_{i3}; $i = 1, 2, 3$, are the elements of a unitary matrix; that is,

$$\sum_{i=1}^{3} g_{is}\,g_{it} = \delta_{st}\,. \tag{5.3.8}$$

The sum of the rotational strengths for the perturbed transition is given by

$$\operatorname{Im}\sum_{i=1}^{3}(\langle\psi_G|\,\boldsymbol{\mu}V\,|\Theta_i\rangle\cdot\langle\Theta_i|\,\mathbf{m}\,|\psi_G\rangle) = -\beta[(xV)_X + (yV)_Y + (zV)_Z]. \tag{5.3.9}$$

In general this sum does not vanish, as is demonstrated by the $\mathcal{O}$ symmetry complex above and the material to be presented below.

With the use of a system of point charges, dipoles, and higher order multipoles it is possible to successively approximate any desired field. By this method any of the circular dichroism patterns in Figure 5.10 may be obtained. This merely represents all possible types of behavior for a triply degenerate system in the fixed nuclei approximation. Vibronic effects often lead to many more extrema. Curves resembling the first six examples are often encountered, particularly the forms shown in Figure 5.10*a* and *b*. The curve of Figure 5.10*g* has never been observed, for reasons to be discussed below.

Several properties of the matrix elements implicit in (5.3.7) can be readily deduced. For any reasonable perturbation the off diagonal terms $V_{XY}, \ldots,$ are quite small because integrals like

$$\iint \phi_{xy}(1)\phi_{x^2-y^2}(1)[V(1) + V(2)]\phi_{yz}(2)\phi_{y^2-z^2}(2)\,d\tau_1\,d\tau_2$$

are zero for one electron operators. These quantities must be found by the use of V^2 terms, and they will generally be much smaller than the diagonal elements. When all three diagonal elements are identical to lowest order, the small splitting may be ignored, and the rotation is given by (5.3.9). In general the rotations for the individual bands will be given by

$$R_X = -\beta(xV)_X \tag{5.3.10a}$$

$$R_Y = -\beta(yV)_Y \tag{5.3.10b}$$

$$R_Z = -\beta(zV)_Z\,. \tag{5.3.10c}$$

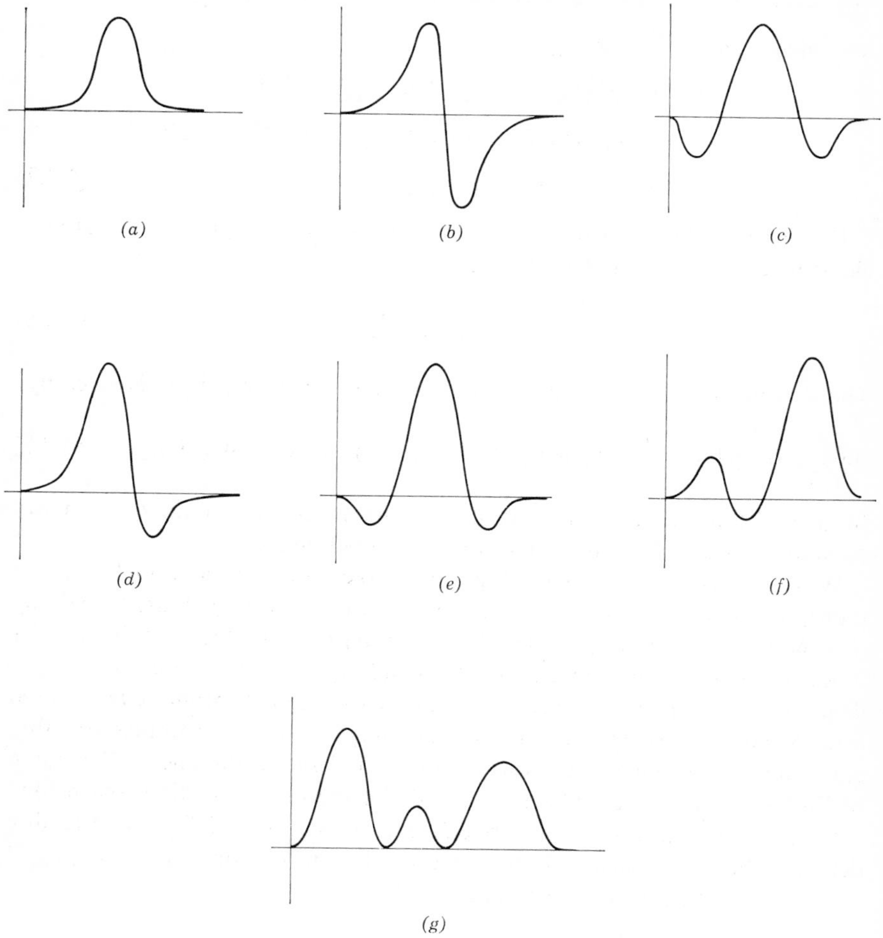

Figure 5.10 Possible CD curves for transition metal complexes.

This result is only true so long as an approximate octahedral configuration is retained.

A second important result is the vanishing of (5.3.9) for the spherically symmetrical basis function $xyf(r)$, $(x^2 - y^2)f(r)$, etc.; for

$$\int [xyz(x^2 - y^2) + xyz(y^2 - z^2) + xyz(z^2 - x^2)]f^2(r)V(x, y, z)\,d\tau = 0. \tag{5.3.11}$$

This result also applies to any coulombic integrals involving such spherical functions, since

$$\iint \phi_{xy}(1)\phi_{x^2-y^2}(1)V_{12}\chi^2(2)\,d\tau_1\,d\tau_2 = \int \phi_{xy}(1)\phi_{x^2-y^2}(1)V(1)\,d\tau_1.$$

The simplest $\mathcal{O}_h$ basis set for which (5.3.11) does not occur is

$$\phi'_{xy} = xyz^2 f(r) \tag{5.3.12a}$$

$$\phi'_{x^2-y^2} = (x^2 - y^2)z^2 f(r). \tag{5.3.12b}$$

Within the framework of crystal field theory the simple dichroism curves displayed by D_3 complexes would have to be explained by the destruction of spherical symmetry. Pictorially speaking, this amounts to a flattening of the *d*-orbitals in their respective planes. To produce the extremely high rotations observed for these compounds it would take an unrealistically high field.

There is one attractive alternative, which may well provide the key to this whole question. The great interpenetration of metal and ligand orbitals has led to the extensive and successful employment of ligand field theory in dealing with these complexes. In the usual presentation the six ligand orbitals are divided into linear combinations having A_{1g}, T_{1u}, and E_g symmetry:

$$\chi_{A_{1g}} = \phi_A + \phi_B + \phi_C + \phi_D + \phi_E + \phi_F \tag{5.3.13a}$$

$$\chi^{(1)}_{T_{1u}} = \phi_A - \phi_B \tag{5.3.13b}$$

$$\chi^{(2)}_{T_{1u}} = \phi_C - \phi_D \tag{5.3.13c}$$

$$\chi^{(3)}_{T_{1u}} = \phi_E - \phi_F \tag{5.3.13d}$$

$$\chi^{(1)}_{E_g} = \phi_E + \phi_F - \phi_A - \phi_B - \phi_C - \phi_D \tag{5.3.13e}$$

$$\chi^{(2)}_{E_g} = \phi_A + \phi_B - \phi_C - \phi_D. \tag{5.3.13f}$$

This symmetry classification strictly applies only so long as the ligands are identical; however, the form of the functions is largely preserved for any derivatives.

The six ligand bonding orbitals are formed by linearly combining $\chi_{A_{1g}}$ with ϕ_{4s}, $\chi^{(1)}_{T_{1u}}$ with ϕ_{4p_x}, etc., $\chi^{(1)}_{E_g}$ with $\phi_{2z^2-x^2-y^2}$, etc. The antibonding orbitals are obtained with the opposite sign. Then the 12 ligand electrons are placed in the six bonding orbitals, and the six *d*-electrons are placed in the T_{2g} ϕ_{xy} orbitals as in crystal field theory. The energy levels are such that the lowest excited orbital is the E_g ligand antibonding. Thus, the formalism closely parallels the crystal field approach.

One of the simplest ways to take advantage of this intimacy of charge clouds is to recognize that in a bridged complex the ligand bonds are not directed exactly along the **i**, **j**, and **k** axes. Both acute and obtuse angles between ligand bonds to bridged atoms are possible. For simplicity it will be assumed that the two bridged ligands are pulled toward one another. The situation is shown in Figure 5.11.

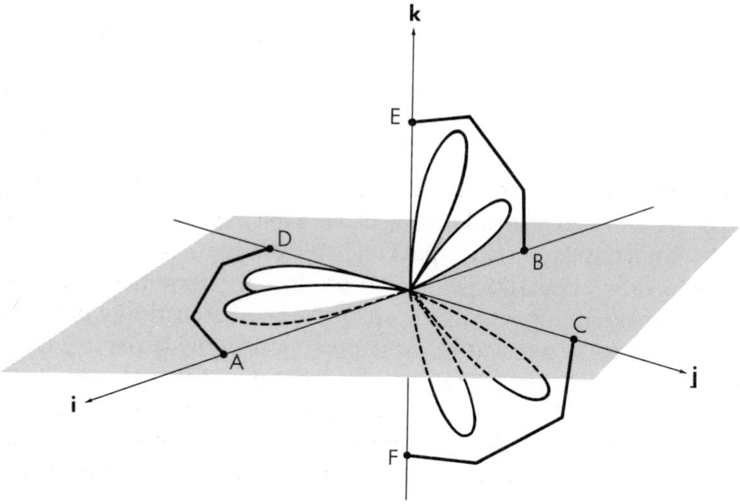

Figure 5.11. The distortion of $\mathcal{O}_h$ symmetry by bridging.

The zeroth order functions for calculation will be taken as the distorted ligand bonding orbitals with the undistorted T_{2g} nonbonding and E_g antibonding; furthermore, the E_g orbitals will be approximated by the original $\phi_{x^2-y^2}$ functions. It is realized that a more sophisticated treatment would perform a variation calculation on all the orbitals to obtain the best ground and excited state functions; but we are here mainly interested in pointing the way toward proper explanation rather than presenting a detailed definitive method.

The appropriate ligand field wave functions are

$$\Theta_G = \frac{1}{\sqrt{18!}} |\chi_{A_{1g}}(1) \cdots \bar{\chi}_{E_g}(12)\phi_{xy}(13) \cdots \bar{\phi}_{xz}(18)| \tag{5.3.14a}$$

$$\Theta_X = \frac{1}{\sqrt{18!}} |\chi_{A_{1g}}(1) \cdots \bar{\chi}_{E_g}(12)\phi_{xy}(13) \cdots \phi_{yz}(17)\bar{\phi}_{y^2-z^2}(18)| \tag{5.3.14b}$$

$$\Theta_Y = \frac{1}{\sqrt{18!}} |\chi_{A_{1g}}(1) \cdots \bar{\chi}_{E_g}(12)\phi_{xy}(13) \cdots \phi_{xz}(17)\bar{\phi}_{z^2-x^2}(18)| \tag{5.3.14c}$$

$$\Theta_Z = \frac{1}{\sqrt{18!}} |\chi_{A_{1g}}(1) \cdots \bar{\chi}_{E_G}(12)\phi_{yz}(13) \cdots \phi_{xy}(17)\bar{\phi}_{x^2-y^2}(18)|. \tag{5.3.14d}$$

If the electric moments are computed, the nonexchange contributions are zero, but the single exchange terms do not vanish:

$$(\mu_x)_X = -e \iint \chi_{A_{1g}}(1)\phi_{yz}(1)(x_1 + x_2)\chi_{A_{1g}}(2)\phi_{y^2-z^2}(2)\, d\tau_1\, d\tau_2$$
$$-(\text{exchange integrals with } \chi_{T_{1u}}\text{'s and } \chi_{E_g}\text{'s}). \quad (5.3.15)$$

The other moments are obtained by cyclic permutation.

The bending of the ligand orbital ϕ_A (Figure 5.11) imparts to it an xy component in addition to its original x component. If one takes care to make all contributions to the orbitals positive in the various octants, the lowest order terms required are

$$\chi_{A_{1g}} = \phi_{A_x} + \phi_{B_x} + \phi_{C_y} + \phi_{D_y} + \phi_{E_z} + \phi_{F_z} - (xy + yz + xz)f(r)$$
$$+ (xy^2 - x^2y + yz^2 - y^2z + zx^2 - z^2x)g(r). \quad (5.3.16)$$

The ϕ_{A_x}, etc., are the octahedrally oriented orbitals, which make no contribution to (5.3.15); the remaining terms take into account the distortion caused by bridging. The substitution of (5.3.16) into (5.3.15) gives

$$(\boldsymbol{\mu}_x)_X = e\left[\int yz\phi_{yz} f(r)\, d\tau\right]\left[\int x^2(y^2 - z^2)\phi_{y^2-z^2} g(r)\, d\tau\right] = eQ.$$

The other two terms are found to give the exact same results:

$$(\mu_x)_X = eQ \quad (5.3.17a)$$

$$(\mu_y)_Y = eQ \quad (5.3.17b)$$

$$(\mu_z)_Z = eQ. \quad (5.3.17c)$$

It is particularly notable that the exchange contributions to the three electric moments do not sum to zero for spherically symmetric basis functions, as do the coulombic terms. When the degeneracy is significantly split by heterosubstitution the situation is markedly changed. Let us consider but one of the several possibilities. The great cancellation which helped to minimize the values of the coulombic terms no longer occurs.

One of the simplest such examples is $Co[(en)_2\,NH_3\,X]$, where X is a substituent like Cl^-, which differs markedly from NH_3. The NH_3 ligand is considered to differ little from the $-NH_2$ groups in ethylene diammine. In Figure 5.11 let the X group be at A and NH_3 at D. Let us further make the plausible assumption that because of the steric interactions and hybridization effects the ligand orbitals ϕ_A and ϕ_D are still distorted as shown.

In analogy to the above exchange calculation the resultant coulombic potential of the ligand orbitals may be written

$$V = -a(yz + xz) - a'xy + b(yz^2 - y^2z + zx^2 - z^2x) + b'(xy^2 - x^2y). \quad (5.3.18)$$

The lowest order nonvanishing terms are $(\mu_x V^2)_X$, etc. The appropriate terms are

$$V^2 = \cdots + (ab' - a'b)xyz(x^2 - y^2) + \cdots . \tag{5.3.19}$$

This leads to the result

$$(\mu_x V^2)_X = -T \tag{5.3.20a}$$

$$(\mu_y V^2)_Y = -T \tag{5.3.20b}$$

$$(\mu_z V^2)_Z = 2T, \tag{5.3.20c}$$

where

$$T = (ab' - a'b) \int xyz^2(x^2 - y^2)\phi_{xy}\,\phi_{x^2-y^2}\,d\tau.$$

The field responsible for splitting the degeneracy is approximately C_{4v}. The Θ_X state is split in energy from the Θ_Y and Θ_Z states, which remain nearly degenerate. This gives a $(-T)$ contribution to the Θ_X state and a $(2T - T = T)$ contribution to the Θ_Y, Θ_Z state. It is by no means obvious from this outline that the heterosubstituted coulombic terms are larger than the exchange. This will be assumed to complete the rationalization of this intricate problem, inasmuch as a curve more resembling Figure 5.10*b* than 5.10*d* is observed.

Other complexes have given CD curves similar to Figure 5.10*d*, indicating a comparable magnitude of the exchange and coulombic terms. If this is the correct explanation for the properties of these complexes, then it is not likely that the behavior of Figure 5.10*g* will be observed; since the coulombic terms must nearly sum to zero.

CHAPTER 6

The Faraday Effect

6.1. General Considerations on Dissymmetric Scattering

It appears that important spectroscopic information can be obtained by placing a molecule in a constant magnetic field and directing plane polarized light along the axis. The phenomena observed have yet to be interpreted in a comprehensive manner; but it is generally agreed that this tool will greatly aid in the characterization of transitions, even though it may play a somewhat minor role in structure determination.

The phenomenon described is variously called magnetooptical activity or the Faraday effect. It occurs when any substance, atomic or molecular, is simultaneously subjected to radiation and constant magnetic fields. When the light beam and the magnetic field are parallel, one observes pure magneto-optical activity, characterized by a difference in the complex indices of refraction for left and right circularly polarized light. This leads to the rotation of the plane of polarization [magnetic optical rotatory dispersion (MORD)] and a difference in extinction coefficients [magnetic circular dichroism (MCD)]. The graphical representation is completely analogous to the corresponding quantities in natural optical activity, optical rotatory dispersion (ORD) and circular dichroism (CD).

When the light beam is perpendicular to the magnetic field, pure magnetic birefringence results, and the medium behaves like an optically inactive anisotropic crystal. Vibrational components parallel and perpendicular to the magnetic field axis are transmitted with different phase velocities. If the initial plane of polarization contains $\mathbf{H}_0$, the magnetic vector, or is perpendicular to it, it will remain so as it traverses the medium. When the electric vector $\mathbf{E}$ makes an arbitrary angle θ with $\mathbf{H}_0$, it will be resolved into components transmitted with different phase velocities. Initially the components are in phase, as they would be for plane polarization. After an appropriate distance of travel the components are 90° out of phase with maximum elliptical polarization. When the components are 180° out of phase plane polarization again results, but the plane makes an angle of 2θ with the original direction. For intermediate phase differences a continuum of elliptical polarizations results with principal axes making angles between $+\theta$ and $-\theta$ with the magnetic vector. This cycle is repeated at regular intervals as the wave traverses the medium. The situation is illustrated in Figure 6.1 for the variation from 0° to 180° phase difference.

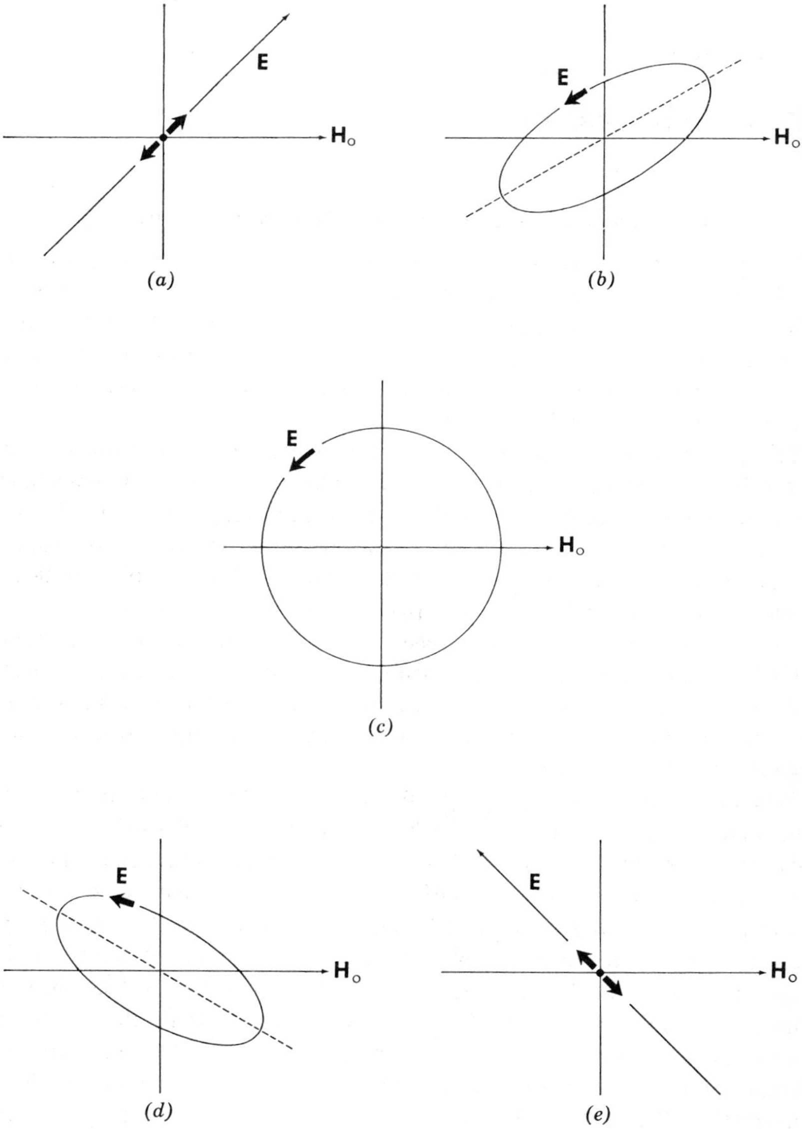

Figure 6.1. Successive polarization in a birefringent medium. (*a*) 0°; (*b*) ~45°; (*c*) 90°; (*d*) ~135°; (*e*) 180°.

Since any anisotropic medium is capable of converting incident plane polarized light into elliptical polarization, an instrument which merely measures the difference between incident and emergent angles of polarization will be incapable of distinguishing between birefringence and optical activity, unless several measurements are made for different path lengths. The problem is considerably more complex when the direction of the light beam makes an arbitrary angle with the magnetic vector. The effects of birefringence and optical activity are superimposed. Experimentally they are difficult to separate, which is one reason why optically active crystals have received relatively little attention.

If the circular dichroism is measured by a method which is independent of the emergent polarization, it will be found that both senses of polarization will have identical absorption coefficients for the purely birefringent case, unlike optical activity. Since it is difficult enough to interpret conventional MORD and MCD data with parallel magnetic field and light beam, little effort has been made to study magnetic birefringence.

6.2. The Classical Theory

As with natural optical activity, it is instructive to briefly develop a classical theory. The situation is even simpler for the Faraday effect, because a precise classical theory may be presented without resorting to artificial constraints. If the incident wave vector is along the z-axis, the motion of charge in an isotropic medium will be confined to the xy-plane. Let the constant magnetic vector also be directed along the z-axis. The perturbing force on a moving charge will be $(e/c)(d\mathbf{r}/dt) \times \mathbf{H}_0$, which is also in the xy-plane.

Consider an isotropically bound electron with force constant $k = \omega_0^2 m$, where $\nu_0 = \omega_0/2\pi$ is the natural vibrational frequency. The equation of motion in the presence of an oscillating electric field $\mathbf{E}$ and a constant magnetic field $\mathbf{H}_0$ is

$$\frac{d^2\mathbf{r}}{dt^2} + \omega_0^2 \mathbf{r} = \frac{e}{m}\left(\mathbf{E} + \frac{1}{c}\frac{d\mathbf{r}}{dt} \times \mathbf{H}_0\right). \tag{6.2.1}$$

Since $\mathbf{E}$ is in the xy-plane and $\mathbf{H}_0$ is perpendicular to it, this reduces to the pair of simultaneous equations

$$\ddot{x} + \omega_0^2 x = \frac{e}{m} E_x + \frac{eH_0}{mc} \dot{y} \tag{6.2.2a}$$

$$\ddot{y} + \omega_0^2 y = \frac{e}{m} E_y - \frac{eH_0}{mc} \dot{x}. \tag{6.2.2b}$$

The oscillatory field will have the form

$$\mathbf{E} = \mathbf{E}_0 e^{-i\omega t},$$

and the steady state solutions to (6.2.2) will consist of forced oscillations with frequency ω:

$$x = x_0 e^{-i\omega t} \tag{6.2.3a}$$

$$y = y_0 e^{-i\omega t}. \tag{6.2.3b}$$

The substitution of these forms into (6.2.2) gives

$$(\omega_0^2 - \omega^2)x + i\omega \frac{eH_0}{mc} y = \frac{e}{m} E_{0x} \tag{6.2.4a}$$

$$-i\omega \frac{eH_0}{mc} x + (\omega_0^2 - \omega^2)y = \frac{e}{m} E_{0y}. \tag{6.2.4b}$$

The solutions to this set of linear algebraic equations are

$$x = \frac{\begin{vmatrix} \frac{e}{m} E_{0x} & i\omega \frac{eH_0}{mc} \\ \frac{e}{m} E_{0y} & \omega_0^2 - \omega^2 \end{vmatrix}}{\begin{vmatrix} \omega_0^2 - \omega^2 & i\omega \frac{eH_0}{mc} \\ -i\omega \frac{eH_0}{mc} & \omega_0^2 - \omega^2 \end{vmatrix}} \tag{6.2.5a}$$

$$y = \frac{\begin{vmatrix} \omega_0^2 - \omega^2 & \frac{e}{m} E_{0x} \\ -i\omega \frac{eH_0}{mc} & \frac{e}{m} E_{0y} \end{vmatrix}}{\begin{vmatrix} \omega_0^2 - \omega^2 & i\omega \frac{eH_0}{mc} \\ -i\omega \frac{eH_0}{mc} & \omega_0^2 - \omega^2 \end{vmatrix}}. \tag{6.2.5b}$$

For the low magnetic intensities required $|\omega e H_0/mc| \ll \omega_0^2 - \omega^2$ outside of the resonance region. The polarization may accordingly be written

$$\mathbf{P} = Ne(\mathbf{i}x + \mathbf{j}y)$$

$$= Ne\left\{\mathbf{i}\left[\frac{e}{m} E_{0x} \frac{1}{\omega_0^2 - \omega^2} - i\omega \frac{e^2 H_0 E_{0y}}{m^2 c(\omega_0^2 - \omega^2)^2}\right]\right.$$

$$\left. + \mathbf{j}\left[\frac{e}{m} E_{0y} \frac{1}{\omega_0^2 - \omega^2} + i\omega \frac{e^2}{m^2 c} \frac{H_0 E_{0x}}{(\omega_0^2 - \omega^2)^2}\right]\right\}. \tag{6.2.6}$$

For propagation along the z-axis the wave equation is

$$\frac{\partial^2 \mathbf{E}}{\partial z^2} = \frac{1}{c^2} \frac{\partial^2 \mathbf{D}}{\partial t^2}. \tag{6.2.7}$$

In the usual manner one assumes that all vectors have the phase factor $e^{-i\omega(t - nz/c)}$, from which it follows that

$$n^2 \mathbf{E} = \mathbf{D} = \mathbf{E} + 4\pi\mathbf{P}. \tag{6.2.8}$$

The types of waves transmitted by such a medium will be determined by combining (6.2.6) and (6.2.8) and solving for the components of $\mathbf{E}_0$. The result is

$$\left[(n^2 - 1) - \frac{4\pi N e^2}{m(\omega_0^2 - \omega^2)}\right] E_{0x} + \frac{4\pi i N e^3}{m^2 c} \frac{\omega H_0}{(\omega_0^2 - \omega^2)^2} E_{0y} = 0 \tag{6.2.9a}$$

$$-\frac{4\pi i N e^3}{m^2 c} \frac{\omega H_0}{(\omega_0^2 - \omega^2)^2} E_{0x} + \left[(n^2 - 1) - \frac{4\pi N e^2}{m(\omega_0^2 - \omega^2)}\right] E_{0y} = 0. \tag{6.2.9b}$$

This pair of homogeneous equations has solutions only if the determinant of the coefficients vanishes. The resulting equation has the form

$$n^2 - \bar{n}^2 = \pm 2\Delta n, \tag{6.2.10}$$

where $\bar{n}^2 = 1 + [4\pi N e^2/m(\omega_0^2 - \omega^2)]$ is the classical index of refraction for a dilute gas of isotropic oscillators and $\Delta n = (2\pi N e^3/m^2 c)[\omega/(\omega_0^2 - \omega^2)^2] H_0$. The two positive solutions to (6.2.10) are

$$n_\pm = \bar{n} \pm \frac{\Delta n}{\bar{n}}.$$

In Chapter 1 it has been shown that the upper sign corresponds to left and the lower to right circularly polarized light. The circular components of incident plane polarized light will be propagated with different phase velocities leading to a rotation per unit path length of

$$\theta = \frac{\pi(n_+ - n_-)}{\lambda} = \frac{\pi(\bar{n}^2 - 1)^2}{2Ne\bar{n}\lambda^2} H_0. \tag{6.2.11}$$

By a simple calculation this can be put into the form originated by Becquerel:

$$\theta = \frac{e}{2mc^2}\,\omega\,\frac{dn}{d\omega}. \tag{6.2.12}$$

The above model applies to a diamagnetic monatomic gas and agrees fairly well with experiment. Outside the absorption region a negative rotation is predicted. It is strongly emphasized that we have used the chemist's convention based on the point of view of the observer, whereas many earlier calculations in the literature have used the opposite signed physicist's convention.

In summary one may say that an oscillatory electric field along the x-axis produces an out of phase component along the y-axis because of the velocity dependence of the magnetic perturbation. This is the same situation encountered in natural optical activity with the resultant rotation of plane polarized light. There is, however, a major difference in mechanism. In the latter case the electron had to undergo a spiral motion in three dimensions; for the Faraday effect the electron need only move in a plane.

6.3. The Quantum Theory

If there are no serious objections to sacrificing a certain amount of rigor, much of the quantum mechanical development of the Faraday effect may be obtained from equations developed in Chapter 2. In the course of determining the properties of waves in optically active media it was necessary to obtain the average values of induced electric and magnetic moments. These in turn led to a solution of the wave equation in which it was found that only circularly polarized waves were propagated for a nonabsorbing medium.

A general relation for the expectation value of an observable in an electromagnetic field is provided by (2.4.19). For isotropic media averaging over all molecular orientations with respect to the fixed electromagnetic field vectors was performed without weighting, leading to the results of (2.4.22). This is not permissible in the presence of a constant magnetic field, for the isotropy has been destroyed. The wave functions are now orientation dependent, and a special type of averaging is required.

It will be important to recognize that, in addition to the perturbation of the molecular wave functions, there will be an alteration of the statistical distribution function. These two effects lead to substantially different behavior. The first occurs for all substances, paramagnetic and diamagnetic, whereas the second is only of importance for paramagnetic substances or those with appreciably populated degenerate states.

One is on firmest ground by treating the diamagnetic effect, in which the perturbation of the wave functions is considered. The paramagnetic case is more complex; and there is a possibility that the more precise relativisitic formulations of quantum theory may be required to properly describe all the various spin dependent phenomena.

The assumption to be made is that (2.4.19) still holds in the presence of a magnetic field $\mathbf{H}_0$, provided that the magnetically perturbed wave functions are used in the averaging process. Strictly speaking, one should use second order time dependent perturbation theory from the start. Since this procedure is somewhat laborious and leads to the same result, as so often happens, the simpler combination of first order time dependent and first order time independent theory will be employed.

In the absence of radiation the magnetic field introduces a term $-\mathbf{H}_0 \cdot \mathbf{m}$ to the Hamiltonian. The ground and excited state functions to be used in the averaging process are

$$\psi_n' = \psi_n + \sum_{s \neq n} \frac{(\mathbf{H}_0 \cdot \mathbf{m})_{sn} \psi_s}{E_s - E_n} \tag{6.3.1a}$$

$$\psi_0' = \psi_0 + \sum_{t \neq 0} \frac{\mathbf{H}_0 \cdot \mathbf{m}_{t0} \psi_t}{E_t - E_0}. \tag{6.3.1b}$$

In (2.4.19) let $Q \to \boldsymbol{\mu}$. A typical term in the averaging is [cf. (2.4.19*a*)]

$$\mathrm{Re}(i\langle o|\boldsymbol{\mu}|n\rangle'\langle n|\boldsymbol{\mu}|0\rangle') \cdot \dot{\mathbf{E}}$$

$$= \mathrm{Re}\, i\Bigg[\boldsymbol{\mu}_{0n}\boldsymbol{\mu}_{n0} + \sum_{s \neq n} \frac{\boldsymbol{\mu}_{0n}(\mathbf{H}_0 \cdot \mathbf{m}_{ns})\boldsymbol{\mu}_{s0} + \boldsymbol{\mu}_{0s}(\mathbf{H}_0 \cdot \mathbf{m}_{sn})\boldsymbol{\mu}_{n0}}{E_s - E_n}$$
$$+ \sum_{t \neq 0} \frac{\boldsymbol{\mu}_{0n}\boldsymbol{\mu}_{nt}(\mathbf{H}_0 \cdot \mathbf{m}_{t0}) + (\mathbf{H}_0 \cdot \mathbf{m}_{0t})\boldsymbol{\mu}_{tn}\boldsymbol{\mu}_{n0}}{E_t - E_0}\Bigg] \cdot \dot{\mathbf{E}} \tag{6.3.2}$$

The relations

$$\langle(\mathbf{A}_1 \cdot \mathbf{B}_1)(\mathbf{A}_2 \cdot \mathbf{B}_2)(\mathbf{A}_3 \cdot \mathbf{B}_3)\rangle_{\mathrm{av}} = \tfrac{1}{6}(\mathbf{A}_1 \cdot \mathbf{A}_2 \times \mathbf{A}_3)(\mathbf{B}_1 \cdot \mathbf{B}_2 \times \mathbf{B}_3)$$

and

$$\langle \mathbf{A}_1(\mathbf{A}_2 \cdot \mathbf{B}_2)(\mathbf{A}_3 \cdot \mathbf{B}_3)\rangle_{\mathrm{av}} = \tfrac{1}{6}(\mathbf{A}_1 \cdot \mathbf{A}_2 \times \mathbf{A}_3)(\mathbf{B}_2 \times \mathbf{B}_3)$$

have been discussed in Chapter 1, where the two sets of vectors define coordinate systems with arbitrary relative orientation. The application of the second formula to (6.3.2) gives

$$\langle \mathrm{Re}(i\langle 0|\boldsymbol{\mu}|n\rangle'\langle n|\boldsymbol{\mu}|0\rangle') \cdot \dot{\mathbf{E}}\rangle_{\mathrm{av}}$$
$$= -\tfrac{1}{6}\mathrm{Im}\Bigg[\sum_{s \neq n} \frac{\boldsymbol{\mu}_{0n} \cdot \mathbf{m}_{ns} \times \boldsymbol{\mu}_{s0} + \boldsymbol{\mu}_{0s} \cdot \mathbf{m}_{sn} \times \boldsymbol{\mu}_{n0}}{E_s - E_n}$$
$$+ \sum_{t \neq 0} \frac{-(\boldsymbol{\mu}_{0n} \cdot \boldsymbol{\mu}_{nt} \times \mathbf{m}_{t0} + \mathbf{m}_{0t} \cdot \boldsymbol{\mu}_{tn} \times \boldsymbol{\mu}_{n0})}{E_t - E_0}\Bigg]. \tag{6.3.3}$$

The term $\langle i\boldsymbol{\mu}_{0n}\boldsymbol{\mu}_{n0} \cdot \dot{\mathbf{E}}\rangle_{av}$ vanishes because it is pure imaginary for nondegenerate functions.

The application of these methods in the averaging of (2.4.19) for $\boldsymbol{\mu}$ and $\mathbf{m}$ gives

$$\langle\boldsymbol{\mu}\rangle_{\text{av}} = (\alpha\mathbf{E} + f_1\mathbf{H}_0 \times \mathbf{E}) + f_2\,\mathbf{H}_0 \times \dot{\mathbf{E}} + (\gamma\mathbf{B} + f_3\,\mathbf{H}_0 \times \mathbf{B}) + \left(-\frac{\beta}{c}\dot{\mathbf{B}} + f_4\mathbf{H}_0 \times \dot{\mathbf{B}}\right) \qquad (6.3.4a)$$

$$\langle\mathbf{m}\rangle_{\text{av}} = (\kappa\mathbf{B} + f'_1\mathbf{H}_0 \times \mathbf{B}) + f'_2\,\mathbf{H}_0 \times \dot{\mathbf{B}} + (\gamma\mathbf{E} + f'_3\,\mathbf{H}_0 \times \mathbf{E}) + \left(\frac{\beta}{c}\dot{\mathbf{E}} + f'_4\,\mathbf{H}_0 \times \dot{\mathbf{E}}\right), \qquad (6.3.4b)$$

where

$$\alpha = \frac{2}{3h}\sum_n \frac{\nu_{0n}\,|\boldsymbol{\mu}_{0n}|^2}{\nu_{0n}^2 - \nu^2},$$

$$\kappa = \frac{2}{3h}\sum_n \frac{\nu_{0n}\,|\mathbf{m}_{0n}|^2}{\nu_{0n}^2 - \nu^2},$$

$$\gamma = \frac{2}{3h}\sum_n \frac{\nu_{0n}\,\text{Re}(\boldsymbol{\mu}_{0n}\cdot\mathbf{m}_{n0})}{\nu_{0n}^2 - \nu^2},$$

$$\beta = \frac{c}{3\pi h}\sum_n \frac{\text{Im}(\boldsymbol{\mu}_{0n}\cdot\mathbf{m}_{n0})}{\nu_{0n}^2 - \nu_2^2},$$

are the terms encountered in the isotropic theory of natural optical activity [(2.4.22)] and

$$f_1 = \frac{1}{3h}\sum_n \frac{\nu_{0n}}{\nu_{0n}^2 - \nu^2}\,\text{Re}(Q_{\boldsymbol{\mu}n})$$

$$f_2 = -\frac{1}{6\pi h}\sum_n \frac{1}{\nu_{0n}^2 - \nu^2}\,\text{Im}(Q_{\boldsymbol{\mu}n})$$

$$f_3 = \frac{1}{3h}\sum_n \frac{\nu_{0n}}{\nu_{0n}^2 - \nu^2}\,\text{Re}(W_n)$$

$$f_4 = -\frac{1}{6\pi h}\sum_n \frac{1}{\nu_{0n}^2 - \nu^2}\,\text{Im}(W_n)$$

$$f'_1 = \frac{1}{3h}\sum_n \frac{\nu_{0n}}{\nu_{0n}^2 - \nu^2}\,\text{Re}(Q_{\mathbf{m}n})$$

$$f'_2 = -\frac{1}{6\pi h}\sum_n \frac{1}{\nu_{0n}^2 - \nu^2}\,\text{Im}(Q_{\mathbf{m}n})$$

$$f'_3 = -f_3$$

$$f'_4 = f_4$$

$$Q_{\mu n} = \left(\sum_{s\neq n} \frac{\boldsymbol{\mu}_{0n}\cdot\mathbf{m}_{ns}\times\boldsymbol{\mu}_{s0} + \boldsymbol{\mu}_{0s}\cdot\mathbf{m}_{sn}\times\boldsymbol{\mu}_{n0}}{E_s - E_n} - \sum_{t\neq 0} \frac{\boldsymbol{\mu}_{0n}\cdot\boldsymbol{\mu}_{nt}\times\mathbf{m}_{t0} + \mathbf{m}_{0t}\cdot\boldsymbol{\mu}_{tn}\times\boldsymbol{\mu}_{n0}}{E_t - E_0}\right)$$

$$= 2i\,\mathrm{Im}\left(\sum_{s\neq n} \frac{\boldsymbol{\mu}_{0n}\cdot\mathbf{m}_{ns}\times\boldsymbol{\mu}_{s0}}{E_s - E_n} - \sum_{t\neq 0} \frac{\boldsymbol{\mu}_{0n}\cdot\boldsymbol{\mu}_{nt}\times\mathbf{m}_{t0}}{E_t - E_0}\right)$$

$$Q_{\mathbf{m}n} = \left(\sum_{s\neq n} \frac{\mathbf{m}_{0n}\cdot\mathbf{m}_{ns}\times\mathbf{m}_{s0} + \mathbf{m}_{0s}\cdot\mathbf{m}_{sn}\times\mathbf{m}_{n0}}{E_s - E_n} - \sum_{t\neq 0} \frac{\mathbf{m}_{0n}\cdot\mathbf{m}_{nt}\times\mathbf{m}_{t0} + \mathbf{m}_{0t}\cdot\mathbf{m}_{tn}\times\mathbf{m}_{n0}}{E_t - E_0}\right)$$

$$= 2i\,\mathrm{Im}\left(\sum_{s\neq n} \frac{\mathbf{m}_{0n}\cdot\mathbf{m}_{ns}\times\mathbf{m}_{s0}}{E_s - E_n} - \sum_{t\neq 0} \frac{\mathbf{m}_{0n}\cdot\mathbf{m}_{nt}\times\mathbf{m}_{t0}}{E_t - E_0}\right)$$

$$W_n = \left(\sum_{s\neq n} \frac{\boldsymbol{\mu}_{0n}\cdot\mathbf{m}_{ns}\times\mathbf{m}_{s0} + \boldsymbol{\mu}_{0s}\cdot\mathbf{m}_{sn}\times\mathbf{m}_{n0}}{E_s - E_n} - \sum_{t\neq 0} \frac{\boldsymbol{\mu}_{0n}\cdot\mathbf{m}_{nt}\times\mathbf{m}_{t0} + \mathbf{m}_{0t}\cdot\boldsymbol{\mu}_{tn}\times\mathbf{m}_{n0}}{E_t - E_0}\right).$$

As has been discussed in Chapters 1 and 2, the electromagnetic field vectors **E** and **B** must be derivable from a single vector potential, which describes the effective field acting on the molecule. It is assumed that there is a linear relation between this field and the average field $\mathbf{A}_{av}$, in terms of which wave propagation is discussed. The necessary relations are

$$\mathbf{E}_{av} = -\frac{1}{c}\dot{\mathbf{A}}_{av} \quad (a) \qquad \mathbf{B}_{av} = \nabla\times\mathbf{A}_{av} \quad (b)$$
$$\mathbf{E}_{eff} = -\frac{S}{c}\dot{\mathbf{A}}_{av} \quad (c) \qquad \mathbf{B}_{eff} = S\nabla\times\mathbf{A}_{av}, \quad (d) \tag{6.3.5}$$

where it is understood that the quantities in (6.3.4) are effective field vectors.

The propagation of waves is governed by (1.4.2*b*) with $\mathbf{J}_{mac} = 0$:

$$\nabla\times\mathbf{B} = \frac{1}{c}\dot{\mathbf{E}} + \frac{4\pi}{c}\mathbf{P} + 4\pi\nabla\times\boldsymbol{\mu}. \tag{6.3.6}$$

The substitution of the relations $\mathbf{P} = N\langle\mathbf{p}\rangle_{\text{av}}$ and $\mathbf{M} = N\langle\mathbf{m}\rangle_{\text{av}}$ from (6.3.4) with $\mathbf{A}$ as the average potential and $S\mathbf{A}$ as the effective potential gives

$$-(1 - 4\pi NS\kappa)\nabla^2\mathbf{A} = -\frac{1}{c^2}(1 + 4\pi NS\alpha)\ddot{\mathbf{A}}$$

$$-\left(\frac{8\pi NS\beta}{c}\right)\nabla \times \ddot{\mathbf{A}} + 4\pi NS\left[-\left(\frac{f_2}{c^2}\right)\mathbf{H}_0 \times \ddot{\mathbf{A}} - f'_2(\mathbf{H}_0 \cdot \nabla)\nabla \times \dot{\mathbf{A}}\right.$$

$$+\left(\frac{1}{c}\right)(f'_3 - f_3)(\mathbf{H}_0 \cdot \nabla)\dot{\mathbf{A}} + \left(\frac{1}{c}\right)(f'_4 - f_4)(\mathbf{H}_0 \cdot \nabla)\ddot{\mathbf{A}} + \left(\frac{f_3}{c}\right)\nabla(\dot{\mathbf{A}} \cdot \mathbf{H}_0)$$

$$\left. + \left(\frac{f_4}{c}\right)\nabla(\ddot{\mathbf{A}} \cdot \mathbf{H}_0)\right], \qquad (6.3.7)$$

where standard vector identities and the radiation gauge assumption $\nabla \cdot \mathbf{A} = 0$ have been used.

It is only necessary to use complex wave functions when the ground or excited state is degenerate. For real wave functions f_1, f'_1, f_4, and f'_4, vanish. A basis set of degenerate functions may always be taken to be real. In the presence of a magnetic field the solution to the secular determinant leads to linear combinations with complex coefficients $\psi_n = \sum_i C_{ni}\phi_i$, where ϕ_i are real and the C_{ni} are complex. A term such as $\boldsymbol{\mu}_{0n} \cdot \mathbf{m}_{ns} \times \boldsymbol{\mu}_{s0}$ will become

$$\sum_n \boldsymbol{\mu}_{0n} \cdot \mathbf{m}_{ns} \times \boldsymbol{\mu}_{s0} = \sum_n \sum_i \sum_j C_{ni} C^*_{nj}$$

$$\boldsymbol{\mu}_{0i} \cdot \mathbf{m}_{js} \times \boldsymbol{\mu}_{s0} = \sum_i \boldsymbol{\mu}_{0i} \cdot \mathbf{m}_{is} \times \boldsymbol{\mu}_{s0}, \qquad (6.3.8)$$

where

$$\boldsymbol{\mu}_{0n} = \langle\psi_0|\,\boldsymbol{\mu}\,|\psi_n\rangle,$$

$$\boldsymbol{\mu}_{0i} = \langle\psi_0|\,\boldsymbol{\mu}\,|\phi_i\rangle.$$

The last step occurs because, in view of the orthogonality of the ψ_n, $\sum_n C_{ni} C_{nj} = \delta_{ij}$.

In the above argument we have neglected the splitting of the degeneracy in the dispersion terms $\nu_{0n} - \nu^2$. A more exact analysis would lead to a higher order term in the frequency splitting, which is always much smaller than the lowest order nonvanishing terms arising from degeneracy to be discussed below. The most important application is when $\mathbf{H}_0$ is parallel to the direction of wave propagation. In this case $\mathbf{A} \cdot \mathbf{H}_0 = 0$, and the last two terms in (6.3.7) vanish, leaving only terms in f_2, f'_2, and $f'_3 - f_3$. The substitution of the trial function $\mathbf{A} = \mathbf{A}_0 e^{-i\omega(t-nz/c)}$, with $\mathbf{H}_0 = H_0\mathbf{k}$, gives

$$[(n^2 - \bar{n}^2) + 8\pi NSH_0 f_3 n]\mathbf{A}_0 = i\left[\frac{8\pi NS\beta\omega n}{c}\right.$$

$$\left. - 4\pi NS\omega H_0(f_2 + n^2 f'_2)\right]\mathbf{k} \times \mathbf{A}_0, \qquad (6.3.9)$$

where $\bar{n} = \sqrt{1 + 4\pi NS\alpha}$ is the average index of refraction for zero field with $\kappa \simeq 0$.

This equation should be compared with (1.7.22), to which it reduces when $H_0 = 0$. By reasoning similar to the derivation of (1.7.15) one concludes that to the first approximation the effects of natural and magnetically induced optical activity are additive with the rotation in radians per unit length given by

$$\phi = \phi_{\text{ORD}} + \phi_{\text{MORD}} = \frac{16\pi^3 \nu^2 NS\beta}{c^2} + \frac{8\pi^3 \nu^2 NS}{c} H_0 \left(\bar{n} f_2' - \frac{f_2}{\bar{n}} \right). \quad (6.3.10)$$

The small correction to $\bar{n}$ proportional to f_3 has been negelected.

In derivatives based on the Lorentz effective field the factor $[(n^2 + 2/3)]^2$ often appears in the dispersion. It is emphasized that such expressions do not have a sound theoretical basis and should be used only as an empirical aid. Unlike natural optical activity, magnetic and electric dipole transitions do not play equivalent roles, as can be seen from the form of the parameters f_2 and f_2. The ratio of these two quantities is proportional to the square of the ratio of a magnetic dipole to an electric dipole moment, which we know to be quite small. This presents a fairly good prima facia case for neglecting f_2' in comparison with f_2 even for forbidden transition. This does not necessarily apply to triplet transitions. From the form of f_2 it follows that electric and magnetic moments do not play equivalent roles as is the case with the natural optical activity parameters $\beta = \text{Im}\, \boldsymbol{\mu}_{0n} \cdot \mathbf{m}_{n0}$.

The preceding formulas break down when there is degeneracy. One must then return to (2.4.19) and use degenerate perturbation theory. As has been mentioned, the correct linear combinations of degenerate functions in the presence of a magnetic field are complex. Consider a set of such functions ψ_{ni}, $i = 1, 2, \ldots$. One should also include the possibility of a degenerate ground state ψ_{0j}. Such levels are split by the magnetic field in such a manner that

$$E_n(i) - E_0(j) = h\nu_{0n}(ji) = h\bar{\nu}_{0n} + \mathbf{H}_0 \cdot [\mathbf{m}_0(jj) - \mathbf{m}_n(ii)], \quad (6.3.11)$$

where $\bar{\nu}_{0n}$ is the unperturbed frequency of the band. In general $\mathbf{m}_{00} - \mathbf{m}_{nn}$ differs from one component of the band to another.

From the preceding development of the nondegenerate case it follows that only the term in $\langle \boldsymbol{\mu} \rangle$ proportional to $\mathbf{E}$ need be considered. Equation 2.4.19 gives

$$\langle \boldsymbol{\mu} \rangle = -\frac{1}{\pi h} \sum_{i,j} \frac{\text{Im}[\boldsymbol{\mu}_{0n}(ji)\boldsymbol{\mu}_{n0}(ij)] \cdot \dot{\mathbf{E}}}{\nu_{0n}^2(ji) - \nu^2}. \quad (6.3.12)$$

A Taylor series expansion of the denominator gives

$$\frac{1}{\nu_{0n}^2(ji) - \nu^2} = \frac{1}{\bar{\nu}_{0n}^2 - \nu^2} - \frac{2[\nu_{0n}(ji) - \bar{\nu}_{0n}]\bar{\nu}_{0n}}{(\bar{\nu}_{0n}^2 - \nu^2)^2}. \quad (6.3.13)$$

The averaging of the first term gives

$$\mathrm{Im}\left[\frac{\langle \boldsymbol{\mu}_{0n}(ji)\boldsymbol{\mu}_{n0}(ij)\cdot\dot{\mathbf{E}}\rangle_{\mathrm{av}}}{\bar{\nu}_{0n}^2-\nu^2}\right]=\frac{1}{3(\bar{\nu}_{0n}^2-\nu^2)}\,\mathrm{Im}[\boldsymbol{\mu}_{0n}(ji)]^2\,\dot{\mathbf{E}}=0. \quad (6.3.14)$$

From the second term is obtained

$$\begin{aligned}\langle\boldsymbol{\mu}\rangle_{\mathrm{av}}&=\frac{2\bar{\nu}_{0n}}{\pi h(\bar{\nu}_{0n}^2-\nu^2)^2}\left\langle\sum_{i,j}\mathrm{Im}\{[\nu_{0n}(ji)-\bar{\nu}_{0n}]\boldsymbol{\mu}_{0n}(ji)\boldsymbol{\mu}_{n0}(ij)\cdot\dot{\mathbf{E}}\}\right\rangle_{\mathrm{av}}\\&=-\frac{2\bar{\nu}_{0n}}{\pi h^2(\bar{\nu}_{0n}^2-\nu^2)^2}\left\langle\sum_{i,j}\mathrm{Im}\{\boldsymbol{\mu}_{0n}(ji)\mathbf{H}_0\cdot[\mathbf{m}_n(ii)-\mathbf{m}_0(jj)]\boldsymbol{\mu}_{n0}(ij)\cdot\dot{\mathbf{E}}\}\right\rangle_{\mathrm{av}}\\&=\frac{\nu_{0n}}{3\pi h^2(\nu_{0n}^2-\nu^2)^2}\,\mathrm{Im}\left\{\sum_{ij}\boldsymbol{\mu}_{0n}(ji)\times\boldsymbol{\mu}_{n0}(ij)\cdot[\mathbf{m}_n(ii)-\mathbf{m}_0(jj)]\right\}\mathbf{H}_0\times\dot{\mathbf{E}}\\&=f_2(\mathrm{degen})\mathbf{H}_0\times\dot{\mathbf{E}},\end{aligned} \quad (6.3.15)$$

where (6.3.11) has been used for $\nu_{0n}(ji)$.

From the intrinsic properties of spherical harmonics it can be shown from this equation that diamagnetic atoms always give positive rotations on the long wave length region for positive H_0. This comprises a quantum mechanical derivation of the Becquerel equation derived classically in Section 6.2.

A further reduction of (6.3.15) is possible. We shall confine ourselves to representational degeneracy where the set of functions spans a single representation of the overall symmetry group. The term "accidental degeneracy" refers to the case where two or more functions of different symmetry have the same energy. The terms "representation" and "accidental" will also be used to describe cases of approximate degeneracy as well.

By analogy with the spherical harmonic hydrogen functions the states may be arranged in pairs leading to magnetic moments with equal values and opposite sign. If the degree of degeneracy is odd, one of the functions will not be affected by the magnetic field (cf. the $2p_x$, $2p_y$, $2p_z$ functions in a field along the z-axis). Such a state will make no contribution to (6.3.15).

Let ψ_1 and ψ_2 be two appropriately paired degenerate functions. For spherical symmetry the secular determinant automatically leads to such a pairing. For lower symmetry the result is only approximate. The only possible case where a problem might arise here is in the $\mathscr{I}$ group with five-fold degeneracy. The pairing will be exact for all other point groups. The secular equations are

$$c_1(V_{11}-\Delta E)+c_2V_{12}=0 \quad (6.3.16a)$$

$$c_1V_{21}+c_2(V_{22}-\Delta E)=0, \quad (6.3.16b)$$

where $V = -\mathbf{H}_0 \cdot \mathbf{m}$. Since ψ_1 and ψ_2 may be taken to be real, V_{11} and V_{22} vanish and V_{12} is pure imaginary. From this it follows that the correct linear combinations in the presence of the magnetic field are

$$\Theta_{\pm} = \frac{1}{\sqrt{2}}(\psi_1 \pm i\psi_2), \tag{6.3.17}$$

where the functions have been presumed to be orthogonal

The contribution to (6.3.15) will be given by

$$\begin{aligned} \boldsymbol{\mu}_{0+} \times \boldsymbol{\mu}_{+0} \cdot \mathbf{m}_{++} + \boldsymbol{\mu}_{0-} \times \boldsymbol{\mu}_{0-} \cdot \mathbf{m}_{--} \\ &= \tfrac{1}{4}(\boldsymbol{\mu}_{01} + i\boldsymbol{\mu}_{02}) \times (\boldsymbol{\mu}_{01} - i\boldsymbol{\mu}_{02}) \cdot (2i\mathbf{m}_{12}) \\ &\quad + \tfrac{1}{4}(\boldsymbol{\mu}_{01} - i\boldsymbol{\mu}_{02}) \times (\boldsymbol{\mu}_{01} + i\boldsymbol{\mu}_{02}) \cdot (-2i\mathbf{m}_{12}) \\ &= 2\boldsymbol{\mu}_{01} \times \boldsymbol{\mu}_{02} \cdot \mathbf{m}_{12}, \end{aligned} \tag{6.3.18}$$

where

$$\boldsymbol{\mu}_{0+} = \langle \Psi_0 | \boldsymbol{\mu} | \Theta_+ \rangle, \text{ etc.}$$

Let $\boldsymbol{\mu}_{01}$ and $\boldsymbol{\mu}_{02}$ be in the xy-plane with $\boldsymbol{\mu}_{01} = A\mathbf{i}$. For cylindrical symmetry about the z-axis $\psi_2 = (\partial/\partial\phi)\psi_1$, since $\psi_1 = f(r) \sin \phi$, $\psi_2 = f(r) \cos \phi$ for an allowed transition from a totally symmetric ground state. Let us assume that this holds approximately for the general case, provided that one has not gone out of his way to construct a degenerate but highly noncylindrical system; for example, one would expect the approximation to be good for benzene (I), but not for the aromatic compound (II).

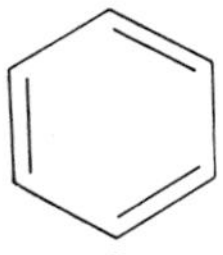

I

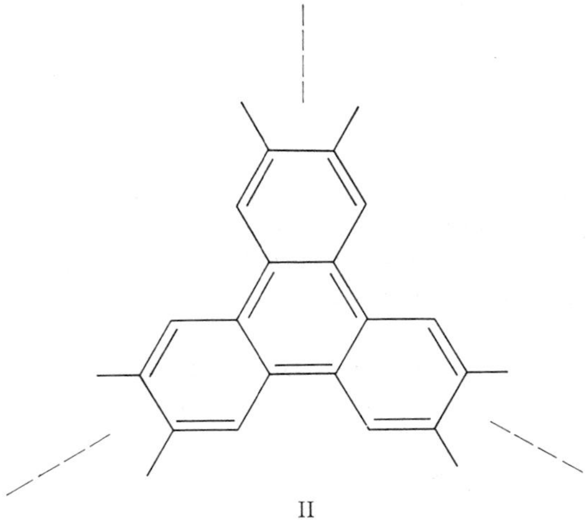

II

Accordingly we write $\psi_2 = (\partial/\partial\phi)\psi_1$, where ϕ is the angle about the z-axis. With the assumption that $\boldsymbol{\mu}_{01}$ is along $\mathbf{i}$ one obtains

$$\boldsymbol{\mu}_{01} = A\mathbf{i} = \mathbf{i}\int \Psi_0\, r \sin\theta \cos\phi\, \psi_1\, d\tau \tag{6.3.19a}$$

$$\boldsymbol{\mu}_{02} = \mathbf{j}\int \Psi_0\, r \sin\theta \sin\phi \frac{\partial}{\partial\phi}\psi_1\, d\tau$$

$$= \mathbf{j}\int \Psi_0\, r \sin\theta \cos\phi\, \psi_1 = -A\mathbf{j}, \tag{6.3.19b}$$

where it has been assumed that the totally symmetric ground state has approximate cylindrical symmetry with $(\partial/\partial\phi)\Psi_0 \simeq 0$. Since $m_z = -i(e\hbar/2mc)(\partial/\partial\phi)$, one obtains

$$\mathbf{m}_{12} = \mathbf{k}\int \psi_1 m_z \frac{\partial}{\partial\phi}\psi_1\, d\tau$$

$$= i\mathbf{k}\left(\frac{e\hbar}{2mc}\right)\int \frac{\partial\psi_1}{\partial\phi}\frac{\partial\psi_1}{\partial\phi}\, d\tau$$

$$= i\mathbf{k}\left(\frac{e\hbar}{2mc}\right)\int \psi_2^2\, d\tau = i\mathbf{k}\left(\frac{e\hbar}{2mc}\right). \tag{6.3.20}$$

The final result is $2\boldsymbol{\mu}_{01} \times \boldsymbol{\mu}_{02} \cdot \mathbf{m}_{12} = -2i\boldsymbol{\mu}_{0_n}^2(e\hbar/2mc)$, where $\bar{\boldsymbol{\mu}}_{0n}$ is the transition moment. This leads to a contribution in (6.3.15):

$$f_2(n) = \frac{-2\bar{\nu}_{0n}(e\hbar/2mc)\boldsymbol{\mu}_{0n}^2}{3\pi h^2(\nu_{0n}^2 - \nu^2)^2}. \tag{6.3.21}$$

Since the electron charge is negative and the rotation is proportional to $-f_2 H_0$, a negative contribution is predicted for positive H_0.

The preceding result is precise for spherical and cylindrical symmetry but only approximate for any other. Since most degenerate systems of interest do have such approximate symmetry, we are led to propose the following rule:

In the long wave region a strongly allowed degenerate transition will make a negative contribution to the magnetic rotatory strength. This will be characterized by both negative dispersion and dichroism curves on the long wave side of the band. The predicted behavior is shown in Figure 6.2.

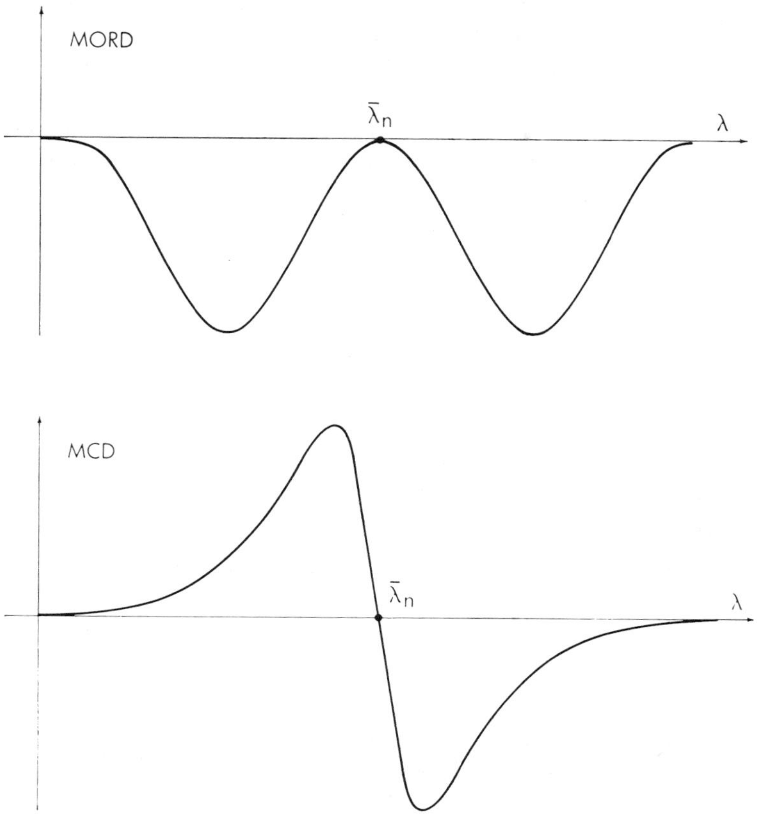

Figure 6.2. Behavior of a degenerate transition.

The terms f_2 in (6.3.4) and f_2 (degen) both describe the diamagnetic contributions to the Faraday effect in an equivalent manner, as can be seen by letting two frequencies in f_2 approach one another:

$$-\frac{1}{6\pi h}\frac{1}{E_s - E_n}\,\mathrm{Im}\left[\frac{1}{v_{0n}^2 - v^2}(\boldsymbol{\mu}_{0n}\cdot\mathbf{m}_{ns}\times\boldsymbol{\mu}_{s0} + \boldsymbol{\mu}_{0s}\cdot\mathbf{m}_{sn}\times\boldsymbol{\mu}_{n0}) - \frac{1}{v_{0s}^2 - v^2}(\boldsymbol{\mu}_{0s}\cdot\mathbf{m}_{sn}\times\boldsymbol{\mu}_{n0} + \boldsymbol{\mu}_{0n}\cdot\mathbf{m}_{ns}\times\boldsymbol{\mu}_{s0})\right]$$

$$\rightarrow \frac{2}{3\pi h^2}\frac{\bar{v}_{0n}}{(\bar{v}_{0n}^2 - v^2)^2}\,\boldsymbol{\mu}_{0n}\times\boldsymbol{\mu}_{0s}\cdot\mathbf{m}_{ns}, \qquad (6.3.22)$$

where $\mathbf{m}_{ns} = -\mathbf{m}_{sn}$, since the functions are real.

This is identical to f_2 (degen) in (6.3.15) with the substitution of the result in (6.3.18). If the whole diamagnetic problem had been treated by a variation procedure with a secular determinant, the result would be written in terms of these two terms. The literature often describes f_2 as the temperature independent paramagnetic term and f_2 (degen) as the diamagnetic term. While there may be some formal grounds for this distinction, it may be preferable to call them nondegenerate and degenerate diamagnetic terms.

When there is a thermally accessible degenerate state, one must take into account the alteration in the molecular distribution function in the presence of the field. Let us write (6.3.12) for a degenerate ground state:

$$\langle \boldsymbol{\mu} \rangle = -\frac{1}{\pi h} \sum_n \sum_i \frac{\text{Im}[\boldsymbol{\mu}_{0n}(i)\boldsymbol{\mu}_{n0}(i)]}{\nu_{0n}^2(i) - \nu^2} \cdot \dot{\mathbf{E}}, \tag{6.3.23}$$

where the summation is over all transitions from the component ground states i to excited states n, which may or may not be degenerate.

The Boltzmann factors for the ground state function ψ_{0i} will be $\exp[-(-\mathbf{H}_0 \cdot \mathbf{m}_{ii})/kT] \simeq 1 + \mathbf{H}_0 \cdot \mathbf{m}_{ii}/kT$. Equation 6.3.23 becomes

$$\begin{aligned} \langle \boldsymbol{\mu} \rangle_{\text{av}} &= -\frac{1}{\pi h k T} \left\langle \text{Im}\left\{ \sum_n \sum_i \frac{[\boldsymbol{\mu}_{0n}(i)\mathbf{H}_0 \cdot \mathbf{m}_{ii}\, \boldsymbol{\mu}_{n0}(i) \cdot \dot{\mathbf{E}}]}{\nu_{0n}^2(i) - \nu^2} \right\} \right\rangle_{\text{av}} \\ &= -\frac{1}{6\pi h k T} \text{Im}\left[\sum_n \sum_i \frac{\boldsymbol{\mu}_{0n}(i) \times \mathbf{m}_{ii} \cdot \boldsymbol{\mu}_{n0}(i)}{\nu_{0n}^2(i) - \nu^2} \right] \mathbf{H}_0 \times \dot{\mathbf{E}}. \end{aligned} \tag{6.3.24}$$

By reasoning similar to the derivation of (6.3.21) it follows that the contribution of this term for transitions to totally symmetric excited states will have the opposite sign to the diamagnetic contributions. Since the total charge distribution of a set of degenerate states has the highest symmetry of the group it is likely that this positive sign will prevail for all significant paramagnetic contributions.

The term just derived is properly called a paramagnetic term, but it should be emphasized that it is on firmest footing for geometrical rather than spin degeneracy. The problem of spin will not be treated in this text. When numerical values are used in the diamagnetic and paramagnetic terms, it is invariably found that the latter are an order of magnitude larger than the former at 300°K.

As with natural optical activity, there are two basic closely related sources of data, dispersion and dichroism. The two curves are connected by a Kronig-

Kramers transform. Historically the magnetic optical rotatory dispersion (MORD) has been reported in terms of a Verdet constant V defined as

$$V = \frac{\phi}{LH_0}, \tag{6.3.25}$$

where L is the path length. Many of the data have been based on the opposite signed convention to the one used here.

If one writes $V = \sum_n V_n/(\nu_{0n}^2 - \nu^2)$, it will follow that $\sum_n V_n = 0$, since all the contributions to the Verdet constant are obtained by suitable averages of the dyads $\boldsymbol{\mu}_{0n}\boldsymbol{\mu}_{n0}$. Regardless of what values the wave functions have, real or complex, it will be true that

$$\mathrm{Im} \sum_{n \neq 0} \boldsymbol{\mu}_{0n}\boldsymbol{\mu}_{n0} = \mathrm{Im}[(\boldsymbol{\mu}\boldsymbol{\mu})_{00} - \boldsymbol{\mu}_{00}\boldsymbol{\mu}_{00}] = 0, \tag{6.3.26}$$

which proves the sum rule for magnetic rotational strengths.

6.4. The Harmonic Oscillator

Before attempting further reductions of the general formulas it will be profitable to pause in a discussion of a simple quantum mechanical model, the harmonic oscillator. We will consider the three allowed electric dipole transitions from the totally symmetric ground state: (000) → (100), (010), (001), which are polarized along the x, y, and z-axes. Equation 6.3.4. becomes

$$f_2(n) = \frac{2}{6\pi h} \frac{1}{\nu_{0n}^2 - \nu^2} \mathrm{Im}\left(\sum_{s \neq n} \frac{\boldsymbol{\mu}_{0n} \times \boldsymbol{\mu}_{s0} \cdot \mathbf{m}_{ns}}{E_s - E_n} + \sum_{t \neq 0} \frac{\boldsymbol{\mu}_{0n} \times \mathbf{m}_{t0} \cdot \boldsymbol{\mu}_{nt}}{E_t - E_0} \right). \tag{6.4.1}$$

For the (000) → (100) transition the only intermediate states which have the necessary nonvanishing matrix elements are (010) and (001) for the excited state and (110) and (101) for the ground state. This leads to the expression

$$f_2(100) = \frac{2}{6\pi h^2} \frac{1}{\nu_1^2 - \nu^2} \mathrm{Im}\left(\frac{\boldsymbol{\mu}_{01} \times \boldsymbol{\mu}_{20} \cdot \mathbf{m}_{12}}{\nu_2 - \nu_1} + \frac{\boldsymbol{\mu}_{01} \times \boldsymbol{\mu}_{30} \cdot \mathbf{m}_{13}}{\nu_3 - \nu_1} \right.$$
$$\left. + \frac{\boldsymbol{\mu}_{01} \times \mathbf{m}_{40} \cdot \boldsymbol{\mu}_{14}}{\nu_1 + \nu_3} + \frac{\boldsymbol{\mu}_{01} \times \mathbf{m}_{50} \cdot \boldsymbol{\mu}_{15}}{\nu_1 + \nu_2} \right), \tag{6.4.2}$$

where $\psi_0 = (000)$, $\psi_1 = (100)$, $\psi_2 = (010)$, $\psi_3 = (001)$, $\psi_4 = (101)$, and $\psi_5 = (110)$.

The electric and magnetic dipole moments have already been determined in (3.2.11) with the results

$$\boldsymbol{\mu}_{01} = ea_1\sqrt{\tfrac{1}{2}}\,\mathbf{i}, \qquad \boldsymbol{\mu}_{02} = ea_2\sqrt{\tfrac{1}{2}}\,\mathbf{j}, \qquad \boldsymbol{\mu}_{03} = ea_3\sqrt{\tfrac{1}{2}}\,\mathbf{k},$$

$$\boldsymbol{\mu}_{14} = ea_3\sqrt{\tfrac{1}{2}}\,\mathbf{k}, \qquad \boldsymbol{\mu}_{15} = ea_2\sqrt{\tfrac{1}{2}}\,\mathbf{j},$$

$$\mathbf{m}_{12} = i\,\frac{e\hbar}{2mc}\,\frac{1}{2}\left(\frac{a_1^2 + a_2^2}{a_1 a_2}\right)\mathbf{k}$$

$$\mathbf{m}_{13} = -i\,\frac{e\hbar}{2mc}\,\frac{1}{2}\left(\frac{a_1^2 + a_3^2}{a_1 a_3}\right)\mathbf{j}$$

$$\mathbf{m}_{40} = i\,\frac{e\hbar}{2mc}\,\frac{1}{2}\left(\frac{a_3^2 - a_1^2}{a_1 a_3}\right)\mathbf{j}$$

$$\mathbf{m}_{50} = i\,\frac{e\hbar}{2mc}\,\frac{1}{2}\left(\frac{a_1^2 - a_2^2}{a_1 a_2}\right)\mathbf{k}$$

where

$$a_i = \frac{1}{2\pi}\left(\frac{h}{m\nu_i}\right)^{1/2}.$$

This leads to the result

$$f_2(100) = -e^2\left(\frac{e\hbar}{2mc}\right)\frac{1}{6\pi h^2}\,\frac{1}{\nu_1^2 - \nu^2}\left(\frac{\nu_1 a_1^2 + \nu_2 a_2^2}{\nu_2^2 - \nu_1^2} + \frac{\nu_1 a_1^2 + \nu_3 a_3^2}{\nu_2^2 - \nu_1^2}\right). \qquad (6.4.3)$$

The terms for the other two transitions are obtained by cyclic permutation. If (100) is the lowest excited state, this predicts a negative contribution to the Verdet constant. It can also be shown that when ν_1, ν_2, and ν_3 are equal the sum $f_2(100) + f_2(010) + f_2(001)$ approaches the Becquerel equation. The sign of the highest transition is positive.

6.5. Approximate Summation of Perturbation Terms

By employing the summation techniques outlined in the previous chapter it is possible to obtain a great deal more information on the behavior of the lowest transitions. The parameter f_2 will be proportional to

$$F_{\mu n} = \sum_{s \neq n} \frac{\boldsymbol{\mu}_{0n} \cdot \mathbf{m}_{ns} \times \boldsymbol{\mu}_{s0}}{E_s - E_n} - \sum_{t \neq 0} \frac{\boldsymbol{\mu}_{0n} \cdot \boldsymbol{\mu}_{nt} \times \mathbf{m}_{t0}}{E_t - E_0}. \qquad (6.5.1)$$

Before proceeding it will be prudent to investigate the requirement of origin invariance. In the expression for the natural optical rotatory parameter a relatively simple situation was encountered where each zeroth order term was invariant and the higher order terms were invariant in pairs. Equation 6.5.1 is only invariant when summed over all intermediate states, which greatly detracts from its usefulness. The invariance is demonstrated by writing (6.5.1) in the form

$$F_{\mu n} = \sum_{s \neq n,\, 0} \frac{\boldsymbol{\mu}_{0n} \cdot \mathbf{m}_{ns} \times \boldsymbol{\mu}_{s0}}{E_s - E_n} - \sum_{t \neq n,\, 0} \frac{\boldsymbol{\mu}_{0n} \cdot \boldsymbol{\mu}_{nt} \times \mathbf{m}_{t0}}{E_t - E_0} + \frac{\boldsymbol{\mu}_{0n} \times \mathbf{m}_{n0} \cdot (\boldsymbol{\mu}_{nn} - \boldsymbol{\mu}_{00})}{E_n - E_0}. \tag{6.5.2}$$

So long as $s \neq 0$, $\boldsymbol{\mu}_{s0}$ is independent of origin, as is $\boldsymbol{\mu}_{nt}$ for $t \neq n$; $\boldsymbol{\mu}_{nn}$ and $\boldsymbol{\mu}_{00}$ depend on origin, but $\boldsymbol{\mu}_{nn} - \boldsymbol{\mu}_{00}$ does not. This leaves $\mathbf{m}_{ns}$ and $\mathbf{m}_{t0}$ as origin dependent terms.

Let $F_{\mu n}$ be evaluated for an arbitrary origin; then make the transformation $\mathbf{r}' = \mathbf{R} + \mathbf{r}$. With the aid of the standard quantum relation

$$\mathbf{p}_{ns} = \frac{im}{e\hbar}(E_n - E_s)\boldsymbol{\mu}_{ns}, \tag{6.5.3}$$

where $\mathbf{p}$ is the momentum operator, $F'_{\mu n}$ in the new coordinate system may be written

$$\begin{aligned} F'_{\mu n} = F_{\mu n} + \frac{im}{e\hbar}\Big[&- \sum_{s \neq n,\, 0} \boldsymbol{\mu}_{0n} \cdot (\mathbf{R} \times \boldsymbol{\mu}_{ns}) \times \boldsymbol{\mu}_{s0} \\ &- \sum_{t \neq n,\, 0} \boldsymbol{\mu}_{0n} \cdot \boldsymbol{\mu}_{nt} \times (\mathbf{R} \times \boldsymbol{\mu}_{t0}) \\ &+ \boldsymbol{\mu}_{0n} \times (\mathbf{R} \times \boldsymbol{\mu}_{n0}) \cdot (\boldsymbol{\mu}_{nn} - \boldsymbol{\mu}_{00})\Big] \\ = F_{\mu n} + \frac{im}{e\hbar}\{ &-[\boldsymbol{\mu}_{0n} \cdot ((\mathbf{R} \times \boldsymbol{\mu}) \times \boldsymbol{\mu})_{n0} \\ &- \boldsymbol{\mu}_{0n} \cdot (\mathbf{R} \times \boldsymbol{\mu}_{nn}) \times \boldsymbol{\mu}_{n0} - \boldsymbol{\mu}_{0n} \cdot (\mathbf{R} \times \boldsymbol{\mu}_{n0})\boldsymbol{\mu}_{00}] \\ &- [\boldsymbol{\mu}_{0n} \cdot (\boldsymbol{\mu} \times (\mathbf{R} \times \boldsymbol{\mu}))_{n0} - \boldsymbol{\mu}_{0n} \cdot \boldsymbol{\mu}_{nn} \times (\mathbf{R} \times \boldsymbol{\mu}_{n0}) \\ &- \boldsymbol{\mu}_{0n} \cdot \boldsymbol{\mu}_{n0} \times (\mathbf{R} \times \boldsymbol{\mu}_{00})]\} = F_{\mu n}. \end{aligned} \tag{6.5.4}$$

The summations over $s \neq n, 0$ and $t \neq n, 0$ have been replaced by summations over all states with the subtraction of the omitted terms.

Any approximate summation technique must be careful to preserve this invariance. Symmetry groups may be classed as centric or axial with the exception of C_1 and C_{1h}. A centric group has a unique origin characterized by either a center of inversion or the simultaneous existence of certain symmetry operations which prevent any components of $\boldsymbol{\mu}$ from being in the totally symmetric representation. Molecules belonging to these groups have zero permanent dipole moments and their magnetic transition moments are independent of origin. This class comprises the groups C_i, C_{nh} $(n \neq 1)$, S_n, D_n, D_{2d}, D_{3d}, D_{nh}, T, $\mathcal{O}$, $\mathcal{O}_h$, T_d, $\mathcal{I}$, and $\mathcal{I}_h$.

The axial groups $C_n (n \neq 1)$ and C_{nv} have a single symmetry axis with no center of inversion. Only the component of $\boldsymbol{\mu}$ along this axis belongs to the totally symmetric representation, which implies that the permanent dipole moment must lie on the symmetry axis. The groups C_1 and C_{1h} are neither axial nor centric. The error in origin dependent terms will be greatest in treating these two groups. Below a method will be developed which avoids this difficulty.

It will be convenient to use the momentum matrix elements $\mathbf{p}_{0n}$ rather than $\boldsymbol{\mu}_{0n}$. Since the dominant f_2 term is derived by averaging the expression $\boldsymbol{\mu}_{0n}\boldsymbol{\mu}_{n0} \cdot \dot{\mathbf{E}}$ it follows from (6.5.3) that one may replace $\boldsymbol{\mu}$ with $\mathbf{p}$ in all the resulting expressions upon multiplication by the factor $e^2\hbar^2/m^2(E_n - E_0)^2]$. This leads to a consideration of the sum

$$F_{\mathbf{p}n} = \sum_{q \neq n} \frac{\mathbf{p}_{0n} \cdot \mathbf{m}_{nq} \times \mathbf{p}_{q0}}{E_q - E_n} - \sum_{q \neq 0} \frac{\mathbf{p}_{0n} \cdot \mathbf{p}_{nq} \times \mathbf{m}_{q0}}{E_q - E_0}. \tag{6.5.5}$$

The desired form can be obtained as a sum of origin dependent and invariant terms by writing

$$\begin{aligned} \mathbf{m}_{nq} &= \frac{1}{2mc} \sum_s \boldsymbol{\mu}_{ns} \times \mathbf{p}_{sq} \\ &= \frac{1}{2mc} \left(\sum_{s \neq n} \boldsymbol{\mu}_{ns} \times \mathbf{p}_{sq} + \boldsymbol{\mu}_{nn} \times \mathbf{p}_{nq} \right). \end{aligned} \tag{6.5.6}$$

The summation is invariant and the origin dependence of $\mathbf{m}_{nq}$ is given by the single term $\boldsymbol{\mu}_{nn} \times \mathbf{p}_{nq}$. This also constitutes a proof of the invariance of $\mathbf{m}_{nq}$ for centric groups, since $\boldsymbol{\mu}_{nn} = 0$.

Equation 6.5.5. becomes

$$\begin{aligned} F_{\mathbf{p}n} = \frac{\mathbf{p}_{0n}}{2mc} \cdot \Bigg[&\sum_{q \neq n} \sum_{s \neq n} \frac{(\boldsymbol{\mu}_{ns} \times \mathbf{p}_{sq}) \times \mathbf{p}_{q0}}{E_q - E_n} \\ &+ \sum_{q \neq 0} \sum_{s \neq 0} \frac{\mathbf{p}_{nq} \times (\mathbf{p}_{qs} \times \boldsymbol{\mu}_{s0})}{E_q - E_0} \\ &+ \sum_{q \neq n} \frac{(\boldsymbol{\mu}_{nn} \times \mathbf{p}_{nq}) \times \mathbf{p}_{q0}}{E_q - E_n} + \sum_{q \neq 0} \frac{\mathbf{p}_{nq} \times (\mathbf{p}_{q0} \times \boldsymbol{\mu}_{00})}{E_q - E_0} \Bigg]. \end{aligned} \tag{6.5.7}$$

With the aid of (6.5.3) the last two terms may be written

$$\sum_{q\neq n}\frac{(\boldsymbol{\mu}_{nn}\times\mathbf{p}_{nq})\times\mathbf{p}_{q0}}{E_q-E_n}+\sum_{q\neq 0}\frac{\mathbf{p}_{nq}\times(\mathbf{p}_{q0}\times\boldsymbol{\mu}_{00})}{E_q-E_0}$$

$$=\frac{im}{e\hbar}\left[-\sum_{q\neq n}(\boldsymbol{\mu}_{nn}\times\boldsymbol{\mu}_{nq})\times\mathbf{p}_{q0}+\sum_{q\neq 0}\mathbf{p}_{nq}\times(\boldsymbol{\mu}_{q0}\times\boldsymbol{\mu}_{00})\right]$$

$$=\frac{im}{e\hbar}[\boldsymbol{\mu}_{nn}(\boldsymbol{\mu}\cdot\mathbf{p})_{n0}-(\boldsymbol{\mu}\mathbf{p})_{n0}\cdot\boldsymbol{\mu}_{nn}-\boldsymbol{\mu}_{00}(\mathbf{p}\cdot\boldsymbol{\mu})_{n0}+\boldsymbol{\mu}_{00}\cdot(\mathbf{p}\boldsymbol{\mu})_{n0}]$$

$$=\frac{im}{e\hbar}[(\boldsymbol{\mu}_{nn}-\boldsymbol{\mu}_{00})(\boldsymbol{\mu}\cdot\mathbf{p})_{n0}-(\boldsymbol{\mu}\mathbf{p})_{n0}\cdot(\boldsymbol{\mu}_{nn}-\boldsymbol{\mu}_{00})], \tag{6.5.8}$$

where the matrix summation rule has been applied along with the relations

$$(\mu_x p_x)_{n0}=(p_x\mu_x)_{n0}, \text{ etc.}$$

The scalar product of this term with $\mathbf{p}_{0n}$ is invariant to an origin change, because

$$\operatorname{Im}\{i\mathbf{p}_{0n}\cdot[(\boldsymbol{\mu}_{nn}-\boldsymbol{\mu}_{00})\mathbf{R}\cdot\mathbf{p}_{n0}-\mathbf{R}\mathbf{p}_{n0}\cdot(\boldsymbol{\mu}_{nn}-\boldsymbol{\mu}_{00})]\}=0. \tag{6.5.9}$$

The individual terms in the first two summations are independent of origin. The summation over s now gives

$$\frac{1}{2mc}\sum_{s\neq n}\boldsymbol{\mu}_{ns}\times\mathbf{p}_{sq}=\mathbf{m}_{nq}-\frac{1}{2mc}\boldsymbol{\mu}_{nn}\times\mathbf{p}_{nq}. \tag{6.5.10}$$

This suggests that the most convenient origin for evaluating the excited state terms is the center of the ψ_n charge cloud with a similar consideration for the ground state. In general (6.5.8) does not vanish and must be added to the individual terms in the first part of (6.5.7).

So far no approximations have been made, and we have arrived at a practicable method for an invariant term by term evaluation of (6.5.5). Let it be assumed that the only state with energy lower than E_n making a contribution to the summations is ψ_0. In the first summation of (6.5.7) $E_q - E_n$ will be positive for all terms because $\mathbf{p}_{00} = 0$. Using an average denominator one may write

$$\frac{1}{2mc}\sum_{q\neq n}\sum_{s\neq n}\frac{(\boldsymbol{\mu}_{ns}\times\mathbf{p}_{sq})\times\mathbf{p}_{q0}}{E_q-E_n}$$

$$\simeq\frac{1}{\bar{E}_n-E_n}\frac{1}{2mc}\sum_{q\neq n}\sum_{s\neq n}(\boldsymbol{\mu}_{ns}\times\mathbf{p}_{sq})\times\mathbf{p}_{q0}$$

$$=\frac{1}{\bar{E}_n-E_n}\left\{(\mathbf{m}\times\mathbf{p})_{n0}-\frac{1}{2mc}[(\boldsymbol{\mu}_{nn}\times\mathbf{p})\times\mathbf{p}]_{n0}-\mathbf{m}_{nn}\times\mathbf{p}_{n0}\right\}. \tag{6.5.11}$$

A similar result is obtained for the ground state sum. When the preceding results are combined (6.5.7) becomes

$$F_{\mathbf{p}n} = \mathbf{p}_{0n} \cdot \left\{ \frac{i}{2e\hbar c} [(\boldsymbol{\mu}_{nn} - \boldsymbol{\mu}_{00})(\boldsymbol{\mu} \cdot \mathbf{p})_{n0} - (\boldsymbol{\mu}\mathbf{p})_{n0} \cdot (\boldsymbol{\mu}_{nn} - \boldsymbol{\mu}_{00})] \right.$$
$$+ \frac{1}{\bar{E}_n - E_n} \left[(\mathbf{m} \times \mathbf{p})_{n0} - \frac{1}{2mc} ((\boldsymbol{\mu}_{nn} \times \mathbf{p}) \times \mathbf{p})_{n0} \right]$$
$$\left. + \frac{1}{\bar{E}_0 - E_0} \left[-(\mathbf{p} \times \mathbf{m})_{n0} - \frac{1}{2mc} (\mathbf{p} \times (\mathbf{p} \times \boldsymbol{\mu}_{00}))_{n0} \right] \right\}. \qquad (6.5.12)$$

If one evaluates the $(\mathbf{m} \times \mathbf{p})_{n0}$ term with an origin at the center of charge of ψ_n ($\boldsymbol{\mu}_{nn} = 0$), the $(\boldsymbol{\mu}_{nn} \times \mathbf{p}) \times \mathbf{p})_{n0}$ term may be dropped; similarly one should evaluate $(\mathbf{p} \times \mathbf{m})_{n0}$ with an origin for which $\boldsymbol{\mu}_{00} = 0$.

With these considerations $F_{\mathbf{p}n}$ may be written in the form

$$F_{\mathbf{p}n} = \mathbf{p}_{0n} \cdot \left\{ \frac{i}{2e\hbar c} [(\boldsymbol{\mu} \times (\boldsymbol{\mu}_{nn} - \boldsymbol{\mu}_{00})) \times \mathbf{p}]_{n0} \right.$$
$$\left. + \frac{1}{\bar{E}_n - E_n} (\mathbf{m} \times \mathbf{p})_{n0} - \frac{1}{\bar{E}_0 - E_0} (\mathbf{p} \times \mathbf{m})_{n0} \right\}. \qquad (6.5.13)$$

For centric groups the first term is zero and the remaining two will be independent of origin.

There is a useful commutation relation between the operators $\mathbf{m} \times \mathbf{p}$ and $\mathbf{p} \times \mathbf{m}$. One first obtains

$$\mathbf{m} \times \mathbf{p} = \frac{e}{2mc} (\mathbf{r} \cdot \mathbf{pp} - \mathbf{rp}^2) \qquad (6.5.14a)$$

$$\mathbf{p} \times \mathbf{m} = \frac{e}{2mc} [\mathbf{p}(\mathbf{r}) \cdot \mathbf{p} - \mathbf{p} \cdot \mathbf{rp}]$$
$$= \frac{e}{2mc} [(\mathbf{rp}^2 - i\hbar\mathbf{p}) - (\mathbf{r} \cdot \mathbf{pp} - 3i\hbar\mathbf{p})], \qquad (6.5.14b)$$

where $\mathbf{p}(\mathbf{r}) \cdot \mathbf{p}$ means that $\mathbf{p}$ operates on $\mathbf{r}$, but the scalar product is taken between the two $\mathbf{p}$ vectors. It then follows that

$$\mathbf{m} \times \mathbf{p} + \mathbf{p} \times \mathbf{m} = \frac{2ie\hbar}{2mc} \mathbf{p}. \qquad (6.5.15)$$

This result emphasizes the fact that $\mathbf{m} \times \mathbf{p}$, $\mathbf{p} \times \mathbf{m}$, and $\mathbf{p}$ have the same symmetry properties. For an electrically forbidden transition the matrix elements $(\mathbf{m} \times \mathbf{p})_{n0}$ and $(\mathbf{p} \times \mathbf{m})_{n0}$ are also zero.

If the transition originates from a totally symmetric orbitals in the ground state $(\mathbf{p} \times \mathbf{m})_{n0}$ will be smaller than $(\mathbf{m} \times \mathbf{p})_{n0}$, because a totally symmetric orbital comes closer to being represented by $f(r)$ than a nontotally symmetric one and $\mathbf{m}f(r) = 0$. For centric groups the dominant term will be in this case

$$\frac{1}{\bar{E}_n - E_n}(\mathbf{m} \times \mathbf{p})_{n0} \simeq \frac{1}{E_n - E_n} 2i\left(\frac{e\hbar}{2mc}\right)\mathbf{p}_{n0},$$

which leads to a negative Verdet constant in agreement with the oscillator model. If the excited orbital is totally symmetric $(\mathbf{p} \times \mathbf{m})_{n0} > (\mathbf{m} \times \mathbf{p})_{n0} \simeq 2i(e\hbar/2mc)\mathbf{p}_{n0}$. It follows from (6.5.13) that an opposite signed Verdet constant will result. If the orbitals are totally symmetric, both $(\mathbf{m} \times \mathbf{p})_{n0}$ and $(\mathbf{p} \times \mathbf{m})_{n0}$ will be quite small.

In practice most transitions correspond to neither of these extremes, and generalizations about the sign of (6.5.13) are not possible. When $\mathbf{p}_{0n}$ vanishes to the first approximation (6.5.13) must be subjected to further treatment. The methods of Chapter 5 may again be used to obtain an expression which depends only on the ground and excited state functions along with the perturbations.

Consider the term $(\boldsymbol{\mu}_{nn} - \boldsymbol{\mu}_{00})(\boldsymbol{\mu} \cdot \mathbf{p})_{n0}$ in (6.5.12). Even though $\boldsymbol{\mu}_{nn} - \boldsymbol{\mu}_{00}$ may be large, it may be in an unfavorable direction; one should therefore calculate its perturbation term. This leads to the result

$$\boldsymbol{\mu}'_{nn} - \boldsymbol{\mu}'_{00} = \boldsymbol{\mu}_{nn} - \boldsymbol{\mu}_{00} + 2\left(\sum_{s \neq n} \frac{V_{ns}\boldsymbol{\mu}_{sn}}{E_n - E_s} - \sum_{s \neq 0} \frac{\boldsymbol{\mu}_{0s} V_{s0}}{E_0 - E_s}\right)$$

$$\simeq \boldsymbol{\mu}_{nn} - \boldsymbol{\mu}_{00} + 2\left[\frac{(\boldsymbol{\mu}V)_{nn} - V_{nn}\boldsymbol{\mu}_{nn}}{E_n - \bar{E}'_n} - \frac{(\boldsymbol{\mu}V)_{00} - V_{00}\boldsymbol{\mu}_{00}}{E_0 - \bar{E}'_0}\right] \qquad (6.5.16a)$$

$$(\boldsymbol{\mu} \cdot \mathbf{p})'_{n0} = (\boldsymbol{\mu} \cdot \mathbf{p})_{n0} + \sum_{s \neq n} \frac{V_{ns}(\boldsymbol{\mu} \cdot \mathbf{p})_{s0}}{E_n - E_s}$$

$$+ \sum_{s \neq 0} \frac{(\boldsymbol{\mu} \cdot \mathbf{p})_{ns} V_{s0}}{E_0 - E_s} \simeq (\boldsymbol{\mu} \cdot \mathbf{p})_{n0} + \frac{(V\boldsymbol{\mu} \cdot \mathbf{p})_{n0} - V_{nn} - (\boldsymbol{\mu} \cdot \mathbf{p})_{n0}}{E_n - \bar{E}'_n}$$

$$+ \frac{(\boldsymbol{\mu} \cdot \mathbf{p}V)_{n0} - (\boldsymbol{\mu} \cdot \mathbf{p})_{n0} V_{00}}{E_0 - \bar{E}'_0}. \qquad (6.5.16b)$$

When $\mathbf{p}_{0n} = 0$ to zeroth order the term in brackets in (6.5.12) will also vanish. One must determine both terms of the scalar product to first order with a resulting second order expression. The evaluation of the perturbation terms, as in (6.5.16), makes the following contribution to (6.5.12):

$$
\begin{aligned}
F_{\mathbf{p}n}^{(2)} = {} & \left[\frac{(V\mathbf{p})_{0n}}{\bar{E}_0 - E_0} + \frac{(\mathbf{p}V)_{0n}}{\bar{E}_n - E_n}\right] \cdot \left\{\frac{i}{2e\hbar c}\left[(\boldsymbol{\mu}_{nn} - \boldsymbol{\mu}_{00})\left(\frac{(V\boldsymbol{\mu}\cdot\mathbf{p})_{n0} - V_{nn}(\boldsymbol{\mu}\cdot\mathbf{p})_{n0}}{\bar{E}_n - E_n}\right.\right.\right. \\
& + \left.\frac{(\boldsymbol{\mu}\cdot\mathbf{p}V)_{n0} - (\boldsymbol{\mu}\cdot\mathbf{p})_{n0}V_{00}}{\bar{E}_0 - E_0}\right) \\
& + 2\left(\frac{(\boldsymbol{\mu}V)_{nn} - V_{nn}\boldsymbol{\mu}_{nn}}{\bar{E}_n - E_n} - \frac{(\boldsymbol{\mu}V)_{00} - V_{00}\boldsymbol{\mu}_{00}}{\bar{E}_0 - E_0}\right)(\boldsymbol{\mu}\cdot\mathbf{p})_{n0} \\
& - \left(\frac{(V\boldsymbol{\mu}\mathbf{p})_{n0} - V_{nn}(\boldsymbol{\mu}\mathbf{p})_{n0}}{\bar{E}_n - E_n} + \frac{(\boldsymbol{\mu}\mathbf{p}V)_{n0} - (\boldsymbol{\mu}\mathbf{p})_{n0}V_{00}}{\bar{E}_0 - E_0}\right)\cdot(\boldsymbol{\mu}_{nn} - \boldsymbol{\mu}_{00}) \\
& \left. - 2(\boldsymbol{\mu}\mathbf{p})_{n0}\cdot\left(\frac{(\boldsymbol{\mu}V)_{nn} - V_{nn}\boldsymbol{\mu}_{nn}}{\bar{E}_n - E_n} - \frac{(\boldsymbol{\mu}V)_{00} - V_{00}\boldsymbol{\mu}_{00}}{\bar{E}_0 - E_0}\right)\right] \\
& + \frac{1}{\bar{E}_n - E_n}\left[\frac{(V\mathbf{m}\times\mathbf{p})_{n0} - V_{nn}(\mathbf{m}\times\mathbf{p})_{n0}}{\bar{E}_n - E_n}\right. \\
& + \frac{(\mathbf{m}\times\mathbf{p}V)_{n0} - V_{00}(\mathbf{m}\times\mathbf{p})_{n0}}{\bar{E}_0 - E_0} - \frac{1}{2mc}\left(\frac{(V\mathbf{p}\mathbf{p})_{n0} - V_{nn}(\mathbf{p}\mathbf{p})_{n0}}{\bar{E}_n - E_n}\right. \\
& + \left.\frac{(\mathbf{p}\mathbf{p}V)_{n0} - V_{00}(\mathbf{p}\mathbf{p})_{n0}}{\bar{E}_0 - E_0}\right)\cdot\boldsymbol{\mu}_{nn} - \frac{1}{2mc}(\mathbf{p}\mathbf{p})_{n0} \\
& \cdot\left(\frac{(\boldsymbol{\mu}V)_{nn} - V_{nn}\boldsymbol{\mu}_{nn}}{\bar{E}_n - E_n}\right) + \frac{1}{2mc}\left(\frac{(V\mathbf{p}^2)_{n0} - V_{nn}(\mathbf{p}^2)_{n0}}{\bar{E}_n - E_n}\right. \\
& + \left.\left.\frac{(\mathbf{p}^2V)_{n0} - V_{00}(\mathbf{p}^2)_{n0}}{\bar{E}_0 - E_0}\right)\boldsymbol{\mu}_{nn} + \frac{1}{2mc}(\mathbf{p}^2)_{n0}\left(\frac{(\boldsymbol{\mu}V)_{nn} - V_{nn}\boldsymbol{\mu}_{nn}}{\bar{E}_n - E_n}\right)\right] \\
& + \frac{1}{\bar{E}_0 - E_0}\left[-\frac{(V\mathbf{p}\times\mathbf{m})_{n0} - V_{nn}(\mathbf{p}\times\mathbf{m})_{n0}}{\bar{E}_n - E_n}\right. \\
& - \frac{(\mathbf{p}\times\mathbf{m}V)_{n0} - V_{00}(\mathbf{p}\times\mathbf{m})_{n0}}{\bar{E}_0 - E_0} - \frac{1}{2mc}\left(\frac{(V\mathbf{p}\mathbf{p})_{n0} - V_{00}(\mathbf{p}\mathbf{p})_{n0}}{\bar{E}_n - E_n}\right. \\
& + \left.\frac{(\mathbf{p}\mathbf{p}V)_{n0} - V_{00}(\mathbf{p}\mathbf{p})_{n0}}{\bar{E}_0 - E_0}\right)\cdot\boldsymbol{\mu}_{00} - \frac{1}{2mc}(\mathbf{p}\mathbf{p})_{n0} \\
& \cdot\left(\frac{(\boldsymbol{\mu}V)_{00} - V_{00}\boldsymbol{\mu}_{00}}{\bar{E}_0 - E_0}\right) + \frac{1}{2mc}\left(\frac{(V\mathbf{p}^2)_{n0} - V_{nn}(\mathbf{p}^2)_{n0}}{\bar{E}_n - E_n}\right. \\
& + \left.\left.\left.\frac{(\mathbf{p}^2V)_{n0} - V_{00}(\mathbf{p}^2)_{n0}}{\bar{E}_0 - E_0}\right)\boldsymbol{\mu}_{00} + \frac{1}{2mc}(\mathbf{p}^2)_{n0}\left(\frac{(\boldsymbol{\mu}V)_{00} - V_{00}\boldsymbol{\mu}_{00}}{\bar{E}_0 - E_0}\right)\right]\right\}.
\end{aligned}
\tag{6.5.17}
$$

This expression is independent of origin and constitutes a fundamental equation for the Verdet constant of a weak or forbidden transition, provided that there are no excited states lower in energy making contributions to the exact equation. When this occurs one must subtract these terms from the numerators in (6.5.17) and evaluate them separately. It will be assumed throughout that the first alternative applies.

Since (6.5.17) will be of practical value only when the zeroth order terms vanish, we may eliminate all the terms which are multiplied by the factors V_{00} or V_{nn}. These merely involve small corrections to the zeroth order terms, when they do not vanish. Next, one may evaluate all the terms with $\bar{E}_n - E_n$ denominators with an origin at the center of charge of ψ_n and all the $\bar{E}_0 - E_0$ terms at the center of ψ_0. With this understanding $\boldsymbol{\mu}_{nn}$ and $\boldsymbol{\mu}_{00}$ may be set equal to zero, but not $\boldsymbol{\mu}_{nn} - \boldsymbol{\mu}_{00}$. Equation 6.5.17 then becomes

$$
\begin{aligned}
F^{(2)}_{\mathbf{p}n} = {} & \left[\frac{(V\mathbf{p})_{0n}}{\bar{E}_0 - E_0} + \frac{(\mathbf{p}V)_{0n}}{\bar{E}_n - E_n}\right] \cdot \left\{\frac{i}{2e\hbar c}\left[(\boldsymbol{\mu}_{nn} - \boldsymbol{\mu}_{00})\left(\frac{(V\boldsymbol{\mu}\cdot\mathbf{p})_{n0}}{\bar{E}_n - E_n}\right.\right.\right. \\
& \left. + \frac{(\boldsymbol{\mu}\cdot\mathbf{p}V)}{\bar{E}_0 - E_0}\right) + 2\left(\frac{(\boldsymbol{\mu}V)_{nn}}{\bar{E}_n - E_n} - \frac{(\boldsymbol{\mu}V)_{00}}{\bar{E}_0 - E_0}\right)(\boldsymbol{\mu}\cdot\mathbf{p})_{n0} \\
& - \left(\frac{(V\boldsymbol{\mu}\mathbf{p})_{n0}}{\bar{E}_n - E_n} + \frac{(\boldsymbol{\mu}\mathbf{p}V)_{n0}}{\bar{E}_0 - E_0}\right)\cdot(\boldsymbol{\mu}_{nn} - \boldsymbol{\mu}_{00}) \\
& \left. - 2(\boldsymbol{\mu}\mathbf{p})_{n0}\cdot\left(\frac{(\boldsymbol{\mu}V)_{nn}}{\bar{E}_n - E_n} - \frac{(\boldsymbol{\mu}V)_{00}}{\bar{E}_0 - E_0}\right)\right] \\
& + \frac{1}{\bar{E}_n - E_n}\left[\frac{(V\mathbf{m}\times\mathbf{p})_{n0}}{\bar{E}_n - E_n} + \frac{(\mathbf{m}\times\mathbf{p}V)_{n0}}{\bar{E}_0 - E_0} - \frac{1}{2mc}(\mathbf{p}\mathbf{p})_{n0}\right. \\
& \left. \cdot\frac{(\boldsymbol{\mu}V)_{nn}}{\bar{E}_n - E_n} + \frac{1}{2mc}(\mathbf{p}^2)_{n0}\frac{(\boldsymbol{\mu}V)_{nn}}{\bar{E}_n - E_n}\right] \\
& + \frac{1}{\bar{E}_0 - E_0}\left[-\frac{(V\mathbf{p}\times\mathbf{m})_{n0}}{\bar{E}_n - E_n} - \frac{(\mathbf{p}\times\mathbf{m}V)_{n0}}{\bar{E}_0 - E_0} - \frac{1}{2mc}(\mathbf{p}\mathbf{p})_{n0}\right. \\
& \left.\left. \cdot\frac{(\boldsymbol{\mu}V)_{00}}{\bar{E}_0 - E_0} + \frac{1}{2mc}(\mathbf{p})^2{}_{n0}\frac{(\boldsymbol{\mu}V)_{00}}{\bar{E}_0 - E_0}\right]\right\}.
\end{aligned}
\tag{6.5.18}
$$

6.6 Vibronic effects

Equation 6.5.18 is somewhat cumbersome, and its usefulness will depend upon the predominance of a few terms over the others. There does not appear to be any general rule for such simplification. Typical specific examples are:

1. For centric groups $\boldsymbol{\mu}_{nn} - \boldsymbol{\mu}_{00} = 0$.

2. For transitions between states of different symmetries $(\boldsymbol{\mu} \cdot \mathbf{p})_{n0}$ and $(\mathbf{p}^2)_{n0}$ are zero.

3. For D_{nh} groups $(\boldsymbol{\mu}\mathbf{p})_{n0}$ and $(\mathbf{pp})_{n0}$ are approximately zero for transitions from a totally symmetric ground state to an excited state with u symmetry (B_{1u}, B_{2u}, etc.).

The last rule follows by writing the diagonal terms as

$$x \frac{\partial}{\partial x} = \frac{1}{3}\left[\mathbf{r} \cdot \nabla + \left(2x \frac{\partial}{\partial x} - y \frac{\partial}{\partial y} - z \frac{\partial}{\partial z}\right)\right], \text{ etc.}$$

Under the stated conditions $(\mathbf{r} \cdot \nabla)_{n0} = 0$ and $[2x(\partial/\partial x) - y(\partial/\partial y) - z(\partial/\partial z)]_{n0}$ is a relatively small term depending on the anisotropy of the system. The off diagonal terms vanish, because they all span g representations. These are but a few of the conditions under which simplification may occur.

There are a number of important molecules for which all three of the above conditions are fulfilled. The B_{1u} and B_{2u} transitions of benzene satisfy all the above conditions. Equation 6.5.18 becomes

$$\begin{aligned} F_{\mathbf{p}n}^{(2)\ddagger} = {} & \left[\frac{(V\mathbf{p})_{0n}}{\bar{E}_0 - E_0} + \frac{(\mathbf{p}V)_{0n}}{\bar{E}_n - E_n}\right] \\ & \cdot \left\{\frac{1}{\bar{E}_n - E_n}\left[\frac{1}{\bar{E}_n - E_n}(V\mathbf{m} \times \mathbf{p})_{n0} + \frac{1}{\bar{E}_0 - E_0}(\mathbf{m} \times \mathbf{p}V)_{n0}\right]\right. \\ & \left. + \frac{1}{\bar{E}_0 - E_0}\left[\frac{1}{\bar{E}_n - E_n}(V\mathbf{p} \times \mathbf{m})_{n0} + \frac{1}{\bar{E}_0 - E_0}(\mathbf{p} \times \mathbf{m}V)_{n0}\right]\right\}. \end{aligned} \quad (6.6.1)$$

For benzene itself V will arise from vibronic effects. For its derivatives V will arise from both vibronic and substitution effects. It is important to recognize the difference between the overall symmetry of a molecule or group and its latent symmetry. Weakly allowed transitions often arise when a higher latent symmetry is present in a molecule of lower overall symmetry. In this case the wave functions of the system with the higher latent symmetry should be used in zeroth order.

A particularly interesting situation arises when the perturbations from the fixed nuclei approximation are comparable to the vibronic perturbations. There is then opportunity for a rich vibronic spectrum including sign changes within a given band. For example, napthalene may fulfill this requirement. This molecule has D_{2h} symmetry and the lowest singlet transitions are weaky allowed, being polarized in the molecular plane. In the Moffit approximation naphthalene is derived from a system with D_{10h} symmetry with a strong interaction between the first and sixth atoms. To zeroth order the transitions are forbidden, but they become allowed by the perturbation. In addition the vibronic interaction terms must be considered. If Q represents for simplicity a single vibrational coordinate, the total perturbing potential may be written

$$V = V_f + QV_v, \tag{6.6.2}$$

where V_f is the fixed nuclei approximation potential and QV_v is the vibronic.

Let the ground and excited state wave functions be written

$$\Theta_0 = \psi_0 \chi_0(Q) \tag{6.6.3a}$$

$$\Theta_n = \psi_n \chi_{ns}(Q), \tag{6.6.3b}$$

where s labels the various excitations. It is possible that the dominant term in (6.6.1) may be

$$\frac{1}{(\bar{E}_n - E_n)^3} (\mathbf{p}V)_{0n} \cdot (V\mathbf{m} \times \mathbf{p})_{n0} \, .$$

The combination of (6.6.1), (6.6.2), and (6.6.3) gives

$$F_{\mathbf{p}ns}^{(2)\ddagger} \simeq \frac{1}{(\bar{E}_n - E_n)^3} \{[(\mathbf{p}V_f)_{0n}\langle\chi_0|\chi_{ns}\rangle + (\mathbf{p}V_v)_{0n}\langle\chi_0|Q|\chi_{ns}\rangle]$$

$$\cdot [(V_f \mathbf{m} \times \mathbf{p})_{n0}\langle\chi_0 \,|\, \chi_{ns}\rangle + (V_v \mathbf{m} \times \mathbf{p})_{n0}\langle\chi_0|Q|\chi_{ns}\rangle]\}.$$

Owing to the variation of this expression through the absorption band as $\langle\chi_0|\chi_{ns}\rangle$ and $\langle\chi_0|Q|\chi_{ns}\rangle$ take on a twofold series of values, sign changes are quite possible when V_0 and $\sqrt{\langle Q^2\rangle_{00}}\, V_v$ are comparable. The interpretation of magnetic rotation data is still in its infancy, and one is entitled to hope that this will become a useful tool in unravelling molecular structures.

CHAPTER 7

Special Topics

7.1. Vibronic Theory

The preceding chapters have been confined almost exclusively to the fixed nuclei approximation. It happens that there are some interesting phenomena which cannot be explained even qualitatively without recourse to a discussion of vibronic effects. First let us review a few fundamental aspects of ordinary absorption. One may divide transitions into three categories in the fixed nuclei approximation: strongly allowed, weakly allowed, and forbidden. The area under the absorption band for the first group may be calculated without recourse to vibronic theory, whereas the forbidden transitions obtain all their intensity from the perturbation of nuclear motion. It is possible for weakly allowed transitions to have comparable contributions from vibronic and fixed geometrical effects.

In all three cases it is generally believed that the dominant mechanism for line shape is vibronic. In order to avoid some possible misconceptions a few remarks on the general nature of UV and visible transitions are worthwhile. The complete wave functions for the stationary states of a molecule are complicated functions of both nuclear and electronic coordinates. The charge distribution of both electrons and nuclei is that of a standing wave. When a system is in one of its stationary states there is no vibration of charge. In the presence of an electromagnetic field the stationary states are not eigenfunctions of the complete Hamiltonian of the system. For relatively low light intensities the state is dominated by the ground state function with a time dependent admixture of excited states depending on the incident frequency. The charge cloud, both nuclear and electronic, undergoes a form of motion.

In the fixed nuclei approximation it is assumed that the change in the position of the nuclei during the high frequency vibrations may be neglected. This is a good approximation for the intensities of strongly allowed transitions. But even in this case the nuclear motion is necessary to account for the broad molecular absorption bands. It has been shown that the next approximation to the total molecular wave function is to replace the infinitely peaked nuclear distribution functions by the finite width Gaussians of the harmonic oscillator.

This comes about by first solving the Schrödinger equation for a continuum of fixed nuclear conformations and minimizing the total energy.

For the case of a single nuclear degree of freedom Q we obtain the familiar curve in Figure 7.1. Owing to the great difference in electronic and nuclear masses, an approximate separation of variables is possible in which the total wave function is written

$$\Theta_{ni}(\mathbf{r}, Q) = \psi_n(\mathbf{r})\chi_i(Q), \tag{7.1.1}$$

where $\psi_n(\mathbf{r})$ is the electronic function for the equilibrium nuclear configuration represented by the well in the figure and $\chi_i(Q)$ is the appropriate Hermite function corresponding to the force constant $\partial^2 E(R_0)/\partial R^2$.

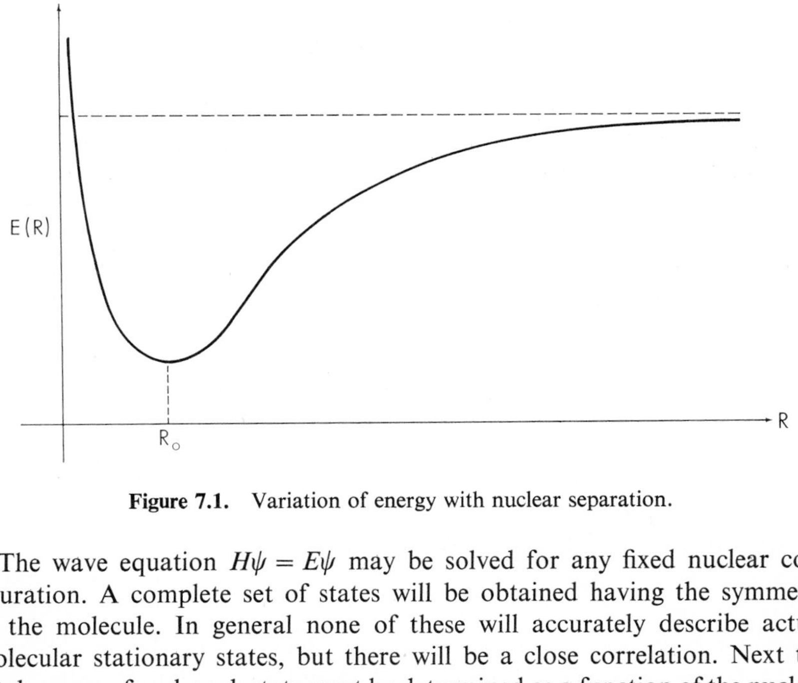

Figure 7.1. Variation of energy with nuclear separation.

The wave equation $H\psi = E\psi$ may be solved for any fixed nuclear configuration. A complete set of states will be obtained having the symmetry of the molecule. In general none of these will accurately describe actual molecular stationary states, but there will be a close correlation. Next the total energy of each such state must be determined as a function of the nuclear coordinates Q_i, leading to the categories:

1. One true minimum.
2. Several minimums.
3. No minimums.

For diatomic molecules only the first and third situations are encountered. Those states with a single minimum will correspond to the stationary states of the total electronic and nuclear Hamiltonian, $H_T = H_E + H_N$, satisfying the boundary conditions $\Theta_{ni}(\infty) = 0$. In polyatomic molecules several minimums separated by barriers may be encountered corresponding to isomers or different conformations. When no minimums exist, it is presumed that the state in the fixed nuclei approximation is not an eigenfunction of H_T satisfying the boundary condition.

An important requirement to be met by any approximate set of functions is orthogonality. The complete set of electronic functions obtained for any fixed nuclear configuration will be orthogonal. In general functions obtained for different configurations will not be orthogonal. In order to preserve this status a special method will be necessary. The total Hamiltonian for a diatomic molecule AB may be written.

$$H_T = H_{\text{el}} + \frac{Z_A Z_B}{R_{AB}} - \frac{\hbar^2}{2\mu}\frac{\partial^2}{\partial R_{AB}^2} + H_{\text{rot}} + H_{\text{trans}}, \tag{7.1.2}$$

where H_{el} describes the interactions of the electrons with the nuclei and with each other and H_{rot} and H_{trans} describe the five rotational and translational degrees of freedom of the two nuclei. Since H_{rot} depends on R_{AB} through the moment of inertia, the equation is separable only in the translational degrees of freedom.

If the wave function is sought in the region not too far removed from the minimum for an excited state A, the Hamiltonian of (7.1.2) may be approximated by

$$H(A) = H_{\text{el}}(Q) - \frac{\hbar^2}{2\mu}\frac{\partial^2}{\partial Q^2} + V_A(Q), \tag{7.1.3}$$

where H_{el} operates on the electronic coordinates but is a function of the normal coordinate Q.

The first reasonable approximation to an eigenfunction of (7.1.3) is

$$\Theta(A;U) = \psi_A(Q)\chi_{AU}(Q) \tag{7.1.4}$$

where $\psi_A(Q)$ is a function of electronic coordinates with Q as a parameter and $\chi_{AU}(Q)$ is a vibrational function of Q and its equilibrium value $Q(A)$. These functions must be chosen so that $\int \psi_A(Q)\psi_{A'}(Q)\,d\tau_{\text{el}} = 0$ for different electronic states. If the equilibrium positions of two states are very far apart the product form in (7.1.4) will not be a valid approximation for both of them. It will be assumed here that this is not the case and (7.1.4) is valid for all excited states of interest.

If one requires that

$$H_{\text{el}}(Q)\psi_A(Q) = E_A(Q)\psi_A(Q) \tag{7.1.5a}$$

$$\left[-\frac{\hbar^2}{2\mu}\frac{\partial^2}{\partial Q^2} + V_A(Q)\right]\chi_{AU}(Q) = E_{AU}\chi_{AU}(Q), \tag{7.1.5b}$$

the energy will be given by

$$\int \Theta(A;U)H(A)\Theta(A;U)\,d\tau_{\mathrm{el}}\,d\tau_{nu} = \int \chi_{AU}^2(Q)E_A(Q)\,dQ + \varepsilon_{AU}$$

$$-\frac{\hbar^2}{2\mu}\int \chi_{AU}^2(Q)\psi_A(Q)\frac{\partial^2}{\partial Q^2}\psi_A(Q)\,d\tau_{\mathrm{el}}\,dQ \simeq \bar{E}_A + \varepsilon_{AU}. \quad (7.1.6)$$

The first term, which depends on the vibrational quantum number, has been replaced by an average value, and it is assumed that ε_{AU} is much more sensitive to the quantum number U than either of the other terms. This point certainly warrants closer examination, but as an introduction to this difficult subject the approximation appears adequate. The last term comprises a small correction to the nuclear kinetic energy due to electronic motion.

We will be interested in the values of

$$\boldsymbol{\mu}_{GA}(U) = \int \psi_G(Q)\boldsymbol{\mu}\psi_A(Q)\chi_{GO}(Q)\chi_{AU}(Q)\,d\tau_{\mathrm{el}}\,dQ$$

and

$$\mathbf{m}_{AG}(U) = \int \psi_A(Q)\mathbf{m}\chi_G(Q)\psi_{GO}(Q)\chi_{AU}(Q)\,d\tau_{\mathrm{el}}\,dQ,$$

where $\psi_G(Q)$ is the ground state electronic function.

The moments for the fixed configuration Q may be defined as

$$\boldsymbol{\mu}_{GA}(Q) = \int \psi_G(Q)\boldsymbol{\mu}\psi_A(Q)\,d\tau_{\mathrm{el}} \quad (7.1.7a)$$

$$\mathbf{m}_{AG}(Q) = \int \psi_A(Q)\mathbf{m}\psi_G(Q)\,d\tau_{\mathrm{el}}. \quad (7.1.7b)$$

It is not possible to develop general formulas for $\boldsymbol{\mu}_{GA}(U)$ and $\mathbf{m}_{AG}(U)$ without further assumptions. First let the moments in (7.1.7) be given by the first few terms of a power series expansion about some conformation $\bar{Q}$:

$$\boldsymbol{\mu}_{GA}(Q) = \boldsymbol{\mu}_{GA}(\bar{Q}) + (Q-\bar{Q})\frac{\partial\boldsymbol{\mu}_{GA}(\bar{Q})}{\partial Q} + \tfrac{1}{2}(Q-\bar{Q})^2\frac{\partial^2\boldsymbol{\mu}_{GA}(\bar{Q})}{\partial Q^2} + \cdots \quad (7.1.8a)$$

$$\mathbf{m}_{AG}(Q) = \mathbf{m}_{AG}(\bar{Q}) + (Q-\bar{Q})\frac{\partial\mathbf{m}_{AG}(\bar{Q})}{\partial Q} + \tfrac{1}{2}(Q-\bar{Q})^2\frac{\partial^2\mathbf{m}_{AG}(\bar{Q})}{\partial Q^2} + \cdots. \quad (7.1.8b)$$

For computing the dipole strength of a symmetry forbidden transition it is convenient to choose the ground state conformation and set $\bar{Q}=0$. Since $\boldsymbol{\mu}_{GA}(0)=0$ in this case, the dipole strength will be determined by

$$\sum_U \boldsymbol{\mu}_{GA}^2(U) = \sum_U \left[\int \boldsymbol{\mu}_{GA}(Q)\chi_{GO}(Q)\chi_{AU}(Q)\,dQ\right]^2. \quad (7.1.9)$$

Since the $\chi_{AU}(Q)$ are a complete set with respect to the coordinate Q, the matrix multiplication rule gives

$$\sum_U \boldsymbol{\mu}_{GA}^2(U) = \langle \chi_{GO}(Q) | \boldsymbol{\mu}_{GA}^2(Q) | \chi_{GO}(Q) \rangle = \left[\frac{\partial \boldsymbol{\mu}_{GA}(\bar{Q})}{\partial Q} \right]^2 \langle \chi_{GO}(Q) | Q^2 | \chi_{GO}(Q) \rangle \tag{7.1.10}$$

to the lowest order. This result also applies to the case of several normal coordinates in the form

$$\sum_{U_1 \cdots U_N} | \boldsymbol{\mu}_{GA}(U_1 \cdots U_N) |^2 = \sum_{i=1}^{N} \langle \chi_{GO}^{(i)}(Q_i) | Q_i^2 | \chi_{GO}^{(i)}(Q_i) \rangle \left[\frac{\partial \boldsymbol{\mu}_{GA}(0 \cdots 0)}{\partial Q_i} \right]^2. \tag{7.1.11}$$

The dipole strength is always a positive quantity, but the dichroism or rotational strength is not. This admits the possibility of sign changes within an absorption band. Since such behavior constitutes the most interesting phase of vibronic optical activity, our discussion will be conducted along these lines. Let it be assumed that $\boldsymbol{\mu}_{GA}(Q) \cdot \mathbf{m}_{AG}(Q)$ changes sign as Q is varied between the ground and excited state equilibrium positions. It will be convenient to select the origin of Q as the null conformation for which $\boldsymbol{\mu}_{GA}(0) \cdot \mathbf{m}_{AG}(0) = 0$. For the transition $GO \to AU$, where G and A refer to the electronic states and O and U refer to the vibrational sublevels, one obtains the rotational strength

$$\begin{aligned}
R_{GA;OU} &= \langle \chi_{GO}(Q) | \boldsymbol{\mu}_{GA}(Q) | \chi_{AU}(Q) \rangle \cdot \langle \chi_{AU}(Q) | \mathbf{m}_{AG}(Q) | \chi_{GO}(Q) \rangle \\
&= \langle \chi_{GO}(Q) | \chi_{AU}(Q) \rangle^2 \boldsymbol{\mu}_{GA}(0) \cdot \mathbf{m}_{AG}(0) + \langle \chi_{GO}(Q) | \chi_{AU}(Q) \rangle \\
&\quad \times \langle \chi_{AU}(Q) | Q | \chi_{GO}(Q) \rangle \left[\boldsymbol{\mu}_{GA}(0) \cdot \frac{\partial \mathbf{m}_{AG}(0)}{\partial Q} + \frac{\partial \boldsymbol{\mu}_{GA}(0)}{\partial Q} \cdot \mathbf{m}_{AG}(0) \right] \\
&\quad + \langle \chi_{GO}(Q) | \chi_{AU}(Q) \rangle \langle \chi_{AU}(Q) | Q^2 | \chi_{GO}(Q) \rangle \\
&\quad \times \left[\boldsymbol{\mu}_{GA}(0) \cdot \frac{\partial^2 \mathbf{m}_{AG}(0)}{\partial Q^2} + \frac{\partial^2 \boldsymbol{\mu}_{GA}(0)}{\partial Q^2} \cdot \mathbf{m}_{AG}(0) \right] \\
&\quad + \langle \chi_{GO}(Q) | Q | \chi_{AU}(Q) \rangle^2 \frac{\partial \boldsymbol{\mu}_{GA}(0)}{\partial Q} \cdot \frac{\partial \mathbf{m}_{AG}(0)}{\partial Q}.
\end{aligned} \tag{7.1.12}$$

If $V_G(Q)$ and $V_A(Q)$ are harmonic potentials centered around the equilibrium positions $\bar{Q}_G$ and $\bar{Q}_A$, the functions $\chi_{Gn}(Q)$ and $\chi_{An}(Q)$ will be given by

$$\chi_{Gn}(Q) = \left(\frac{\sqrt{\beta_G/\pi}}{2^n n!} \right)^{1/2} H_n[\sqrt{\beta_G}(Q - Q_G)] e^{-\beta_G(Q-Q_G)^2/2} \tag{7.1.13a}$$

$$\chi_{An}(Q) = \left(\frac{\sqrt{\beta_A/\pi}}{2^n n!} \right)^{1/2} H_n[\sqrt{\beta_A}(Q - Q_A)] e^{-\beta_A(Q-Q_A)^2/2}, \tag{7.1.13b}$$

where H_n are the Hermite polynominals defined by

$$H_n(y) = (-1)^n e^{y^2}\left(\frac{d}{dy}\right) e^{-y^2}.$$

A great simplification occurs in the evaluation of the integrals $\langle \chi_{GO}(Q) | \chi_{An}(Q) \rangle$ if an average value $\beta = (\beta_G + \beta_A)/2$ is used. With the substitutions $y = \sqrt{\beta}(Q - \bar{Q}_A)$ and $y_0 = \sqrt{\beta}(\bar{Q}_G - \bar{Q}_A)$, the overlap integral becomes

$$\begin{aligned}\langle \chi_{GO}(Q) | \chi_{An}(Q) \rangle &= \left(\frac{1}{2^n n!}\right)^{1/2} \frac{1}{\sqrt{\pi}} \int_{-\infty}^{\infty} H_n(y) e^{-y^2/2} e^{-(y-y_0)^2/2}\, dy \\ &= (-1)^n \left(\frac{1}{2^n n!}\right)^{1/2} \frac{1}{\sqrt{\pi}} e^{-y_0{}^2/2} \int_{-\infty}^{\infty} e^{y_0 y} \left(\frac{d}{dy}\right)^n e^{-y^2}\, dy \\ &= e^{-y_0{}^2/4} \left(\frac{y_0^{2n}}{2^n n!}\right)^{1/2}. \end{aligned} \tag{7.1.14}$$

Since $\sum_n (y_0^{2n}/2^n n!) = e^{y_0{}^2/2}$, this satisfies the necessary relation

$$\sum_n \langle \chi_{GO}(Q) | \chi_{An}(Q) \rangle^2 = 1.$$

The plot of the function in (7.1.14) for integral values of n closely corresponds with typical absorption curves is shown in Figure 7.2.

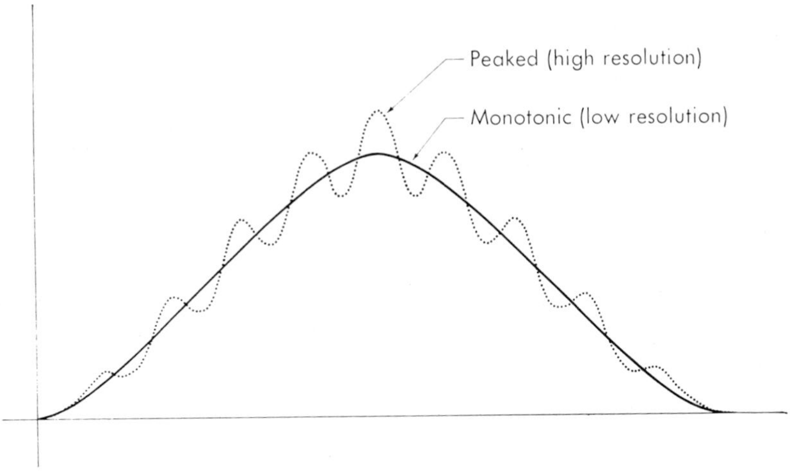

Figure 7.2. Typical absorption curves.

By the substitution $Q_A = Q - \bar{Q}_A$ one may write

$$\langle \chi_{GO}(Q)| Q | \chi_{An}(Q)\rangle = \langle \chi_{GO}(Q)| Q_A + \bar{Q}_A | \chi_{An}(Q)\rangle$$
$$= \bar{Q}_A \langle \chi_{GO}(Q) | \chi_{An}(Q)\rangle + \langle \chi_{GO}(Q)| Q_A | \chi_{An}(Q)\rangle$$

which by use of the matrix multiplication rule gives

$$\langle \chi_{GO}(Q)| Q_A | \chi_{An}(Q)\rangle$$
$$= \sum_m \langle \chi_{GO}(Q) | \chi_{Am}(Q)\rangle\langle \chi_{Am}(Q)| Q_A | \chi_{An}(Q)\rangle$$
$$= \langle \chi_{GO}(Q) | \chi_{An-1}(Q)\rangle\langle \chi_{An-1}(Q)| Q_A | \chi_{An}(Q)\rangle$$
$$+ \langle \chi_{GO}(Q) | \chi_{An+1}(Q)\rangle\langle \chi_{An+1}(Q)| Q_A | \chi_{An}(Q)\rangle$$
$$= e^{-y_0{}^2/4}\left[\left(\frac{y_0^{2(n-1)}}{2^{n-1}(n-1)!}\right)^{1/2}\left(\frac{n}{2\beta}\right)^{1/2} + \left(\frac{y_0^{2(n+1)}}{2^{n+1}(n+1)!}\right)^{1/2}\left(\frac{n+1}{2}\right)^{1/2}\right]$$
$$= \frac{\beta^{n/2}(\bar{Q}_G - \bar{Q}_A)^{n+1}}{\sqrt{2^n n!}} e^{-\beta(\bar{Q}_G - \bar{Q}_A)^2/4}\left[\frac{n}{\beta(\bar{Q}_G - \bar{Q}_A)^2} + \frac{1}{2}\right]. \tag{7.1.15}$$

Equation 7.1.14 and the relation $\langle \chi_{An-1}(Q)| Q - \bar{Q}_A | \chi_{An}\rangle = \sqrt{n/2\beta}$ have been used in the above derivation. The quadratic term is obtained in like manner:

$$\langle \chi_{GO}(Q)| (Q_A + \bar{Q}_A)^2 | \chi_{An}\rangle = \langle \chi_{GO}(Q)| Q_A^2 | \chi_{An}(Q)\rangle$$
$$+ 2\bar{Q}_A\langle \chi_{GO}(Q)| Q_A | \chi_{An}\rangle + \bar{Q}_A^2\langle \chi_{GO}(Q) | \chi_{An}(Q)\rangle \tag{7.1.16}$$

and

$$\langle \chi_{GO}(Q)| Q_A^2 | \chi_{An}(Q)\rangle = \langle \chi_{GO}(Q)| Q_A | \chi_{An-1}(Q)\rangle$$
$$\times \langle \chi_{An-1}(Q)| Q_A | \chi_{An}(Q)\rangle + \langle \chi_{GO}(Q)| Q_A | \chi_{An+1}(Q)\rangle$$
$$\times \langle \chi_{An+1}(Q)| Q_A | \chi_{An}(Q)\rangle, \tag{7.1.17}$$

from which it follows that

$$\langle \chi_{GO}(Q)| Q^2 | \chi_{An}(Q)\rangle = \frac{\beta^{n/2}(\bar{Q}_G - \bar{Q}_A)^n}{\sqrt{2^n n!}} e^{-\beta(\bar{Q}_G - \bar{Q}_A)^2/4}$$
$$\times \left\{\left(\frac{\bar{Q}_G + \bar{Q}_A}{2}\right)^2\left[\frac{n(n-1)}{\beta^2(\bar{Q}_G - \bar{Q}_A)^2} + \frac{2n\bar{Q}_A}{\beta(\bar{Q}_G - \bar{Q}_A)} + \frac{n+\frac{1}{2}}{\beta}\right]\right\} \tag{7.1.18a}$$

$$\langle \chi_{GO}(Q)| Q | \chi_{An}(Q)\rangle = \frac{\beta^{n/2}(\bar{Q}_G - \bar{Q}_A)^n}{\sqrt{2^n n!}} e^{-\beta(\bar{Q}_G - \bar{Q}_A)^2/4}$$
$$\times \left[\tfrac{1}{2}(\bar{Q}_G - \bar{Q}_A) + \frac{n}{(\bar{Q}_G - \bar{Q}_A)\beta}\right]. \tag{7.1.18b}$$

The substitution of these results into (7.1.12) gives

$$
\begin{aligned}
R_{GA;\,On} = {} & \frac{\beta^n(\bar{Q}_G - \bar{Q}_A)^{2n}}{2^n n!} e^{-\beta(\bar{Q}_G - \bar{Q}_A)^2/2} \\
& \times \left\{ \left[\tfrac{1}{2}(\bar{Q}_G + \bar{Q}_A) + \frac{n}{\beta(\bar{Q}_G - \bar{Q}_A)} \right] \left[\boldsymbol{\mu}_{GA}(0) \cdot \frac{\partial \mathbf{m}_{AG}(0)}{\partial Q} \right. \right. \\
& \left. + \frac{\partial \boldsymbol{\mu}_{GA}(0)}{\partial Q} \cdot \mathbf{m}_{AG}(0) \right] + \frac{1}{2} \left[\left(\frac{\bar{Q}_G + \bar{Q}_A}{2} \right)^2 \right. \\
& \left. + \frac{n(n-1)}{\beta^2(\bar{Q}_G - \bar{Q}_A)^2} + \frac{2n\bar{Q}_A}{\beta(\bar{Q}_G - \bar{Q}_A)} + \frac{n + \frac{1}{2}}{\beta} \right] \\
& \times \left[\boldsymbol{\mu}_{GA}(0) \cdot \frac{\partial^2 \mathbf{m}_{AG}(0)}{\partial Q^2} + \frac{\partial^2 \boldsymbol{\mu}_{GA}(0)}{\partial Q^2} \cdot \mathbf{m}_{AG}(0) \right] \\
& \left. + \left[\tfrac{1}{2}(\bar{Q}_G + \bar{Q}_A) + \frac{n}{\beta(\bar{Q}_G - \bar{Q}_A)} \right]^2 \left[\frac{\partial \boldsymbol{\mu}_{GA}(0)}{\partial Q} \cdot \frac{\partial \mathbf{m}_{AG}(0)}{\partial Q} \right] \right\}. \qquad (7.1.19)
\end{aligned}
$$

For several normal coordinates there are cross terms and the formulas become somewhat more complex, but the extension is not difficult conceptually.

To this degree of approximation there is predicted a sum rule stating that the total rotational strength for the band is equal to what would have been obtained for the ground state conformation:

$$
\begin{aligned}
& \sum_n \langle \chi_{GO}(Q) | \boldsymbol{\mu}_{GA}(Q) | \chi_{An}(Q) \rangle \cdot \langle \chi_{An}(Q) | \mathbf{m}_{AG}(Q) | \chi_{GO} \rangle \\
& \qquad = \langle \chi_{GO}(Q) | \boldsymbol{\mu}_{GA}(Q) \cdot \mathbf{m}_{AG}(Q) | \chi_{GO}(Q) \rangle. \qquad (7.1.20)
\end{aligned}
$$

Equation 7.1.19 may be written

$$
R_{GA;\,On} = k \frac{g^h}{n!} (n - a)(n - b). \qquad (7.1.21)
$$

If a and b are complex conjugates, there will be no change of sign as n varies from 0 to ∞. For one positive and one negative root there will be one change of sign, and for two positive roots there will be two changes of sign. For positive k and g the behavior is shown in Figure 7.3. When it is recognized that only the first two terms of a series expansion have been used and only one normal coordinate, the possibility of quite complex behavior by this mechanism seems apparent.

In chromophore-vicinal group language there are two principal ways in which this sign change can come about: either by a change in the relative positions of chromphore and surroundings or by a vibrational distortion of

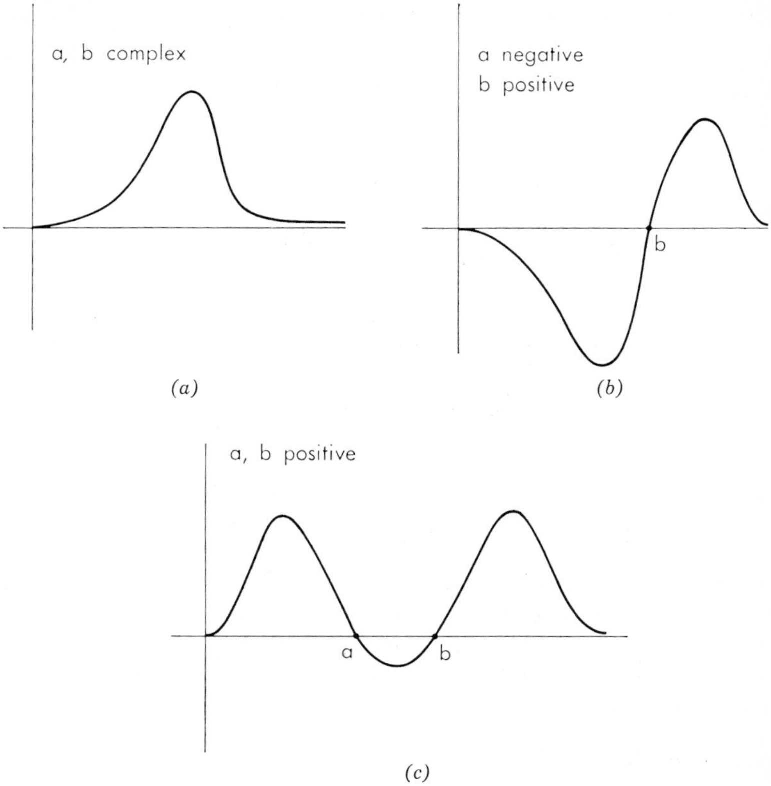

Figure 7.3. Vibronically induced sign changes in CD.

the chromophore. The second seems more likely and leads us to an investigation of weakly allowed transitions where coulombic intramolecular perturbations and vibronic effects can enter on nearly an equal footing.

Consider a chromophore in an arbitrary conformation Q. Let the electric and magnetic moments be zero for the undistorted and unperturbed moiety ($Q = 0$). This will not necessarily be the null conformation and the term $\boldsymbol{\mu}_{GA}(0) \cdot \mathbf{m}_{AG}(0)$ should be included in (7.1.19). In general the perturbing potential will be a function of Q. If ψ_G and ψ_A are the wave functions for the isolated undistorted chromophore, the methods of Chapter 4 give

$$\boldsymbol{\mu}_{GA}(Q) = \frac{[\boldsymbol{\mu} V(Q)]_{GA}}{E_A - \bar{E}_A} + \frac{[V(Q)\boldsymbol{\mu}]_{GA}}{E_G - \bar{E}_G} \tag{7.1.22a}$$

$$\mathbf{m}_{AG}(Q) = \frac{[V(Q)\mathbf{m}]_{AG}}{E_A - \bar{E}_A} + \frac{[\mathbf{m} V(Q)]_{AG}}{E_G - \bar{E}_G}. \tag{7.1.22b}$$

It will be assumed that there is a part of the potential which is insensitive to small variations in Q. This would be arising from the vicinal groups. That portion which depends on Q may be considered to be caused by those vibrational modes which are most effective in distorting the chromophore. In many cases one will be encountering a synergistic effect which cannot be separated this way. Let $V(Q) = V_1(0) + V_2(Q)$, where $V_1(0)$ is the potential field affecting the undistorted chromophore and $V_2(0) = 0$. This gives for the appropriate derivatives when $Q = 0$

$$\boldsymbol{\mu}_{GA}(0) = \frac{[\boldsymbol{\mu} V_1(0)]_{GA}}{E_A - \bar{E}_A} + \frac{[V_1(0)\boldsymbol{\mu}]_{GA}}{E_G - \bar{E}_G} \tag{7.1.23a}$$

$$\frac{\partial \boldsymbol{\mu}_{GA}(0)}{\partial Q} = \frac{\{\boldsymbol{\mu}[\partial V_2(0)/\partial Q]\}_{GA}}{E_A - \bar{E}_A} + \frac{\{[\partial V_2(0)/\partial Q]\boldsymbol{\mu}\}_{GA}}{E_G - \bar{E}_G} \tag{7.1.23b}$$

$$\frac{\partial^2 \boldsymbol{\mu}_{GA}(0)}{\partial Q^2} = \frac{\{\boldsymbol{\mu}[\partial^2 V_2(0)/\partial Q^2]\}_{GA}}{E_A - \bar{E}_A} + \frac{\{[\partial^2 V_2(0)/\partial Q^2]\boldsymbol{\mu}\}_{GA}}{E_G - \bar{E}_G}. \tag{7.1.23c}$$

The potentials $V_1(0)$ and $V_2(Q)$ may be determined by standard methods and the results substituted into vibronic equations like (7.1.19). To this lowest order of approximation all that is required is a good estimate for the ground and excited state electronic wave functions, the appropriate normal coordinates, the force constants, and an estimate of the position of the minimums $\bar{Q}_G$ and $\bar{Q}_A$. When not all these data are forthcoming, we are still in possession of a powerful empirical method for studying vibronic effects.

If by chance the ground and excited states have the same equilibrium positions with different force constants, the same reasoning that required $\boldsymbol{\mu}_{GA} \cdot \mathbf{m}_{AG} = 0$ for a nondissymmetric conformation can be used to show that

$$\langle \chi_{Go}(Q)|\,[\boldsymbol{\mu} V(Q)]_{GA}\,|\chi_{An}(Q)\rangle \cdot \langle \chi_{An}(Q)|\,[V(Q)\mathbf{m}]_{AG}\,|\chi_{Go}(Q)\rangle = 0,$$

when $V(Q)$ arises from a purely vibronic effect. This occurs because $\partial^2 V(Q)/\partial Q^2$ and the even derivatives must span one of the representations of the symmetry group and the terms $\langle \chi_{Go}(Q)|\, Q\, |\chi_{An}(Q)\rangle$ vanish. When the two states do not have the same equilibrium position, the excited state must have two equilibrium positions at $\pm \bar{Q}_A$. The contributions to the sublevel bands $0 - n$ cancel in pairs, leading to zero net rotational strength.

For active molecules the effect from one of the equilibrium positions generally predominates, but to be thorough one should include both in the calculation of (7.1.19). The null conformation will generally lie between $\bar{Q}_G$ and $\bar{Q}_A$ or between $\bar{Q}_G$ and $-\bar{Q}_A$. It appears likely that whenever $\boldsymbol{\mu}_{GA}$ or $\mathbf{m}_{AG}$ for the ground state equilibrium position is quite small, a favorable disposition of vicinal groups can lead to a situation where the vibronic contribution to the small moment is comparable to the vicinal or along a more favorable direction parallel to the large moment. In Figure 7.4 are shown typical situations that might arise for a strong magnetic transition such as the carbonyl $n \rightarrow \pi^*$. Compounds have actually been studied in which this sign change does occur.

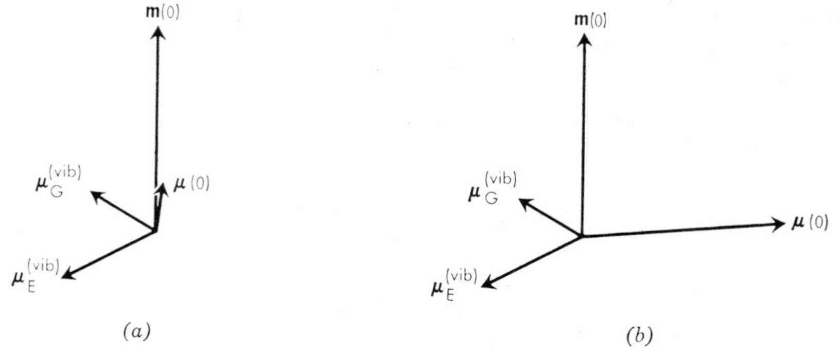

Figure 7.4. Changes in position of vibronic contribution to $\boldsymbol{\mu}$ for the extremes $\boldsymbol{\mu}_G$(vib) and $\boldsymbol{\mu}_E$(vib).

7.2. Exciton Effects

A special type of degeneracy arises when two or more identical groups are present in the same molecule. In most cases this does not lead to symmetry degeneracy, but the results are essentially the same. Of particular interest are helical molecules in which the chromophores are arranged at regular intervals on the periphery of a helix. An infinite system would have screw symmetry. This fact led to the initial treatment of the polypeptide backbone as a one dimensional crystal. Despite certain mathematical irregularities the model led to results which are in qualitative agreement with observation.

Let us consider a closely related planar model, which may be treated in a rigorous manner. In Figure 7.5 is a circular array of vectors indicating the transition moment directions for the individual chromophores. The symmetry of this system is C_n, since the vectors are assumed to be neither perpendicular to the plane nor contained in any dihedral plane passing through the origin. The C_n symmetry groups are Abelian, which means that all operations are generated by the rotation C_n through an angle of $2\pi/n$ radians.

The simplest way to construct the character table is to consider the powers of $\omega = e^{2\pi i/n}$. Each of the sequences $\omega^0, \omega^1 \ldots, \omega^{n-1}$; $\omega^0, \omega^2, \ldots, \omega^{2(n-1)}$; ... ; ω^0, ω^n, ..., $\omega^{n(n-1)}$ leads to a different representation of the group. The sequence ω^n, ω^{2n}, ..., $\omega^{n^2} = 1, 1, \ldots, 1$, comprises the totally symmetric representation A. The sequences ω^0, ω^q, ..., $\omega^{(n-1)q}$ and ω^0, ω^{-q}, ..., $\omega^{-(n-1)q}$

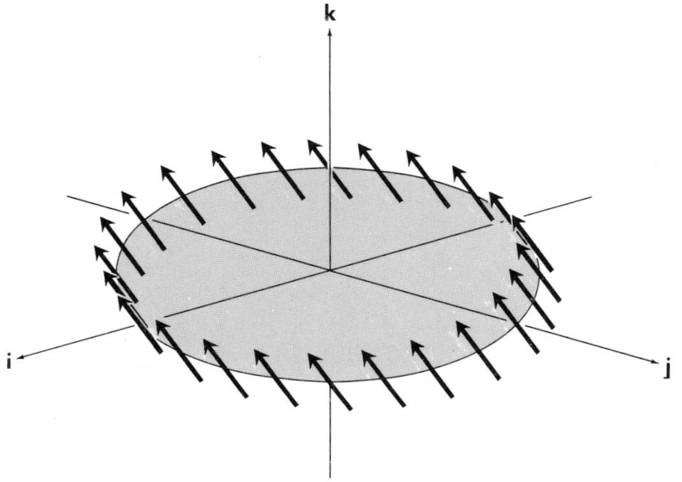

Figure 7.5. Array of oscillators with C_n symmetry.

may be paired to give the doubly degenerate representations E_q. The complex conjugate sequence $\omega^0, \omega^{-q}, \ldots, \omega^{-(n-1)q}$ is obtained by multiplying the appropriate sequence by $\omega^{-n} = 1$. For even numbered groups the sequence $1, \omega^{n/2}, \ldots, \omega^{(n/2)(n-1)} = 1, -1, \ldots, -1$, does not pair with any other and therefore comprises a nondegenerate representation B. It follows that even numbered groups will consist of the one dimensional representations A and B as well as $(n/2 - 1)$ two dimensional representations E_q; whereas odd numbered groups will have the single representation A and $(n-1)/2$ degenerate ones. The character table for n even is shown in Table 7.1.

The z-components of $\boldsymbol{\mu}$ and $\mathbf{m}$ belong to the totally symmetric representation A and the perpendicular components belong to the first of the doubly degenerate representations, because a rotation through $2\pi/n$ radians has the matrix $\begin{bmatrix} \cos 2\pi/n & \sin 2\pi/n \\ -\sin 2\pi/n & \cos 2\pi/n \end{bmatrix}$, with character $2 \cos 2\pi/n = \omega + \omega^{-1}$. If g_s and e_s represent the ground and excited state functions of group s, the sums will have the indicated symmetry

$$\chi_A(g) = \frac{1}{\sqrt{n}} \sum_{s=0}^{n-1} g_s \tag{7.2.1a}$$

$$\chi_A(e) = \frac{1}{\sqrt{n}} \sum_{s=0}^{n-1} e_s \tag{7.2.1b}$$

$$\left\{\begin{aligned} \chi_{E_1}^{(+)}(e) &= \frac{1}{\sqrt{n}} \sum_{s=0}^{n-1} \omega^{s} e_s &(7.2.1c)\\ \chi_{E_1}^{(-)}(e) &= \frac{1}{\sqrt{n}} \sum_{s=0}^{n-1} \omega^{-s} e_s &(7.2.1d) \end{aligned}\right.$$

$$\vdots$$

$$\chi_{E_q}^{(+)}(e) = \frac{1}{\sqrt{n}} \sum_{s=0}^{n-1} \omega^{qs} e_s \qquad (7.2.1e)$$

$$\chi_{E_q}^{(-1)}(e) = \frac{1}{\sqrt{n}} \sum_{s=0}^{n-1} \omega^{-qs} e_s . \qquad (7.2.1f)$$

TABLE 7.1

Character Table for the Group C_n (n even)

	C_n	E	C_n	C_n^2	$\cdots$	C_n^s	$\cdots$	C_n^{n-1}
μ_z, m_z	A	1	1	1	$\cdots$	1	$\cdots$	1
	B	1	-1	1	$\cdots$	$(-1)^s$	$\cdots$	-1
(μ_x, μ_y)	E_1	1	ω	ω^2	$\cdots$	ω^s	$\cdots$	$\omega^{(n-1)}$
(m_x, m_y)		1	ω^{-1}	ω^{-2}	$\cdots$	ω^{-s}	$\cdots$	$\omega^{-(n-1)}$
	E_2	1	ω^2	ω^4	$\cdots$	ω^{2s}	$\cdots$	$\omega^{2(n-1)}$
		1	ω^{-2}	ω^{-4}	$\cdots$	ω^{-2s}	$\cdots$	$\omega^{-2(n-1)}$
	$\vdots$	$\vdots$	$\vdots$	$\vdots$		$\vdots$		$\vdots$
	E_q	1	ω^q	ω^{2q}	$\cdots$	ω^{qs}	$\cdots$	$\omega^{q(n-1)}$
		1	ω^{-q}	ω^{-2q}	$\cdots$	ω^{-qs}	$\cdots$	$\omega^{-q(n-1)}$
	$\vdots$	$\vdots$	$\vdots$	$\vdots$		$\vdots$		$\vdots$
	$E_{(n-2)/2}$	1	$\omega^{(n-2)/2}$	$\omega^{2(n-2)/2}$		$\omega^{(n-2)s/2}$		$\omega^{(n-2)(n-1)/2}$
					$\cdots$		$\cdots$	
		1	$\omega^{-(n-2)/2}$	$\omega^{-2(n-2)/2}$		$\omega^{-(n-2)s/2}$		$\omega^{-(n-2)(n-1)/2}$
					$\cdots$		$\cdots$	

For simplicity consider the g_s functions as containing a single electron with the composite system having n electrons. If only nearest neighbor interactions are considered, one is led, as in the benzene problem, to a secular determinant

$$\begin{vmatrix} H_{11}-E & \beta & \cdot & \cdot & \cdot & \beta \\ \beta & H_{11}-E & \cdot & \cdot & \cdot & \cdot \\ \cdot & \beta & \cdot & \cdot & \cdot & \cdot \\ \cdot & \cdot & \cdot & \cdot & \cdot & \cdot \\ \cdot & \cdot & \cdot & \cdot & \cdot & \cdot \\ \cdot & \cdot & \cdot & \cdot & \cdot & \beta \\ \beta & \cdot & \cdot & \cdot & \cdot & H_{11}-E \end{vmatrix} = 0. \qquad (7.2.2)$$

The eigenvalues of such a cyclic matrix are given by

$$E_k = H_{11} + 2\beta \cos \frac{2\pi k}{n}. \tag{7.2.3}$$

This leads to a set of levels symmetrically centered around H_{11}.

The n electrons will be placed in the lowest $\chi(g)$ orbitals. It will next be necessary to find all determinantal functions with A and E_1 symmetry formed by promoting one electron from a $\chi(g)$ orbital to a $\chi(e)$ orbital. By reference to Table 7.1 the group multiplication table may be formed. The results are in Table 7.2.

TABLE 7.2

Group Multiplication Table for C_n

$E_q \times E_{q'} = E_{q+q'}$ mod$(n-2)/2$	$+\ E_{q-q'}$
$E_q \times E_q = E_{2q}$ mod$(n-2)/2$	$+\ 2A$
$A \times B = B$	
$A \times A = A$	
$B \times B = A$	
$A \times E_q = E_q$	
$B \times E_q = E_{q+1}$ mod$(n-2)/2$	

An exhaustive treatment of all possible cases would be somewhat intricate, and we will follow a suggestive line of argument to outline the general result; for example, if $n = 6$ the six electrons will be in the $\chi_A(g)$ and $\chi_{E_1}(g)$ orbitals. Promotion from the $\chi_A(g)$ orbital to the $\chi_A(e)$ and $\chi_{E_1}(e)$ orbitals gives states with A and E_1 symmetry; promotion from the $\chi_{E_1}(g)$ orbital to the $\chi_{A_1}(e)$, $\chi_{E_1}(e)$, and $\chi_{E_2}(e)$ orbitals gives states with E_1, $E_2 + 2A$, and $E_1 + E_2$ symmetry. This makes a total of three A and three E_1 states.

Let us neglect the change in energy of the $\chi(g)$ orbitals and only consider the $\chi(e)$ orbitals. The energies are

$$\begin{aligned} E_A &= H_{11} + 2\beta \ (a) \qquad & E_{E_1} &= H_{11} + \beta \quad (b) \\ E_{E_2} &= H_{11} - \beta \quad (c) \qquad & E_B &= H_{11} - 2\beta \quad (d) \end{aligned} \tag{7.2.4}$$

This leads to an average value of $H_{11} + 4\beta/3$ for the A states and $H_{11} + 2\beta/3$ for the E_1 states. The complete treatment will lead to the result that the net rotational strengths of these two sets are equal and opposite in sign.

Returning to the general case, we will demonstrate this general result by concentrating on the transitions $\chi_A(g) \to \chi_A(e)$ and $\chi_A(g) \to \chi_{E_1}(e)$. Let the phases be chosen so that the transition moments are obtained from $\boldsymbol{\mu}_0$ by rotation through multiples of $2\pi/n$ radians. If $\boldsymbol{\mu}_0 = a\mathbf{i} + b\mathbf{j} + c\mathbf{k}$, then $\boldsymbol{\mu}_s = a\mathbf{i}_s + b\mathbf{j}_s + c\mathbf{k}$, where

$$\mathbf{i}_s = \mathbf{i}\cos\frac{2\pi s}{n} + \mathbf{j}\sin\frac{2\pi s}{n} \tag{7.2.5a}$$

$$\mathbf{j}_s = -\mathbf{i}\sin\frac{2\pi s}{n} + \mathbf{j}\cos\frac{2\pi s}{n}. \tag{7.2.5b}$$

Since $\cos 2\pi s/n = (\omega^s + \omega^{-s})/2$ and $\sin 2\pi s/n = (\omega^s - \omega^{-s})/2i$, the electric dipole moment at the sth position may be written

$$\boldsymbol{\mu}_s = \left[\frac{a(\omega^s + \omega^{-s})}{2} - \frac{b(\omega^s - \omega^{-s})}{2i}\right]\mathbf{i} + \left[\frac{a(\omega^s - \omega^{-s})}{2i} + \frac{b(\omega^s + \omega^{-s})}{2}\right]\mathbf{j} + c\mathbf{k}. \tag{7.2.6}$$

The magnetic moment of the tth transition relative to the origin in Figure 7.4 is given by

$$\mathbf{m}_s = \frac{e}{2mc} R\mathbf{i}_s \times \mathbf{p}_s = 2\pi i m \nu_0 \frac{1}{2mc} R\mathbf{i}_s \times \boldsymbol{\mu}_s, \tag{7.2.7}$$

where the standard quantum relation between $\boldsymbol{\mu}$ and $\mathbf{p}$ has been used and ν_0 is the unperturbed frequency of an individual oscillator with R the radius of the circle.

By use of the relation $\sum_{s=0}^{n-1} \omega^s = 0$, the electric and magnetic moments are found to be

$$\langle\chi_A(g)|\,\boldsymbol{\mu}\,|\chi_{E_1}^{+}(e)\rangle = \frac{1}{n}\sum_{s=0}^{n-1} \omega^s \boldsymbol{\mu}_s = \tfrac{1}{2}[(a - ib)\mathbf{i} + (ia + b)\mathbf{j}] \tag{7.2.8a}$$

$$\langle\chi_{E_1}^{+}(e)|\,\mathbf{m}\,|\chi_A(g)\rangle = \frac{1}{n}\sum_{s=0}^{n-1} \omega^{-s}\mathbf{m}_s = \frac{2\pi i m}{2mc}\nu_0 R(-c)\tfrac{1}{2}(i\mathbf{i} + \mathbf{j}) \tag{7.2.8b}$$

$$\langle\chi_A(g)|\,\boldsymbol{\mu}\,|\chi_A(e)\rangle = \frac{1}{n}\sum_{s=0}^{n-1} \boldsymbol{\mu}_s = c\mathbf{k}. \tag{7.2.8c}$$

$$\langle\chi_A(e)|\,\mathbf{m}\,|\chi_A(g)\rangle = \frac{1}{n}\sum_{s=0}^{n-1} \mathbf{m}_s = \frac{2\pi i m}{2mc}\nu_0 R b\mathbf{k}. \tag{7.2.8d}$$

This leads to the rotational strengths

$$R_{AA} = \frac{\pi R \nu_0}{c} \mu_Y \mu_Z \qquad (7.2.9a)$$

$$R_{AE_1{}^+} = -\frac{1}{2}\frac{\pi R \nu_0}{c} \mu_Y \mu_Z, \qquad (7.2.9b)$$

where μ_Y and μ_Z are the moments perpendicular to the dihedral planes and perpendicular to the xy-plane. The E_1^- state makes a contribution identical to that of the E_1^+, which leads to the asserted conclusion that parallel and perpendicular bands make equal and opposite signed contributions.

In the preceding section it was shown how the width of molecular absorption bands is governed by vibronic effects. As yet little has been done with the vibronic theory of group degeneracy. It has been suggested that the observed S-shaped circular dichroism curves for such systems be considered to be a limiting form of

$$\theta(\nu) = kR_{AA}[\delta(\nu - \nu_0) - \delta(\nu - \nu_0 - \Delta\nu)], \qquad (7.2.10)$$

where $\delta(\nu - \nu_0)$ is the Dirac delta function and $\Delta\nu$ is the so-called exciton splitting. This has led to the fitting of the data with the difference between two displaced Gaussian curves and the interpretation of the difference in frequency as the exciton splitting. Within the framework of the simple theory here outlined this leads to a number which should increase with increasing intergroup distance. For the time being it is probably best to use empirical equations which fit the data and relate calculated quantities to more well-defined parameters such as the area of half the dichroism curve or the difference between the extrema.

A word of caution is in order concerning the simple exciton theory. One of its principal shortcomings is the inability to explain the changes in total intensity of absorption which so often occur in these compounds. The above procedure leads to a total intensity of n times the individual monomer absorption in disagreement with experiment. One method has resorted to a higher order borrowing from other transitions with the result that one transition gains intensity at the expense of another with the total unchanged. A second mechanism not fully investigated is the change in effective field caused at the position of one chromophore by the oscillations of another at the identical frequency. Before this question is answered one can only expect limited success in exciton theory.

7.3. Anisotropic Media

A brief word is in order on the subject of anisotropy. Initially in Chapters 1 and 2 we developed expressions relating the observed rotational strengths of isotropic media to molecular parameters. In Chapter 6 we relaxed this isotropy condition slightly by introducing a constant magnetic field, which caused the averaging over molecular orientations to be performed in a special manner. When the orientation of each molecule is fixed, a complication arises which often makes the interpretation of dissymmetry data difficult.

The averaging process used to obtain (2.4.22) may no longer be carried out in a simple manner, nor may a Boltzmann factor be used. It should further be recognized that it is not necessary for the individual molecules or ions of a crystal to be dissymmetric in order that the substance be optically active. Many crystals such as $NaClO_3$ are active by virtue of the relative arrangement of the individual inactive fragments. Since this is true, one is put on his guard against attempting a simple correlation of liquid or vapor phase data with the solid state. In general interactions which tend to cancel out for random orientations do not do so in the crystalline state. It cannot be expected that the average rotational strength for all orientations of a crystal formed by optically active molecules will equal the vapor phase value.

There exists for each crystal a set of axes called the principal dielectric axes, for which the average polarization per unit volume **P** is parallel to the average field **E**. This also implies that $\mathbf{D} = \mathbf{E} + 4\pi\mathbf{P}$ is also parallel to **E**. The disposition of the effective fields and individual electric dipole moments is another matter, which has not yet been satisfactorily formulated for radiation fields. In phenomenological discussions there is some merit to using the dielectric displacement vector **D**. For nonmagnetic media Maxwell's equations take the form [cf. (1.4.2)]

$$\nabla \times \mathbf{E} = -\frac{1}{c}\frac{\partial \mathbf{H}}{\partial t} \tag{7.3.1a}$$

$$\nabla \times \mathbf{H} = \frac{1}{c}\frac{\partial \mathbf{D}}{\partial t}. \tag{7.3.1b}$$

A linear relation between **D** and **E** is presupposed:

$$\mathbf{D} = \boldsymbol{\varepsilon}\mathbf{E}, \tag{7.3.2}$$

where $\boldsymbol{\varepsilon}$ is a tensor. For inactive nondissipative media $\boldsymbol{\varepsilon}$ is symmetrical and real. For the other cases $\boldsymbol{\varepsilon}$ will be complex in general. When the diagonal components of $\boldsymbol{\varepsilon}$ are complex an exponential attentuation factor appears in the solutions to (7.3.1) corresponding to absorption. If the off diagonal components comprise a pure imaginary skew symmetric tensor, optical activity is implied.

By taking the curl of (7.3.1a) and the time derivative of (7.3.1b) the standard wave equation is obtained:

$$\frac{1}{c^2}\boldsymbol{\varepsilon}\frac{\partial^2}{\partial t^2}\mathbf{E} = -\nabla \times \nabla \times \mathbf{E}. \tag{7.3.3}$$

It is important to recognize that $\nabla \cdot \mathbf{E} = 0$ only for isotropic media and that $\nabla \cdot \mathbf{D}$ always vanishes in the absence of net charges. Therefore it is not worthwhile to attempt a further reduction of $\nabla \times \nabla \times \mathbf{E}$. If a solution is assumed of the form

$$\mathbf{E} = \mathbf{E}_0 e^{-i\omega(t - n\mathbf{k}\cdot\mathbf{r}/c)}, \tag{7.3.4}$$

one is led to the equation

$$-\frac{\omega^2}{c^2}\,\boldsymbol{\varepsilon}\mathbf{E}_0 = \frac{\omega^2 n^2}{c^2}\,\mathbf{k} \times (\mathbf{k} \times \mathbf{E}_0) = \frac{\omega^2 n^2}{c^2}\,[\mathbf{k}(\mathbf{k}\cdot\mathbf{E}_0) - \mathbf{E}_0]. \tag{7.3.5}$$

This is a set of homogeneous equations in the components of $\mathbf{E}_0$. In order to obtain a solution, the determinant of the coefficients must be set equal to zero. By using the fact that $\mathbf{k} \cdot \mathbf{D} = 0$ the sixth degree equation in n can be reduced to a quartic. The result is that for an arbitrarily selected propagation direction $\mathbf{k}$ there will be two waves propagated with different phase velocities. By suitable manipulation of (7.3.5) and related equations, the phenomenological theory of biaxial crystals and birefringence may be developed.

We will content ourselves with a brief summary of the overall features of crystal optics. There will exist two unique directions in an anisotropic crystal called the optic axes, for which the velocity of propagation is independent of the direction of polarization. Only for propagation along these directions may the effects of dissymmetry be observed directly without complications from the birefringence phenomenon discussed in Chapter 6. The best results on the experimental side have been obtained for uniaxial crystals such as quartz where the two directions coincide. There appears to be no simple relation between molecular parameters and observed CD data even for propagation along optic axes. Much work is needed in this field.

7.4. The Kerr Effect

An isotropic fluid may be given the optical features of a uniaxial crystal by subjecting it to a constant electric field, the direction of which becomes the single optic axis. If the medium is inactive, it will remain so, unlike the case when a constant magnetic field is applied. This phenomenon is known as the Kerr effect. In order that molecules may be preferentially oriented in an electric field it is necessary that they be anisotropic. If $\boldsymbol{\mu}_{00}$ is the permanent electric dipole moment for the ground state and $\boldsymbol{\alpha} = \alpha_1 \mathbf{b}_1 \mathbf{b}_1 + \alpha_2 \mathbf{b}_2 \mathbf{b}_2 + \alpha_3 \mathbf{b}_3 \mathbf{b}_3$ is the polarizability tensor in the principal axis system of the molecule, the additional terms to the Hamiltonian will be

$$H' = -\boldsymbol{\mu}_{00} \cdot \mathbf{E}_0 - \mathbf{E}_0 \cdot \boldsymbol{\alpha} \cdot \mathbf{E}_0. \tag{7.4.1}$$

This will lead to a Boltzmann factor for the ground state

$$\exp \frac{(\boldsymbol{\mu}_{00} \cdot \mathbf{E}_0 + \mathbf{E}_0 \cdot \boldsymbol{\alpha} \cdot \mathbf{E}_0)}{kT} \approx 1 + \frac{\boldsymbol{\mu}_{00} \cdot \mathbf{E}_0}{kT} + \mathbf{E}_0 \cdot \boldsymbol{\alpha} \cdot \frac{\mathbf{E}_0}{kT}. \quad (7.4.2)$$

Reference to (2.4.19) leads to the evaluation of the expression

$$\langle \boldsymbol{\mu} \rangle_{00} = \Big\langle \sum_{n \neq 0} \frac{2}{\hbar(\omega_{0n}^2 - \omega^2)} \Big[\omega_{0n} \operatorname{Im}(i\boldsymbol{\mu}_{0n} \boldsymbol{\mu}_{n0}) \cdot \mathbf{E}$$

$$+ \frac{\omega_{0n}^2}{\omega^2} \operatorname{Re}(i\boldsymbol{\mu}_{0n} \boldsymbol{\mu}_{n0}) \cdot \dot{\mathbf{E}} + \omega_{0n} \operatorname{Re}(\boldsymbol{\mu}_{0n} \mathbf{m}_{n0}) \cdot \mathbf{B} - \operatorname{Im}(\boldsymbol{\mu}_{0n} \mathbf{m}_{n0}) \cdot \dot{\mathbf{B}} \Big]$$

$$\times \Big[\Big(\frac{1}{kT} \Big) (\boldsymbol{\mu}_{00} \cdot \mathbf{E}_0 + \mathbf{E}_0 \cdot \boldsymbol{\alpha} \cdot \mathbf{E}_0) \Big] \Big\rangle_{\text{av}}. \quad (7.4.3)$$

The averaging formula in Chapter 1 gives

$$\langle \boldsymbol{\mu}_{0n}(\boldsymbol{\mu}_{00} \cdot \mathbf{E}_0)(\boldsymbol{\mu}_{n0} \cdot \mathbf{E}) \rangle = \tfrac{1}{6}(\boldsymbol{\mu}_{0n} \cdot \boldsymbol{\mu}_{00} \times \boldsymbol{\mu}_{n0}) \mathbf{E}_0 \times \mathbf{E} = 0 \quad (7.4.4a)$$

$$\langle \boldsymbol{\mu}_{0n}(\boldsymbol{\mu}_{00} \cdot \mathbf{E}_0)(\mathbf{m}_{n0} \cdot \mathbf{B}) \rangle = \tfrac{1}{6}(\boldsymbol{\mu}_{0n} \cdot \boldsymbol{\mu}_{00} \times \mathbf{m}_{n0}) \mathbf{E}_0 \times \mathbf{B}. \quad (7.4.4b)$$

For the electric field intensity used the predominant effects will come from $\boldsymbol{\mu}\boldsymbol{\mu}$ rather than $\boldsymbol{\mu}\mathbf{m}$ terms. This leads us to investigate the term

$$\langle \boldsymbol{\mu}_{0n}(\mathbf{E}_0 \cdot \boldsymbol{\alpha} \cdot \mathbf{E}_0) \boldsymbol{\mu}_{0n} \cdot \mathbf{E} \rangle_{\text{av}} = \sum_{i=1}^{3} \alpha_i \langle \boldsymbol{\mu}_{0n}(\mathbf{b}_i \cdot \mathbf{E}_0)^2 (\boldsymbol{\mu}_{0n} \cdot \mathbf{E}) \rangle_{\text{av}}. \quad (7.4.5)$$

The fixed coordinate system is determined by the vectors $\mathbf{E}_0$ and $\mathbf{E}$ and the molecular by $\boldsymbol{\mu}_{0n}$ and the $\mathbf{b}_i$. This may be reduced to finding the value of the tensor $\langle \boldsymbol{\mu}_{0n}(\mathbf{b}_i \cdot \mathbf{E}_0)^2 \boldsymbol{\mu}_{0n} \rangle_{\text{av}}$. Let $\mathbf{i}, \mathbf{j}, \mathbf{k}$ be the fixed set of vectors with

$$\mathbf{b}_i = \mathbf{i} \sin\theta \cos\phi + \mathbf{j} \sin\theta \sin\phi + \mathbf{k} \cos\theta. \quad (7.4.6)$$

Let the coordinate system obtained by rotating about $\mathbf{k}$ through the angle ϕ be given by

$$\mathbf{i}^{\ddagger} = \mathbf{i} \cos\phi + \mathbf{j} \sin\phi \quad (7.4.7a)$$

$$\mathbf{j}^{\ddagger} = -\mathbf{i} \sin\phi + \mathbf{j} \cos\phi \quad (7.4.7b)$$

$$\mathbf{k}^{\ddagger} = \mathbf{k}. \quad (7.4.7c)$$

Then let a coordinate system suitable for describing the orientation of $\boldsymbol{\mu}_{0n}$ about $\mathbf{b}_i$ be defined by

$$\mathbf{k}^* = \mathbf{b}_i \quad (7.4.8a)$$

$$\mathbf{j}^* = \mathbf{j}^{\ddagger} \quad (7.4.8b)$$

$$\mathbf{i}^* = \mathbf{j}^* \times \mathbf{k}^* = \mathbf{j}^{\ddagger} \times \mathbf{b}_i. \quad (7.4.8c)$$

The situation is shown in Figure 7.6.

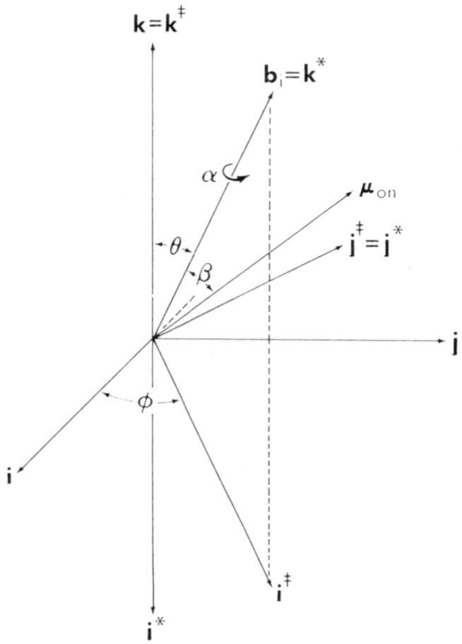

Figure 7.6. The vectors in the averaging process.

In the figure θ and ϕ are the polar and azimuthal angles of the vector $\mathbf{b}_i$, α is the azimuthal angle of $\boldsymbol{\mu}_{0n}$ around $\mathbf{b}_i$, and β is the fixed angle between $\mathbf{b}_i$ and $\boldsymbol{\mu}_{0n}$. If $\mathbf{a}$ is a vector along $\boldsymbol{\mu}_{0n}$, its z-component will be given by

$$a_z = \cos\theta\cos\beta - \sin\theta\sin\beta\cos\alpha. \tag{7.4.9}$$

With the use of the fact that $\int_0^{2\pi}\sin\phi\cos\phi\,d\phi = 0$ and $\int_0^{2\pi}\cos\alpha\,d\alpha = 0$ one is led to the following intermediate stage in the averaging:

$$\begin{aligned}\langle\boldsymbol{\mu}_{0n}\boldsymbol{\mu}_{0n}(\mathbf{E}_0\cdot\mathbf{b}_i)^2\rangle_{\text{av}} &= \frac{1}{8\pi^2}\int_0^{2\pi}d\alpha\int_0^{2\pi}d\phi\int_0^{2\pi}\sin\theta\,d\theta|\boldsymbol{\mu}_{0n}|^2\mathbf{E}_0^2\\ &\times[(\mathbf{ii}\sin^2\theta\cos^2\phi + \mathbf{jj}\sin^2\theta\sin^2\phi + \mathbf{kk}\cos^2\theta)\\ &\times(\cos^2\theta\cos^2\beta + \sin^2\theta\sin^2\beta\cos^2\alpha)].\end{aligned} \tag{7.4.10}$$

The use of such relations as $\int_0^{\pi}\sin^5\theta\,d\theta = \frac{16}{15}$ gives the final result

$$\begin{aligned}\langle\boldsymbol{\mu}_{0n}\boldsymbol{\mu}_{0n}(\mathbf{E}_0\cdot\mathbf{b}_i)^2\rangle_{\text{av}} &= \tfrac{1}{15}|\boldsymbol{\mu}_{0n}|^2E_0^2\\ &[(2-\cos^2\beta)\mathbf{ii} + (2-\cos^2\beta)\mathbf{jj} + (1+2\cos^2\beta)\mathbf{kk}].\end{aligned} \tag{7.4.11}$$

The combination of this result with (7.4.5) gives

$$\begin{aligned}\langle\boldsymbol{\mu}_{0n}(\mathbf{E}_0\cdot\boldsymbol{\alpha}\cdot\mathbf{E}_0)\boldsymbol{\mu}_{0n}\cdot\mathbf{E}\rangle_{\text{av}} &= \tfrac{1}{15}|\boldsymbol{\mu}_{0n}|^2E_0^2\\ &\times\sum_{i=1}^{3}[\alpha_i(2-\cos^2\beta_i)\mathbf{I} + \alpha_i(-1+3\cos^2\beta_i)\mathbf{kk}]\cdot\mathbf{E}.\end{aligned} \tag{7.4.12}$$

If one writes

$$\boldsymbol{\alpha} = \alpha_\perp \mathbf{I} + (\alpha_\parallel - \alpha_\perp)\mathbf{kk},$$

the difference in dielectric constant for waves polarized parallel and perpendicular to the constant field (Figure 7.7) will be governed by the **kk** term

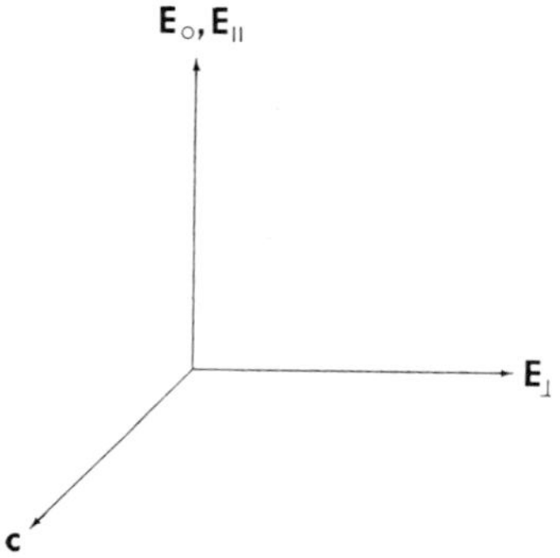

Figure 7.7. The propagation of a wave perpendicular to the constant electric field.

in (7.4.12). For the two directions of polarization $\mathbf{E}_\perp$ and $\mathbf{E}_\parallel$ there will be two dielectric constants and two indices of refraction, $n_\perp = \sqrt{\varepsilon_\perp}$, $n_\parallel = \sqrt{\varepsilon_\parallel}$.

One may write from (7.4.3) and (7.4.12)

$$(n_\perp^2 - n_\parallel^2)_\infty = \text{const.}\,\frac{E_0^2}{kT}\sum_{i=1}^{3}\sum_{n}\frac{\nu_{0n}\boldsymbol{\mu}_{0n}^2}{\nu_{0n}^2 - \nu^2}\,\alpha_i(1 - 3\cos^2\beta_i^{(n)}), \qquad (7.4.13)$$

where the α_i are the principal axis zero frequency polarizabilities of the molecule and $\beta_i^{(n)}$ is the angle between the $\mathbf{b}_i$ principal axis and the transition moment $\boldsymbol{\mu}_{0n}$.

If the three polarizabilities are equal,

$$\sum_{i=1}^{3}\alpha_i(1 - 3\cos^2\beta_i^{(n)}) = 0,$$

since

$$\cos^2\beta_1^{(n)} + \cos^2\beta_2^{(n)} + \cos^2\beta_3^{(n)} = 1,$$

which proves our original assertion that the effect is observed only for anisotropic molecules. In order to obtain all three elements of the polarizability tensor for a molecule with $\boldsymbol{\mu}_{00} = 0$ it is necessary to have three linearly independent relations among the α_i. The average polarizability always provides one:

$$\bar{\alpha} = \tfrac{1}{3}(\alpha_1 + \alpha_2 + \alpha_3). \qquad (7.4.14)$$

If two separate absorption bands with different polarizations are available, it may be possible to obtain the two additional relations from (7.4.13). For example, if two transitions are polarized along $\mathbf{b}_1$ and $\mathbf{b}_2$ respectively the data in these absorption regions would lead to relations of the form

$$(n_\perp^2 - n_\parallel^2)_1 = A_1(-2\alpha_1 + \alpha_2 + \alpha_3) \quad (7.4.15a)$$

$$(n_\perp^2 - n_\parallel^2)_2 = A_2(\alpha_1 - 2\alpha_2 + \alpha_3), \quad (7.4.15b)$$

from which all three components may be obtained with the use of (7.4.14). In practice such ideal situations are difficult to find, and one often treats a molecule as approximately cylindrically symmetrical.

In order to obtain the dependence on $\boldsymbol{\mu}_{00}$, it is necessary to expand (7.4.2) to one more power, which leads us to consider the term $(\boldsymbol{\mu}_{00} \cdot \mathbf{E}_0)^2/2(KT)^2$. Since this expression depends on the tensor $\boldsymbol{\mu}_{00}\boldsymbol{\mu}_{00}$ in just the same way as $\mathbf{E}_0 \cdot \boldsymbol{\alpha} \cdot \mathbf{E}_0$ depends on $\boldsymbol{\alpha}$, it immediately follows in analogy to the derivation of (7.4.13) that a permanent dipole moment makes a contribution

$$(n_1^2 - n_\parallel^2)_{\boldsymbol{\mu}} = \text{const.} \frac{\mathbf{E}_0^2}{2(kT)^2} \sum_n \frac{\nu_{0n}\boldsymbol{\mu}_{0n}^2}{\nu_{0n}^2 - \nu^2} \boldsymbol{\mu}_{00}^2(1 - 3\cos^2\gamma^{(n)}), \quad (7.4.16)$$

where $\gamma^{(n)}$ is the angle between $\boldsymbol{\mu}_{0n}$ and $\boldsymbol{\mu}_{00}$.

The above development is not meant to be an exhaustive treatment of the Kerr effect, but rather a descriptive outline indicating the principal origins of the phenomenon.

CHAPTER 8

Methods of Interpretation

8.1. Empirical Considerations

To conclude this investigation of optical activity it will be fitting to present a cross section of typical data along with some methods of interpretation. This is not intended to be a definitive exposition of correlating theory with experiment, but rather a representative display of what is likely to be encountered by investigators in this field.

The results of theories such as those presented in the preceding chapters have been helpful in formulating general empirical methods for correlating optical activity data. Figure 8.1 is a schematic illustration of a molecule

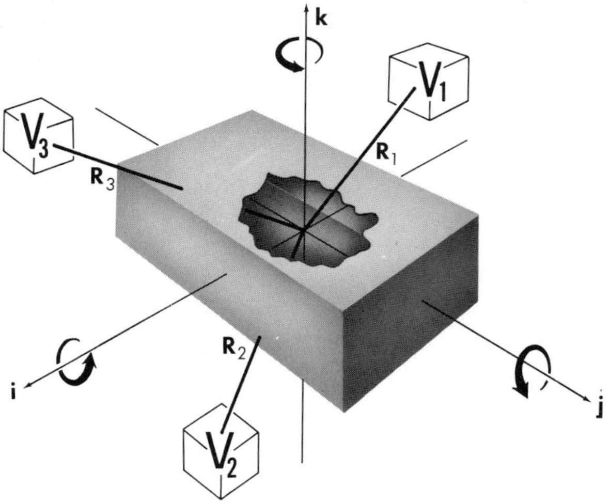

Figure 8.1. D_{2h} chromophore and vicinal groups.

consisting of a single chromophore in the presence of several perturbing groups. A crucial factor in determining the form of the interaction law is the effective symmetry of the chromophore. In the example of the figure,

D_{2h} has been selected. The simplest form of the rotational strength to be tested is

$$R_{0n}^{(\mathrm{SCF})} = K_{0n} \sum_i \gamma_x^{(i)} \gamma_y^{(i)} \gamma_z^{(i)} G^{(i)}(R_i). \tag{8.1.1}$$

In this equation K_{0n} is a constant which depends only on the chromophore and $G^{(i)}(R_i)$ is a function of R_i which depends only on the vicinal group; $\gamma_x^{(i)}$, $\gamma_y^{(i)}$, $\gamma_z^{(i)}$ are the usual direction cosines.

This separation into products of chromophore and vicinal factors has already been encountered in the evaluation of terms like $(\mathbf{p}V)_{0n}$, where V is a multipole expansion of the perturbing charge distribution potential. This separation will probably be valid for a great many forms of V provided that the overlap between the groups is small. Concerning a multipole expansion there is theoretical justification for nearly every inverse power of R. In the example chosen it follows from Chapters 4 and 5 that the lowest power to be tried is $1/R^4$. The possibility of a constant factor for α-substituents should not be overlooked. This suggests that $G^{(i)}$ be written as

$$G(R) = A + \frac{B}{R^4} + \frac{C}{R^5} + \cdots. \tag{8.1.2}$$

This describes the SCF or one electron effects but not electron correlation in general. The coupled oscillator model treated in Chapter 3 provides a suitable empirical foothold on the problem. If $\boldsymbol{\mu}_{0n}$ is the transition moment of the chromophore, the result for the interaction of a cylindrically symmetric vicinal group with the transition $\boldsymbol{\mu}_{0n}$ suggests the form

$$R_{0n}^{(\mathrm{COR})} = S_{0n} \sum_i H_i \frac{\mathbf{b}_1 \cdot \mathbf{b}_{1i} \times \mathbf{b}_i}{R_i^2} [\mathbf{b}_i \cdot \mathbf{b}_1 - 3(\mathbf{b}_1 \cdot \mathbf{b}_{1i})(\mathbf{b}_i \cdot \mathbf{b}_{1i})], \tag{8.1.3}$$

where $\mathbf{b}_1$ = direction of $\boldsymbol{\mu}_{0n}$,
$\mathbf{b}_i$ = axis of approximate cylindrical symmetry of group i,
$\mathbf{b}_{1i}$ = unit vector along $\mathbf{R}_i$,
S_{0n} = chromophore constant,
H_i = vicinal group constant.

It is possible that the same chromophore constant can be used for a variety of vicinal groups; and with a judicious handling of the $G(R)$ functions it may be possible to correlate the vicinal constants for different chromophores. If the chromophore has C_{2v} symmetry, (8.1.1) should be replaced by

$$R_{0n}^{(\mathrm{SCF})} = K_{0n} \sum_i \gamma_x^{(i)} \gamma_y^{(i)} G^{(i)}(R_i), \tag{8.1.4}$$

where z is along the symmetry axis. From the development in Chapters 4 and 5 it follows that theory can suggest a great many intricate mathematical forms for empirical rules. The power of such a procedure lies in the ability to select a small number of dominant terms while discarding the rest. The selection of a rigid model system for the initial investigation is also important, as well as the opportunity for the synthesis of a substantial number of derivatives.

8.2. Typical ORD and CD Data

Owing to their great importance in biochemistry, the peptide and carbonyl chromophores have received a fair amount of attention. Initially attention was concentrated on the so-called exciton effects arising from the interaction of the electric dipole transitions in the identical peptide chromophores of a polypeptide. This constituted a pure electron correlation treatment, which enjoyed a moderate amount of success outside of absorption regions. As experimental techniques become more refined it became evident that not only were $\pi - \pi^*$ transitions contributing but the forbidden $n - \pi^*$ as well. Because of their low intensity it appears that the $n - \pi^*$ contributions to the optical activity of polypeptides are best treated by the SCF terms rather than by exciton theory.

An interesting series of compounds containing the peptide chromophore is typified by the two basic systems shown in Figure 8.2. Both these compounds

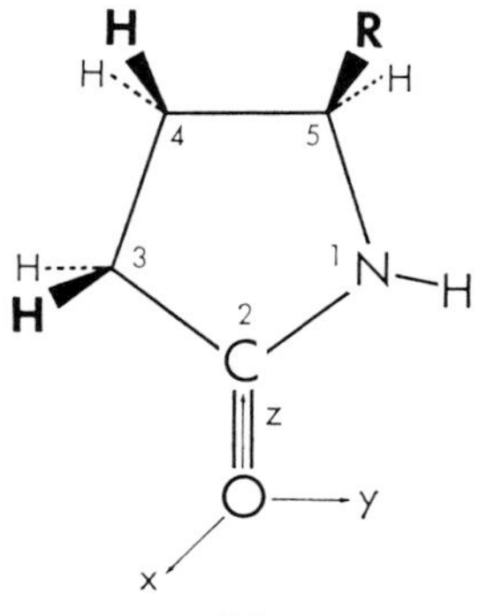

(a)

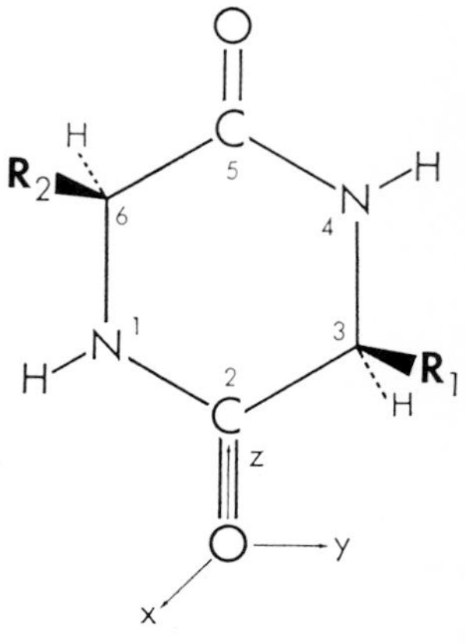

(b)

Figure 8.2. Model compounds for the peptide chromophore: (*a*) L-pyrrolid-2-one; (*b*) L-2,5-diketopiperazine (DKP).

are very nearly planar, and the second one also provides the opportunity for studying the effects of two identical chromophores in the same molecule. Current thinking seems to be that special effects in the case of group degeneracy are only observed for strongly allowed electric dipole transitions.

Another compound of importance to the theory is shown in Figure 8.3. Particularly interesting are the CD curves for the vapor phase and the nonpolar solvent, cyclohexane, shown in Figure 8.4. Outside of a richer fine structure in the gas phase there is little difference between these curves. This

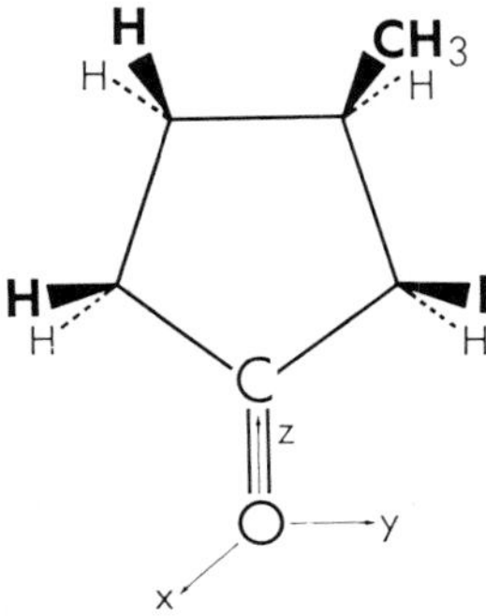

Figure 8.3. 3(+)-Methyl cyclopentanone.

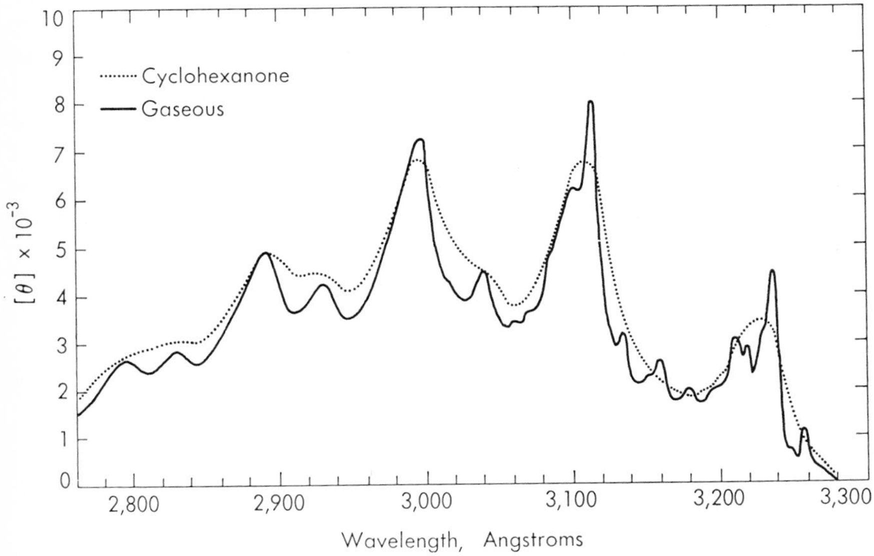

Figure 8.4. The CD curves for 3(+)-methyl cyclopentanone.

would almost indicate that for weakly absorbing isotropic fluids there is little difference between the effective field and the average field discussed in Chapters 1 and 2. There is a qualitative correspondence with the symmetrical curve of Figure 7.1 predicted by theory.

When the 5 position of L-pyrrolid-2-one is substituted, a trend is observed in which increasingly negatively charged groups give larger positive CD maximums. A single term expression of the form (8.1.4) would be written

$$R_{n\pi*} = -K\gamma_x\gamma_y \frac{Q}{R^m}, \tag{8.2.1}$$

where Q is the effective charge of the group. The 5 position in Figure 8.2*a* has both γ_x and γ_y positive. When the 3 position is substituted, γ_x is positive and γ_y is negative. Observation indicates that an increasing positive charge gives increasing negative rotations, which requires a term with the opposite sign from (8.2.1). The data on the L-2,5-diketopiperazines (Figure 8.2*b*) support this conclusion. One is thus led to an equation of the form

$$R_{n\pi*} = \sum_i Q_i \gamma_x^{(i)}\gamma_y^{(i)} \left(\frac{a_i}{R_i^l} - \frac{b_i}{R_i^m}\right). \tag{8.2.2}$$

The constant a_i describes the effect of α-substitution; l can be set equal to zero, because the distance is nearly the same for all substituents and the contribution made by coulombic and exchange integrals can be absorbed into a single geometric factor, $a_i\gamma_x^{(i)}\gamma_y^{(i)}$.

It was found that such a two term expression was capable of correlating the data of the peptide model compounds. Furthermore, the application of the formula to certain polypeptides has shown promising results, which indicate that when properly formulated these simple expressions may provide a useful method for correlating optical activity data with structure. A compound closely related to Figure 8.2*a* is L-homoserine-γ-lactone, shown in Figure 8.5.

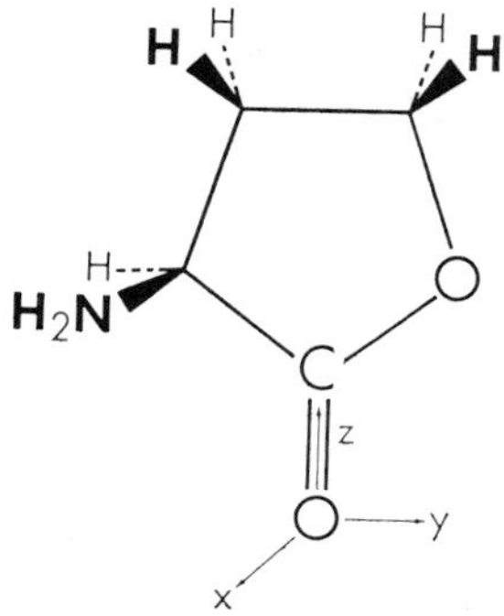

Figure 8.5. L-Homoserine-γ-lactone.

This compound has some of the features of the peptides in that it also has an $n - \pi^*$ transition in about the same region. A notable difference lies in the fact that the sign trends are the opposite to those of the 3-amino-L-pyrrolid-2-one derivative. This indicates that it is not always sufficient to treat these $n-\pi^*$ transitions like those of the carbonyl group. From the empirical standpoint there is no problem, and one may assume an equation with the form of (8.2.2) having different values of the constants.

A particularly interesting vibronic example occurs in poly-L-phenylalanine where in the 2600 Å region sign changes are observed from one vibrational component to the next. The CD extrema have a rough correspondence with those of the absorption curve. Considerable progress has been made in the analysis of data from such compounds.

8.3. Polypeptides

Three well-defined forms of the polypeptide are the helix, random coil, and pleated sheet. When there is a regular interval between identical monomers, as in the helix, the discussion of Section 7.3 indicates the occurrence of a special type of CD curve in which there are two adjacent bands of equal magnitude and opposite sign. If the groups have a relatively unrestricted rotation, this effect disappears. They then behave almost as if they were in two different molecules. This difference in behavior has been used quite intensively as a method for determining percentage helix. We now wish to examine the ramifications of this procedure.

One may state a general rule concerning free rotation about bonds: If the bond joining a vicinal group to a chromophore lies in a plane of symmetry and there is free rotation about this bond, the rotational strength vanishes to first order. This means that to all intents there will be a large difference in rotational strengths of rigid molecules as compared with nonrigid. Figure 8.6 shows the peptide chromophore with the adjacent

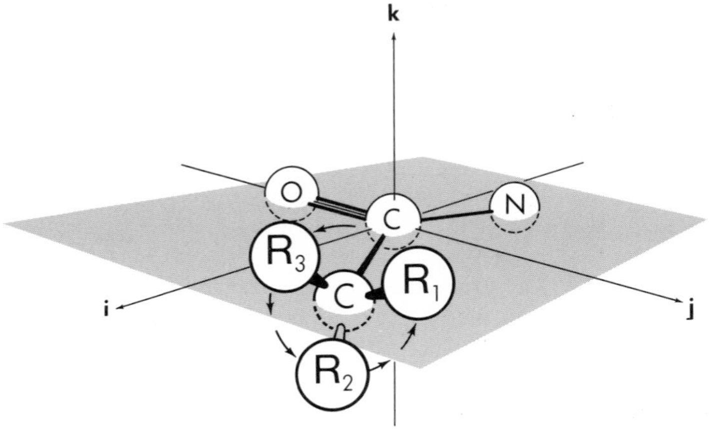

Figure 8.6. Free rotation about a bond.

carbon atom substituted by three different groups. Each position of a group above the *xy*-plane is counteracted by a corresponding one below it.

It should next be recognized that the phenomenon of equal and opposite signed rotational strengths is not confined to helical symmetry. It may occur whenever two or more rigidly oriented identical groups are present in the same molecule. Unless some unmistakable fine structural characteristics are always found to be present for helical conformations, there will be in general no well-defined qualitative difference between the CD curve of a helical protein and some other rigid conformation. Before the era of CD, methods were developed under the assumption that the ORD satisfied an equation of the form

$$\phi_{\text{protein}} = \frac{A_{\text{random}}}{\lambda^2 - \lambda_0^2} + \frac{B_{\text{helix}}}{(\lambda^2 - \lambda_0^2)^2}. \tag{8.3.1}$$

The ratio of the two constants was taken as a measure of percentage helical conformation. Not the least of the assumptions for such a relation to be valid is that the only rigid conformation present is the helix. Perhaps the most questionable aspect of this procedure was the analytical methods for choosing λ_0 and determining the two constants.

Now a far better method comes from the analysis of the CD curve. As the transition from helix to coil occurs, there will be a marked decrease in the intensity of the S-curve. It does not always disappear, but the amount of the change may serve as the basis for a useful empirical method of structure determination.

The characteristic degenerate behavior shows up in many ways. For example, the visible portion of the spectrum is not the only region of interest in transition metal complexes when the ligands have accessible transitions. The ligand portion of the spectrum for the octahedral complex

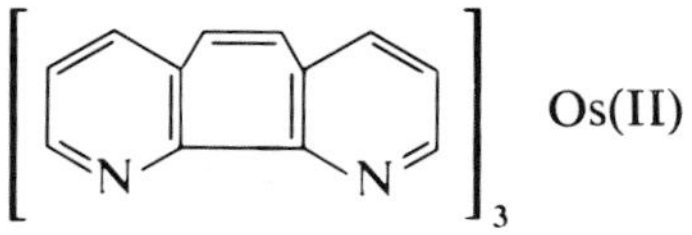

is shown in Figure 8.7. The exciton behavior is in the 2600 Å region, with approximately equal areas in the positive and negative segments. The underlying mechanism behind this has been discussed in Section 7.2. The weaker bands in the UV appear to have some vibronic fine structure, as is often observed with metal complexes.

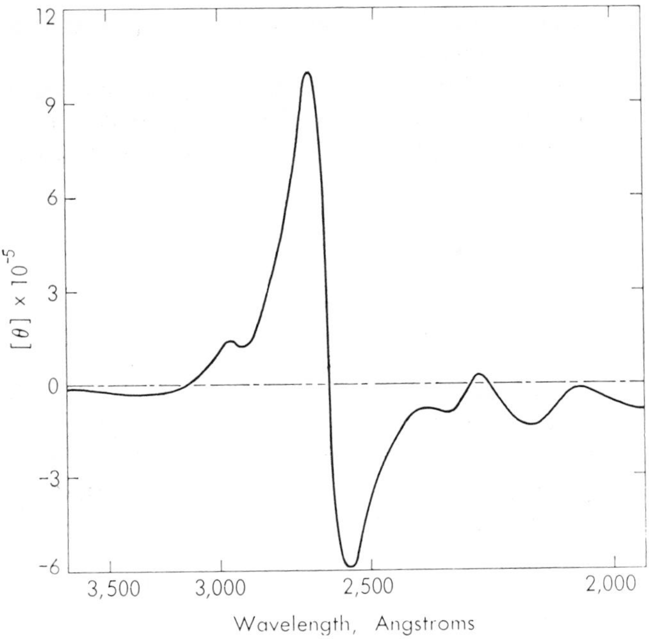

Figure 8.7. CD of the trisphenanthrolene Os(II) complex.

8.4. Skewed Dienes

A fair amount of attention has been focused on what have been termed inherently dissymmetric chromophores. This situation arises when the simplest reasonable zeroth order functions for a chromophore are themselves dissymmetric. As would be expected, the rotational strengths of such compounds are considerably larger than those arising from chromophores whose symmetry is destroyed by longer range interactions with neighboring groups. To date most of the papers have concentrated on conjugated systems. Typical examples of skewed dienes are compounds I and II. In order to

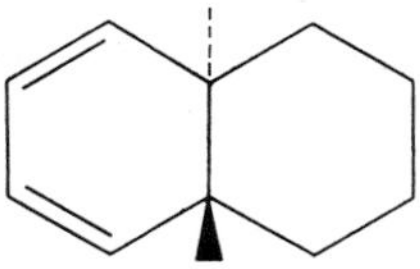

I

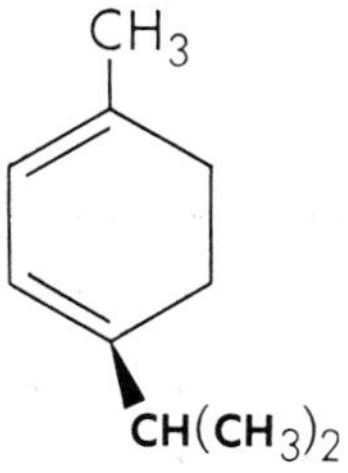

II

maintain approximate tetrahedral bond angles the diene system is twisted out of the planar conformation.

By use of a simple LCAO method it has been possible to explain most of the experimental facets of this system. The basic geometry is illustrated in Figure 8.8. Carbon atom C_1 lies as much above the xy-plane as C_4 lies below

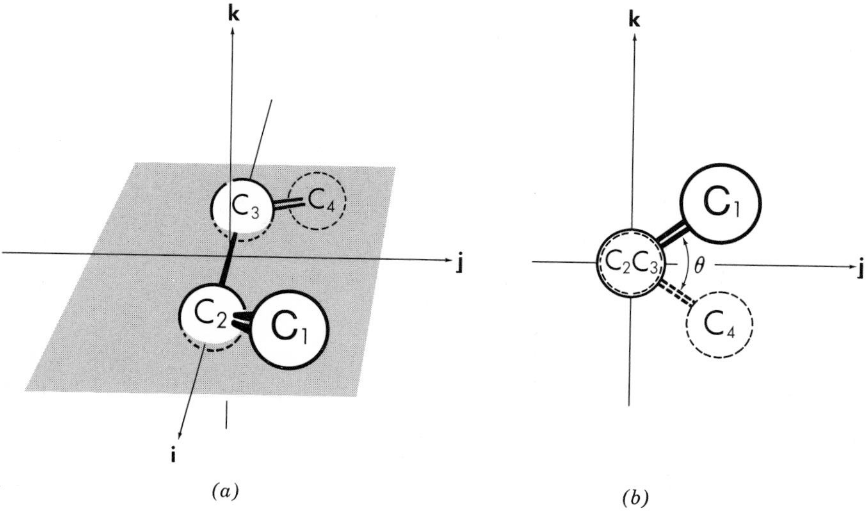

Figure 8.8. Skewed diene system.

it. The cisoid configuration has been illustrated, which occurs when $|\theta| < 90°$; when $|\theta| > 90°$ one has the transoid configuration. For $|\theta| \approx 90°$ there is little distinction between the two, but when $|\theta| \simeq 0°$ or 180°, as is so often the case, the different symmetries of cis and trans butadiene should be borne in mind; cis butadiene ($\theta = 0°$) has C_{2v} symmetry, whereas the trans isomer ($\theta = 180°$) belongs to the C_{2h} group. The character tables of these two groups are given in Table 8.1.

TABLE 8.1

Symmetry Groups C_{2v} and C_{2h}

C_{2v}		E	C_2	σ_v	σ_v'	C_{2h}		E	C_2	σ_h	i
μ_z	A_1	1	1	1	1	m_z	A_g	1	1	1	1
m_z	A_2	1	1	−1	−1	μ_z	A_u	1	1	−1	−1
m_y, μ_x	B_1	1	−1	1	−1	m_x, m_y	B_g	1	−1	−1	1
m_x, μ_y	B_2	1	−1	−1	1	μ_x, μ_y	B_u	1	−1	1	−1

Certain qualitative features can be immediately assessed by reference to Table 8.1. The cis (C_{2v}) isomer may have some of its transitions allowed electrically and magnetically with perpendicular polarizations; whereas the center of symmetry of the trans isomers requires transitions to be allowed either magnetically or electrically, but not both. The twofold rotation axis in Figure 8.8 is the **i**-axis for both cis and trans configurations as well as for the intermediate dissymmetric compounds with C_2 symmetry.

By forming those linear combinations of π-orbitals having A and B symmetry of the C_2 group the secular determinant factors into two second degree components. The appropriate functions and their symmetry are

$$\left.\begin{aligned} \chi_A &= \frac{1}{\sqrt{2}}(\phi_1 + \phi_4) \qquad (8.4.1a) \\ \chi'_A &= \frac{1}{\sqrt{2}}(\phi_2 + \phi_3) \qquad (8.4.1b) \end{aligned}\right\} A$$

$$\left.\begin{aligned} \chi_B &= \frac{1}{\sqrt{2}}(\phi_1 - \phi_4) \qquad (8.4.1c) \\ \chi'_B &= \frac{1}{\sqrt{2}}(\phi_2 - \phi_3) \qquad (8.4.1d) \end{aligned}\right\} B.$$

If H is the effective Hamiltonian of the system, the secular equation is

$$\begin{vmatrix} H_{AA} - E & H_{AA'} & 0 & 0 \\ H_{AA'} & H_{A'A'} - E & 0 & 0 \\ 0 & 0 & H_{BB} - E & H_{BB'} \\ 0 & 0 & H_{BB'} & H_{B'B'} - E \end{vmatrix} = 0. \qquad (8.4.2)$$

The roots are

$$E_A^{(\pm)} = \frac{H_{AA} + H_{A'A'} \pm \sqrt{(H_{AA} - H_{A'A'})^2 + 4H_{AA'}^2}}{2} \qquad (8.4.3a)$$

$$E_B^{(\pm)} = \frac{H_{BB} + H_{B'B'} \pm \sqrt{(H_{BB} - H_{B'B'})^2 + 4H_{BB'}^2}}{2}, \qquad (8.4.3b)$$

and the coefficients may be written

$$\Theta_B^{(\pm)} = \chi_A \cos \varepsilon_A^{(\pm)} + \chi_{A'} \sin \varepsilon_A^{(\pm)} \qquad (8.4.4a)$$

$$\Theta_B^{(\pm)} = \chi_B \cos \varepsilon_B^{(\pm)} + \chi_{B'} \sin \varepsilon_B^{(\pm)}, \qquad (8.4.4b)$$

where

$$\varepsilon_A^{(\pm)} = \tan^{-1}\left[\frac{H_{A'A'} - H_{AA} \pm \sqrt{(H_{A'A'} - H_{AA})^2 + 4H_{AA'}^2}}{2H_{AA'}}\right],$$

$$\varepsilon_B^{(\pm)} = \tan^{-1}\left[\frac{H_{B'B'} - H_{BB} \pm \sqrt{(H_{BB'} - H_{BB})^2 + 4H_{BB'}^2}}{2H_{BB'}}\right].$$

If only integrals between adjacent atoms are considered, the above equations give

$$E_A^{(\pm)} = H_{11} + \tfrac{1}{2}H_{23} \pm \tfrac{1}{2}\sqrt{H_{23}^2 + 4H_{12}^2} \qquad (8.4.5a)$$

$$E_B^{(\pm)} = H_{11} - \tfrac{1}{2}H_{23} \pm \tfrac{1}{2}\sqrt{H_{23}^2 + 4H_{12}^2} \qquad (8.4.5b)$$

$$\varepsilon_A^{(\pm)} = \tan^{-1}\left(\frac{H_{23} \pm \sqrt{H_{23}^2 + 4H_{12}^2}}{2H_{12}}\right) \qquad (8.4.5c)$$

$$\varepsilon_B^{(\pm)} = \tan^{-1}\left(\frac{-H_{23} \pm \sqrt{H_{23}^2 + H_{12}^2}}{2H_{12}}\right), \qquad (8.4.5d)$$

where $H_{12} = H_{34}$ and H_{11}, H_{22}, etc., have all been taken to be equal. It is seen that

$$\varepsilon_B^{(+)} = -\varepsilon_A^{(-)} \quad \text{and} \quad \varepsilon_B^{(-)} = -\varepsilon_A^{(+)}.$$

The energies are in increasing order: $E_A^{(+)}$, $E_B^{(+)}$, $E_A^{(-)}$, $E_B^{(-)}$; and the wave functions may be written,

$$\Theta_B^{(-)} = \frac{1}{\sqrt{2}}(\cos \varepsilon_1 \phi_1 - \sin \varepsilon_1 \phi_2 + \sin \varepsilon_1 \phi_3 - \cos \varepsilon_1 \phi_4) \qquad (8.4.6a)$$

$$\Theta_A^{(-)} = \frac{1}{\sqrt{2}}(\cos \varepsilon_2 \phi_1 + \sin \varepsilon_2 \phi_2 + \sin \varepsilon_2 \phi_3 + \cos \varepsilon_2 \phi_4) \qquad (8.4.6b)$$

$$\Theta_B^{(+)} = \frac{1}{\sqrt{2}}(\cos \varepsilon_2 \phi_1 - \sin \varepsilon_2 \phi_2 + \sin \varepsilon_2 \phi_3 - \cos \varepsilon_2 \phi_4) \qquad (8.4.6c)$$

$$\Theta_A^{(+)} = \frac{1}{\sqrt{2}}(\cos \varepsilon_1 \phi_1 + \sin \varepsilon_1 \phi_2 + \sin \varepsilon_1 \phi_3 + \cos \varepsilon_1 \phi_4), \qquad (8.4.6d)$$

where $\varepsilon_1 = \varepsilon_A^{(+)}$, $\varepsilon_2 = \varepsilon_A^{(-)}$.

Since H_{23} is always somewhat less than H_{12}, one may take

$$\frac{H_{23} \pm \sqrt{H_{23}^2 + 4H_{12}^2}}{2H_{12}} \simeq \pm\frac{\sqrt{H_{23}^2 + 4H_{12}^2}}{2H_{12}};$$

in fact the essential features of the theory would be preserved if H_{23} were set equal to zero and the coefficients became $\pm\frac{1}{2}$. Let us display the system in a more convenient coordinate setting, shown in Figure 8.9 along with the *p*-orbitals.

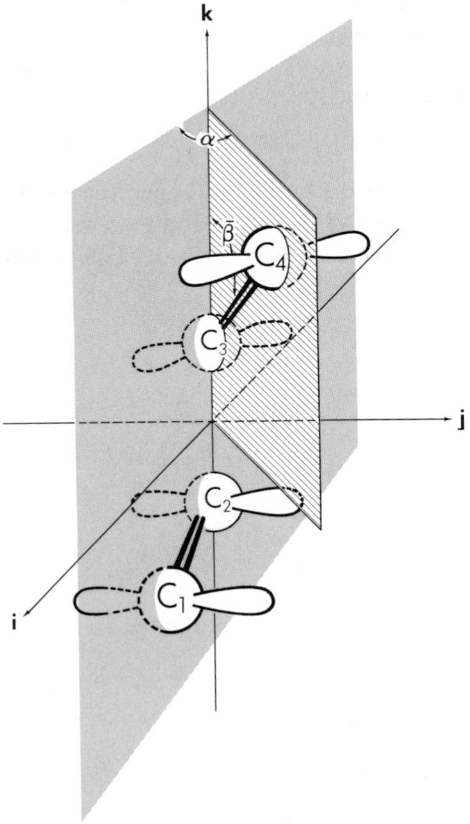

Figure 8.9. The coordinate system for calculating matrix elements. Carbon atoms 1 and 2 are in the *xz*-plane.

The matrix elements will be given in terms of the interatomic quantities $\langle\phi_1|\nabla|\phi_2\rangle$ and $\langle\phi_1|\mathbf{r}\times\nabla|\phi_2\rangle$, where only adjacent atoms are considered and $\langle\phi_i|\nabla|\phi_i\rangle = 0$, $\langle\phi_i|\mathbf{r}\times\nabla|\phi_i\rangle = 0$. The dipole velocity (momentum) matrix elements have been used rather than the electric dipole moments in order to insure an origin independent result.

For simplicity all the adjacent interatomic distances will be taken as equal.

Since the axes of the p-orbitals are perpendicular to the line joining them, only the component of $\mathbf{V}_{12}$ along this line will not vanish. If Q is the value of the integral for parallel orbitals, the value for a skew angle α is

$$\mathbf{V}_{12} = \mathbf{b}_{12}\, Q \cos \alpha, \tag{8.4.7}$$

where $\mathbf{b}_{12}$ is the unit vector from atom 1 to atom 2. Since the derivative of the exponential wave function is negative and a coordinate is introduced which is negative in the region between the two atoms, Q will be positive.

With the origin as shown in Figure 8.9 the angular momentum integral between atoms 1 and 2 may be written

$$(\mathbf{r} \times \mathbf{V})_{12} = \mathbf{R}_2 \times \mathbf{V}_{12} + (\mathbf{r}_2 \times \mathbf{V}_2)_{12}, \tag{8.4.8}$$

where the second term refers to the local operator on atom 2 and $\mathbf{R}_2$ is along $-\mathbf{k}$. For atoms (1, 2) and (3, 4) the second term will vanish but not the first; for atoms (2, 3) the reverse will be true. In Figure 8.10 let the axis of ϕ_2

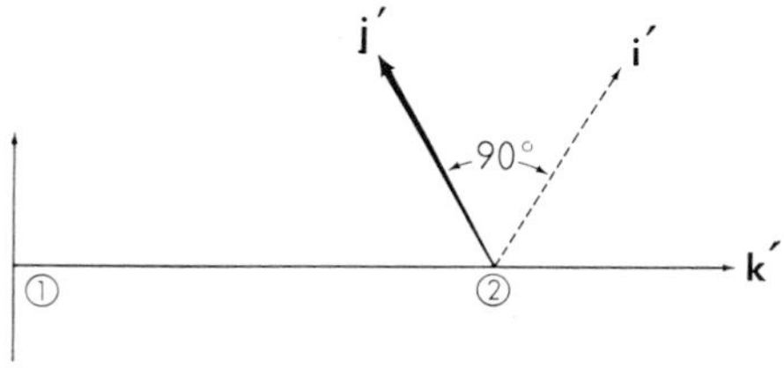

Figure 8.10. The computation of $(\mathbf{r} \times \mathbf{V})_{12}$.

be along $\mathbf{i}'$. Then the result of operating on ϕ_2 is

$$(\mathbf{r}_2 \times \mathbf{V}_2)\phi_{2x'} = \mathbf{j}'\phi_{2z'} - \mathbf{k}'\phi_{2y'}. \tag{8.4.9}$$

Since $\int \phi_1 \phi_{2z'}\, d\tau = 0$, the result is

$$\begin{aligned}(\mathbf{r}_2 \times \mathbf{V}_2)_{12} &= -\mathbf{b}_{12} \int \phi_1 \phi_{2y'}\, d\tau \\ &= -\mathbf{b}_{12}(\mathbf{b}_{12} \times \mathbf{b}_2 \cdot \mathbf{b}_1)S,\end{aligned} \tag{8.4.10}$$

where $\mathbf{b}_1$ and $\mathbf{b}_2$ are along the positive directions of ϕ_1 and ϕ_2, $\mathbf{b}_{12}$ is the unit vector from atom 1 to atom 2, and S is the overlap integral for parallel orbitals.

From the preceding equations and Figure 8.9 the matrix elements are found to be

$$\mathbf{V}_{12} = (\mathbf{k} \cos \bar{\beta} - \mathbf{i} \sin \bar{\beta})Q \tag{8.4.11a}$$

$$\mathbf{V}_{23} = \mathbf{k}Q \cos \alpha \tag{8.4.11b}$$

$$\mathbf{V}_{34} = (\mathbf{i} \sin \bar{\beta} \cos \alpha + \mathbf{j} \sin \bar{\beta} \sin \alpha + \mathbf{k} \cos \bar{\beta})Q \tag{8.4.11c}$$

$$(\mathbf{r} \times \mathbf{V})_{12} = \mathbf{j} aQ \sin \bar{\beta} \tag{8.4.11d}$$

$$(\mathbf{r} \times \mathbf{V})_{23} = \mathbf{k} S \sin \alpha \tag{8.4.11e}$$

$$(\mathbf{r} \times \mathbf{V})_{34} = a(-\mathbf{i} \sin \bar{\beta} \sin \alpha + \mathbf{j} \sin \bar{\beta} \cos \alpha)Q, \tag{8.4.11f}$$

where $a = R/2$ is half the distance between adjacent atoms.

The four possible transitions will be from a ground orbital to an excited one:

$$\Theta_G = C_{G1}\phi_1 + C_{G2}\phi_2 + C_{G3}\phi_3 + C_{G4}\phi_4$$

$$\Theta_E = C_{E1}\phi_1 + C_{E2}\phi_2 + C_{E3}\phi_3 + C_{E4}\phi_4.$$

The desired matrix elements will be written

$$\langle \Theta_G | \mathbf{V} | \Theta_E \rangle = D_{12}\mathbf{V}_{12} + D_{23}\mathbf{V}_{23} + D_{34}\mathbf{V}_{34} \tag{8.4.12a}$$

$$\langle \Theta_E | \mathbf{r} \times \mathbf{V} | \Theta_G \rangle = -[D_{12}(\mathbf{r} \times \mathbf{V})_{12} + D_{23}(\mathbf{r} \times \mathbf{V})_{23} + D_{34}(\mathbf{r} \times \mathbf{V})_{34}], \tag{8.4.12b}$$

where

$$D_{12} = C_{G1}C_{E2} - C_{G2}C_{E1}$$

$$D_{23} = C_{G2}C_{E3} - C_{G3}C_{E2}$$

$$D_{34} = C_{G3}C_{E4} - C_{G4}C_{E3}.$$

The combination of the above three equations gives

$$\begin{aligned}\langle \Theta_G | \mathbf{V} | \Theta_E \rangle \cdot \langle \Theta_E | \mathbf{r} \times \mathbf{V} | \Theta_G \rangle = -[&D_{23}(D_{12} + D_{34})QS \cos \bar{\beta} \sin \alpha \\ &+ 2D_{12}D_{34}aQ \sin^2 \bar{\beta} \sin \alpha \\ &+ D_{23}^2 QS \sin \alpha \cos \alpha].\end{aligned} \tag{8.4.13}$$

With the approximation that $\varepsilon_1 = -\varepsilon_2$ the matrix of the four orbitals becomes

$$\begin{array}{c|cccc} & \phi_1 & \phi_2 & \phi_3 & \phi_4 \\ \hline \Theta_4 & C_1 & -C_2 & C_2 & -C_1 \\ \Theta_3 & C_2 & -C_1 & -C_1 & C_2 \\ \Theta_2 & C_2 & C_1 & -C_1 & -C_2 \\ \Theta_1 & C_1 & C_2 & C_2 & C_1 \end{array}, \tag{8.4.14}$$

where

$$C_1 = \frac{2H_{12}}{\sqrt{H_{23}^2 + 8H_{12}^2}} \tag{8.4.15a}$$

$$C_2 = \sqrt{\frac{H_{23}^2 + 4H_{12}^2}{H_{23}^2 + 8H_{12}^2}}. \tag{8.4.15b}$$

The bottom two rows of (8.4.14) represent the filled orbitals and the upper two the vacant excited orbitals. The values of the D_{ij} terms are given in Table 8.2.

TABLE 8.2

The D_{ij} Coefficients

	$\Theta_2 \to \Theta_3$	$\Theta_2 \to \Theta_4$	$\Theta_1 \to \Theta_3$	$\Theta_1 \to \Theta_4$
D_{12}	$-2C_1C_2$	$-(C_1^2 + C_2^2)$	$-(C_1^2 + C_2^2)$	$-2C_1C_2$
D_{23}	$-2C_1^2$	0	0	$2C_2^2$
D_{34}	$-2C_1C_2$	$(C_1^2 + C_2^2)$	$(C_1^2 + C_2^2)$	$-2C_1C_2$

The rotational strengths of the four transitions will be proportional to

$$K_{23} = \left[\frac{64H_{12}^3\sqrt{\overline{H}_{23}^2 \cos^2\alpha + 4H_{12}^2}}{(\overline{H}_{23}^2 \cos^2\alpha + 8H_{12}^2)^2}\,F + \frac{16H_{12}^2(\overline{H}_{23}^2 \cos^2\alpha + 4H_{12}^2)}{(\overline{H}_{23}^2 \cos^2\alpha + 8H_{12}^2)^2}\,G\right]\sin\alpha$$

$$+ \frac{64H_{12}^4}{(\overline{H}_{23}^2 \cos^2\alpha + 8H_{12}^2)^2}\,H \sin 2\alpha \tag{8.4.16a}$$

$$K_{24} = -G\sin\alpha \tag{8.4.16b}$$

$$K_{13} = -G\sin\alpha, \tag{8.4.16c}$$

where

$$F = QS\cos\bar{\beta},$$
$$G = QR\sin^2\bar{\beta},$$
$$H = \tfrac{1}{2}QS,$$

and $H_{23} = \overline{H}_{23}\cos\alpha$ is the assumed angular dependence of the coupling integral. The highest transition, $\Theta_1 \to \Theta_4$, has been omitted.

The original treatment of this problem assumed that $G \gg F$, $G \gg H$. In this case the magnitude of the $2 \to 3$ transition is approximately equal to that of the $2 \to 4$ or $1 \to 3$ transitions and of opposite sign. In this simple approach the $1 \to 3$ and $2 \to 4$ transitions are accidentally degenerate and give identical contributions of the same sign. Whatever the shortcomings of this theory, there is one important feature that has been overlooked.

When $\alpha = 90°$ all the coefficients become equal to $\pm\frac{1}{2}$. Thus maximum delocalization occurs when $H_{23} = 0$, and a maximum in the rotatory strength is expected at 90°. When it is recognized that for this angle of skew the system behaves in most respects like two isolated ethylene groups, one is led to suspect that the correct wave function is a relatively localized one consisting of a product of ethylene functions centered on the pairs (1, 2) and (3, 4). An important contribution to the rotational strength would then be made by an electron correlation mechanism such as the coupled oscillator theory. One would expect a greatly reduced value as compared with the above theory.

This suggests the use of functions such as

$$\Psi = \sin \alpha \Psi(\text{loc}) + \cos \alpha \Psi(\text{deloc}), \tag{8.4.17}$$

where $\Psi(\text{loc})$ is the ethylenic product function and $\Psi(\text{deloc})$ is the one used in the above exposition. The behavior of these two theories is shown in Figure 8.11. It is thus anticipated that a complete treatment of the problem

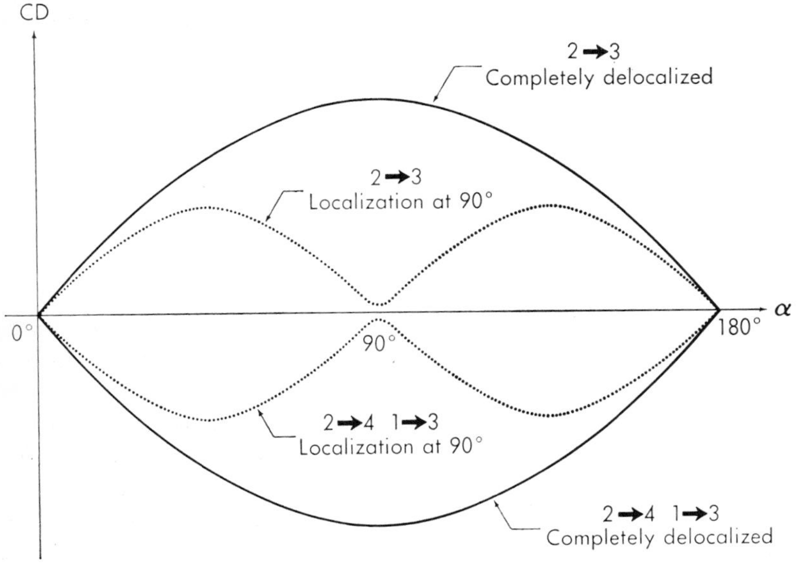

Figure 8.11. Behavior of CD for skew angles from 0° to 180°.

will drastically alter the conclusions for the 90° region. Meanwhile it may be said that much activity in the investigation of coupled chromophores was stimulated by the original publications. The theory predicts that the lowest transition associated with a right-handed skew sense has a positive rotational strength; this has been overwhelmingly supported by observation. Most compounds measured have $\alpha < 30°$, and the quantitative agreement is fairly good. A 90° model compound would be most welcome.

When the conjugated chromophores are sufficiently different, the orbitals for 90° exhibit little mixing and the rotational strength is nearly zero, corresponding to the dotted curve in Figure 8.11.

8.5. Nonconjugated Dienes and Delocalization

In order for special enhancement effects to occur it is not always necessary for unsaturated chromophores to be in conjugation. Considerable work with $\beta\gamma$-unsaturated ketones and similar compounds has provided an interesting and complex situation intermediate between conventional unconjugated and inherently dissymmetric chromophores. Whereas the rotational strengths of inherently dissymmetric systems are one or two orders of magnitude larger than those of the conventional variety, factors of 3–8 generally apply to the intermediate case. Typical molecules are shown in Figure 8.12.

This subject serves as a good review of the various mechanisms of optical activity, because all of them have at one time or another been considered in an attempt to explain the experimental observations. The following summary of the methods for treating this problem may be given:

(A) Line of sight interactions.
  (1) Electrostatic SCF perturbations.
  (2) Pure electron correlation (coupled oscillator).
  (3) Nonzero overlap.
  (4) Charge transfer.
(B) Through bond effects.

The framework for treating any of these theories is at hand in the formalism of Chapter 4. The difference lies in the choice of zeroth order wave function and the perturbation terms evaluated. A convenient choice is the Slater determinant formed from the localized orbitals of the moieties comprising the molecule. The simplest choice is symmetrical orbitals which would prevail in the absence of neighboring interactions. The first two mechanisms of (A) follow from the methods of Chapter 4 by means of the first order pairwise interactions. For reasonable values of the physical parameters a result much lower than observed is invariably obtained.

By calculating exchange perturbation terms some of the effects of nonzero overlap can be included. Through bond effects can be assessed by such expressions as

$$\iiiint \boldsymbol{\mu}_1 \frac{1}{r_{12}} \frac{1}{r_{23}} \frac{1}{r_{34}} \phi_A(1)\phi_A'(1)\phi_B^2(2)\phi_C^2(3)\phi_D^2(4)\, d\tau_1 \cdots d\tau_4 .$$

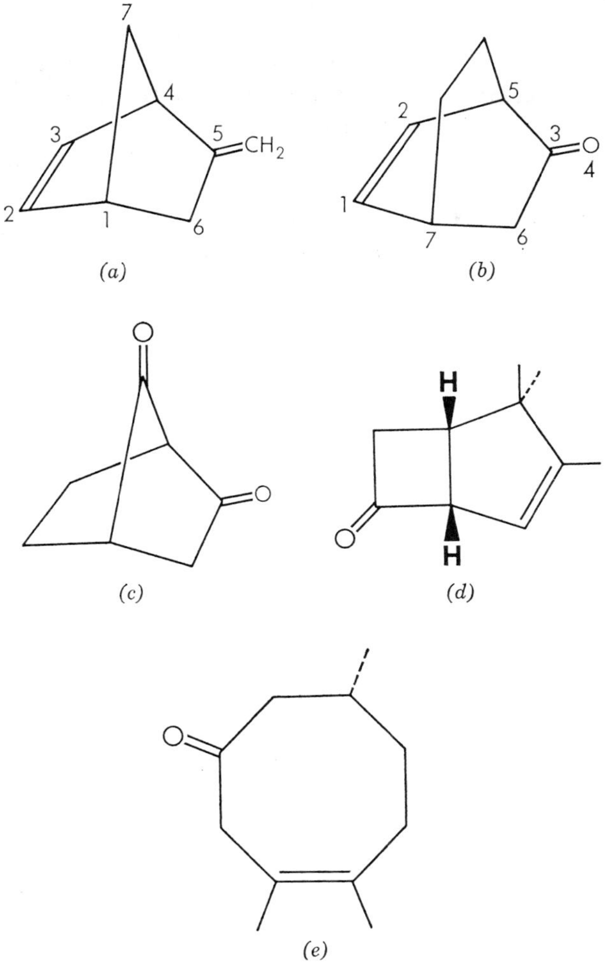

Figure 8.12 Non-Conjugated $\beta\gamma$-unsaturated systems.

Under many circumstances the use of such a chain is more effective in communicating dissymmetry than direct interactions, which tend to taper off quite steeply with distance.

Alternatively one may form single determinants in a general SCF treatment requiring the best single electron orbitals regardless of orthogonality. In general, as has been pointed out in Chapter 4, a transition no longer is described by the promotion of a single electron to an excited orbital. Corresponding orbitals in the ground and excited states are no longer identical.

In many cases one pair of ground and excited orbitals will be nearly orthogonal, with the others consisting of nearly identical pairs.

If the best possible SCF single electron functions have been obtained, the rotational strengths will be obtained from the zeroth order $\mathbf{p}_{0n} \cdot \mathbf{m}_{n0}$ and from the direct and through bond electron correlation terms. Such determinants are difficult to construct, and it is better to proceed from the first type.

Considerable attention has been concentrated on the C=C—C—C=C and C=C—C—C=O systems. The energy level scheme is shown in Figure 8.13. The same principles as used in the previous section with a few sophisti-

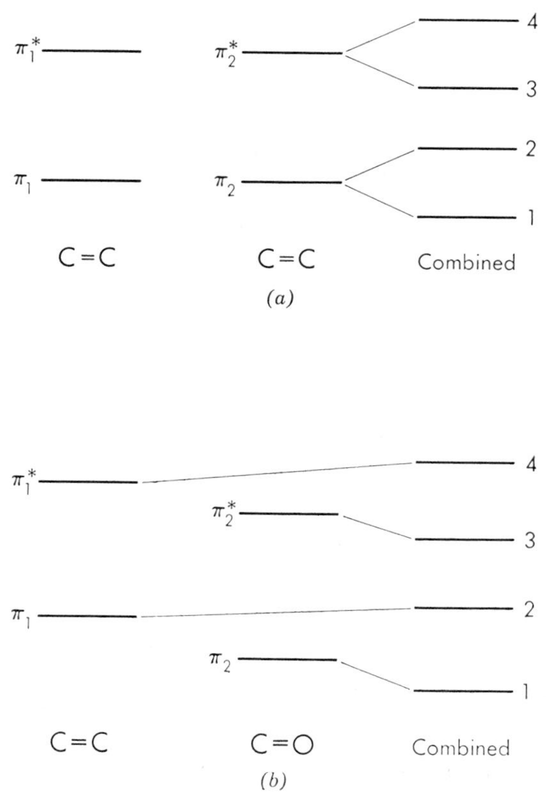

Figure 8.13. Energy levels of coupled unsaturated chromophores.

cated refinements have been employed with apparent success. There are some important points to be made. It is well known that the use of LCAO orbitals is not a suitable method for describing long range interactions. For this reason it was suggested that the valence bond method be used to describe the composite wave function for two reacting molecules at large distances.

Unless careful attention is paid to the complete many electron system one may be led into the same error that besets the four hydrogen atom problem (Figure 8.14). It is true that the ground state for a two electron system would

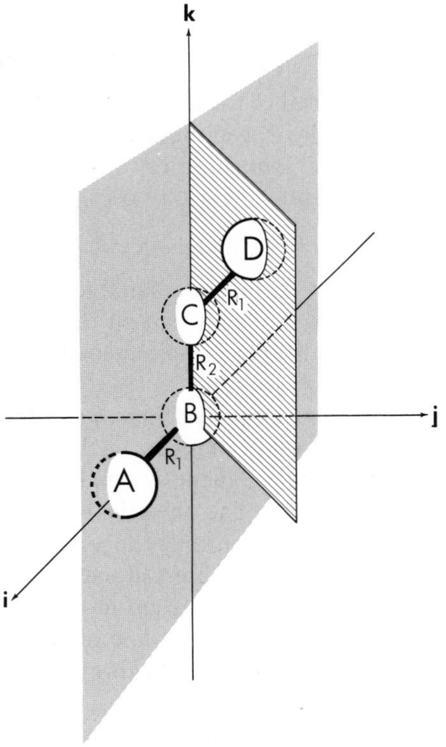

Figure 8.14. Dissymmetric array of hydrogen atoms.

best be approximated by the delocalized orbitals:

$$\Psi_G(\text{deloc}) = |\bar{\chi}_{D1}(1)\chi_{D1}(2)|, \tag{8.5.1}$$

where

$$\chi_{D1} = 1/\sqrt{4}(\phi_A + \phi_B + \phi_C + \phi_D).$$

For the four electron case one is faced with the localized and delocalized extremes:

$$\Psi_G(\text{loc}) = |\chi_{L1}(1)\bar{\chi}_{L1}(2)\chi_{L2}(3)\bar{\chi}_{L2}(4)| \tag{8.5.2a}$$

$$\psi_G(\text{deloc}) = |\chi_{D1}(1)\bar{\chi}_{D1}(2)\chi_{D2}(3)\bar{\chi}_{D2}(4)|, \tag{8.5.2b}$$

where

$$\chi_{L1} = (1/\sqrt{2})(\phi_A + \phi_B) \qquad (8.5.3a)$$

$$\chi_{L2} = (1/\sqrt{2})(\phi_C + \phi_D) \qquad (8.5.3b)$$

$$\chi_{D1} = (1/\sqrt{4})(\phi_A + \phi_B + \phi_C + \phi_D) \qquad (8.5.3c)$$

$$\chi_{D2} = (1/\sqrt{4})(\phi_A + \phi_B - \phi_C - \phi_D). \qquad (8.5.3d)$$

For R_2 beyond a certain distance the delocalized orbital greatly predominates and we have two separate hydrogen molecules.

This suggests that more semiempirical work be done with the use of composite functions such as

$$\Psi_G = \Psi_G(\text{loc}) + \lambda\Psi_G(\text{deloc}). \qquad (8.5.4)$$

The methods of Chapter 4 seem quite suitable for the use of such zeroth order functions. In this way not only can all the geometrical characteristics of each mechanism be combined in a single concerted effort, but self-consistent numerical results may be forthcoming.

The delocalized method is especially suited to give high rotational strengths, since it introduces maximum dissymmetry at the minimum price of energy. It was for this reason that the 1, 3 diene system in Section 8.4 seemed to have its maximum strength at 90°. The investigation of diene and ethylenic-carbonyl systems where the two chromophores are separated by about 8 Å has led to the conclusion that the observed enhancement of absorption and CD persists over many intervening carbon atoms and not merely for β, γ-unsaturation. At these distances a direct line of sight coupling seems rather unlikely, and attention should be given to through bond mechanisms.

8.6. Rotation about Bonds

So far most of our efforts have been concentrated on rigid systems. Needless to say, there are numerous optically active nonrigid molecules, many of importance to biochemistry. In a homologous series of compounds with similar rotational barriers it is sometimes possible to formulate simple rules based on energetically favorable rotamers. A certain amount of success in this field has been achieved with branched hydrocarbon derivatives. The various conformations encountered in this system are shown in Figure 8.15. One now assumes that conformations with adjacent bulky R groups are energetically unfavorable. For example, conformation (*b*) is preferred over (*a*), because R and R' are on opposite sides in (*b*) and adjacent in (*a*). Conformations (*c*) and (*e*) are preferred over (*d*), because it has the particularly crowded array of three adjacent bulky groups. Conformation (*h*) is preferred

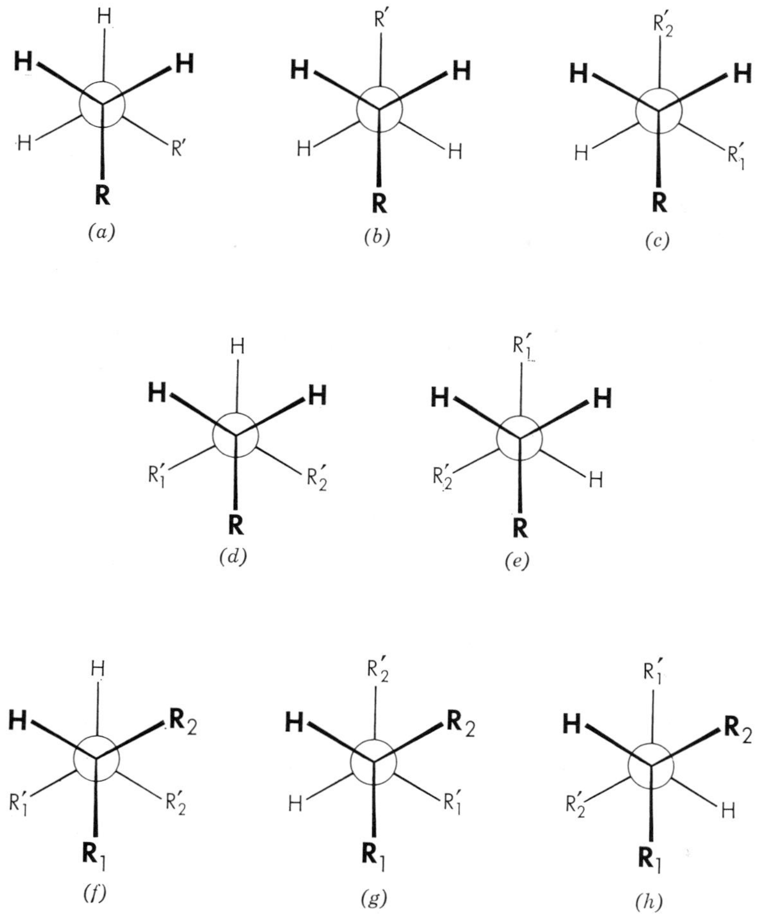

Figure 8.15. Tetrahedral conformations in nonrigid molecules.

over (*f*) and (*g*), because it has no multiply crowded groups, only the pairs (R_1', R_2) and (R_1, R_2').

If such compounds had unrestricted rotation about all bonds, the rotational strength would be negligible, since the contributions from each conformer tend to cancel. The observed rotational strengths arise from the elimination of the crowded conformations in favor of the less crowded. In analogy to the coupled oscillator model one might suppose that the interaction of two groups, 1 and 2, leads to a contribution of $\pm A_1 A_2$. The geometry of the interaction is fixed at two possible mirror image conformations (Figure 8.16). An electron correlation mechanism would give the indicated signs. The third orientation gives zero, because the pair has a plane of symmetry.

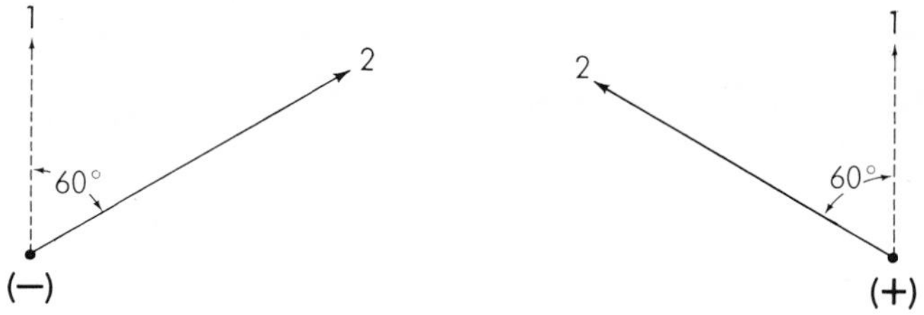

Figure 8.16. Pairwise interaction scheme.

From this it follows that the sum of the six nonvanishing pairwise contributions taken for each of the three rotamers of a given bond is zero. Let us apply this theory to the optically active substituted hydrocarbon, 2-chlorobutane (III). The conformer scheme about the 2—3 bond is shown in Figure 8.17. The crowded conformation (*c*) may be eliminated. Since the

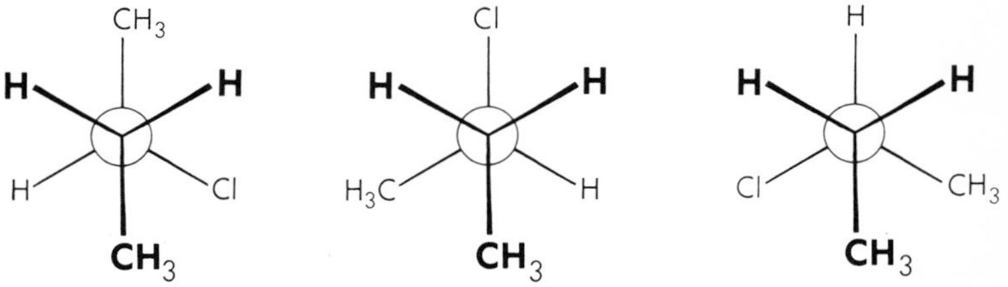

(*a*) (*b*) (*c*)

Figure 8.17. The rotamers of 2-chlorobutane.

sum of (*a*), (*b*), and (*c*) is zero, the rotational strength will be given by the negative of (*c*):

$$R = (A_{CH_3} - A_H)(A_{CH_3} - A_{Cl}). \tag{8.6.1}$$

When a multiply branched compound such as (IV) is encountered, additional

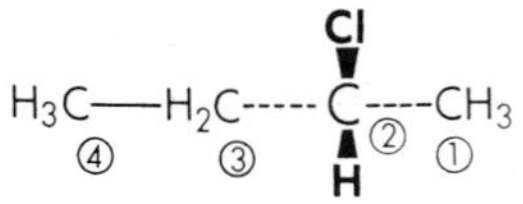

III

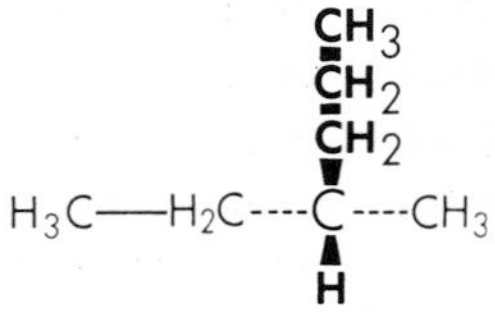

IV

rules are required which employ the simultaneous dependence of the orientation about several bonds. Otherwise one would obtain a zero result; since, if only rotations about bonds joined to the asymmetric center were considered, it would be impossible to distinguish between active and inactive isomers.

This flexibility introduces another set of crowded conformations, the elimination of which leads to a nonvanishing result.

By means of such rules Brewster was able to correlate the Na-D line rotations of a large number of hydrocarbon derivatives by means of a relatively small number of parameters. In complex biomolecules a similar system may well prove to be useful.

8.7. Conclusion

In this concluding chapter we have attempted to give a capsule view of typical problems and methods of interpretation of optical activity data. It is evident that far-reaching general methods are not available. Each chromophore presents its own special problems. It is our belief that most of the qualitative features of CD and ORD curves including vibronic effects can be explained by relatively simple mechanisms which are amenable to a semiempirical calculation.

There are reasons for doubting the validity of most first principles calculations of rotatory parameters in view of the degree of subtlety required in the wave functions. When it is recognized that no single wave function seems to prove adequate for describing all the properties of a molecule, agreement with experiment, when it does occur, must almost be regarded as fortuitous. Over the years a wealth of divergent calculations based on totally different mechanisms has accumulated, which individually seem to account for all the rotatory strength of a given transition.

For the present it appears that the main power of quantum theory in this field will be as a scaffolding to aid in the formulation of the correct methods of correlating CD data with structure. This is by no means meant to discourage further *ab initio* calculations, but merely to put the situation in proper perspective.

References

General Physical and Mathematical

1. Eyring, H., J. Walter, and J. E. Kimball, *Quantum Chemistry*, Wiley, 1944.
2. Landau, L. D., and E. M. Lifshitz, *Electrodynamics of Continuous Media*, Pergamon Press, 1960.
3. Macdonald, J. R., and M. H. Brochman, *Rev. Mod. Phys.*, **28,** 393 (1956).
4. Margenau, H., *Electromagnetic Theory*, McGraw-Hill, 1941.
5. Morse, P. M., and H. Feshbach, *Methods of Theoretical Physics*, McGraw-Hill, 1953.
6. Panofsky, W. K. H., and M. Phillips, *Classical Electricity and Magnetism*, Addison-Wesley, 1955.
7. Pauling, L., and E. B. Wilson, Jr., *Introduction to Quantum Mechanics*, McGraw-Hill, 1935.

8. Sommerfeld, A., *Optics*, Academic Press, 1949.
9. Stratton, J. A., *Electromagnetic Theory*, McGraw-Hill, 1941.

General Optical Activity

1. Condon, E. U., *Rev. Mod. Phys.*, **9,** 432 (1937).
2. Condon, E. U., W. Alter, and H. Eyring, *J. Chem. Phys.*, **5,** 753 (1937).
3. Djerassi, C., *Optical Rotatory Dispersion*, McGraw-Hill, 1960.
4. Kauzmann, W., J. Walter, and H. Eyring, *Chem. Rev.*, **26,** 339 (1940).
5. Lowry, T. M., *Optical Rotatory Power*, Longmans, Green, 1935.
6. Mason, S. F., *Quarterly Review*, **17** (1963).
7. Rosenfeld, L., *Z. Physik*, **52,** 161 (1928).
8. Tinoco, I., *Advances in Chemical Physics*, Vol. IV, Interscience, 1962.
9. Urry, D. W., *Ann. Rev. Phys. Chem.*, **19,** 477 (1968).

Specific Theories

1. Brewster, J. H., *J.A.C.S.*, **81,** 5475, 5483, 5493 (1959).
2. Caldwell, D. J., *J. Chem. Phys.*, **51,** 984 (1969).
3. Charney, E., *Tetrahedron*, **21,** 3127 (1965).
4. Kirkwood, J. G., *J. Chem. Phys.*, **5,** 479 (1937).
5. Kuhn, W., *Naturwiss.*, **19,** 289 (1938).
6. Moffitt, W., *Proc. Natl. Acad. Sci.*, **42,** 736 (1956).
7. Moffitt, W., D. D. Fitts, and J. G. Kirdwood, *Proc. Natl. Acad. Sci.*, **42,** 736 (1957).
8. Moscowitz, A. J., Thesis, Harvard, 1957.
9. Schellman, J. A., *J. Chem. Phys.*, **44,** 55 (1966).
10. *Tetrahedron*, **13,** Nos. 1–3 (1961).
11. Yaris, M., A. Moscowitz, and R. S. Berry, *J. Chem. Phys.*, **49,** 3150 (1968).

Special Topics

1. Groenewege, M. P., *Mol. Phys.*, **5,** 541 (1962).
2. Kramer, H. A., *Proc. Acad. Sci. Amst.*, **33,** 959 (1930).
3. Tobias, I., and W. Kauzmann, *J. Chem. Phys.*, **35,** 538 (1961).

Subject Index